Communication in Healthca

D1423853

DATE DUE

Sociology of Health and Illness Monograph Series

Edited by Hannah Bradby
Department of Sociology
University of Warwick
Coventry
CV4 7AL
UK

Current titles

Communication in Healthcare Settings
Policy, Participation and New Technologies

Edited by

Alison Pilnick, Jon Hindmarsh and Virginia Teas Gill

WILEY-BLACKWELL

A John Wiley & Sons, Ltd., Publication

This edition first published 2010
Chapter © 2010 The Authors
Book compilation © 2010 Foundation for the Sociology of Health & Illness / Blackwell Publishing Ltd

Edition history: originally published as volume 31, issue 6 of *Sociology of Health & Illness*

Blackwell Publishing was acquired by John Wiley & Sons in February 2007. Blackwell's publishing program has been merged with Wiley's global Scientific, Technical, and Medical business to form Wiley-Blackwell.

Registered Office
John Wiley & Sons Ltd, The Atrium, Southern Gate, Chichester, West Sussex, PO19 8SQ, United Kingdom

Editorial Offices
350 Main Street, Malden, MA 02148-5020, USA
9600 Garsington Road, Oxford, OX4 2DQ, UK
The Atrium, Southern Gate, Chichester, West Sussex, PO19 8SQ, UK

For details of our global editorial offices, for customer services, and for information about how to apply for permission to reuse the copyright material in this book please see our website at www.wiley.com/wiley-blackwell.

The right of Alison Pilnick, Jon Hindmarsh and Virginia Teas Gill to be identified as the authors of the editorial material in this work has been asserted in accordance with the UK Copyright, Designs and Patents Act 1988.

Wiley also publishes its books in a variety of electronic formats. Some content that appears in print may not be available in electronic books.

Designations used by companies to distinguish their products are often claimed as trademarks. All brand names and product names used in this book are trade names, service marks, trademarks or registered trademarks of their respective owners. The publisher is not associated with any product or vendor mentioned in this book. This publication is designed to provide accurate and authoritative information in regard to the subject matter covered. It is sold on the understanding that the publisher is not engaged in rendering professional services. If professional advice or other expert assistance is required, the services of a competent professional should be sought.

Library of Congress Cataloging-in-Publication Data

Communication in healthcare settings : policy, participation, and new technologies / edited by Alison Pilnick, Jon Hindmarsh, and Virginia Teas Gill.
        p. ; cm. – (Sociology of health and illness monograph series)
    Includes bibliographical references and index.
    ISBN 978-1-4051-9827-1 (pbk. : alk. paper)   1. Communication in medicine.   I. Pilnick, A.   II. Hindmarsh, Jon.   III. Gill, Virginia Teas.   IV. Series: Sociology of health and illness monograph series.
    [DNLM: 1. Delivery of Health Care.   2. Communication.   3. Professional-Patient Relations. W 84.1 C7338 2010]
    R118.C61857 2010
    610–dc22   2010000772

A catalogue record for this book is available from the British Library.

Set in 9.5/11.5pt Times NR Monotype by Toppan Best-set Premedia Limited

01   2010

Contents

List of Contributors

Carly W. Butler
School of Journalism and Communication
The University of Queensland
Australia

Donald Chand
Department of Information and Process
Management
Bentley University
Waltham MA
USA

Ignasi Clemente
Department of Anthropology
Hunter College CUNY
New York
USA

Susan Danby
School of Early Childhood
Queensland University of Technology
Australia

Gary C. David
Department of Sociology
Bentley University
Waltham MA
USA

Michael Emmison
School of Social Science
University of Queensland
Australia

Angela Cora Garcia
Department of Sociology
Bentley University
Waltham MA
USA

Virginia Teas Gill
Department of Sociology and
Anthropology
Illinois State University
USA

Christian Heath
Department of Management
King's College London
London
UK

Jon Hindmarsh
Department of Management
King's College London
London
UK

Aled Jones
Institute for Health Research
School of Human & Health Sciences
Swansea University
UK

Paul Luff
Department of Management
King's College London
London
UK

Douglas W. Maynard
Department of Sociology
University of Wisconsin, Madison
USA

Ruth Parry
School of Community Health Sciences
University of Nottingham
Nottingham
UK

Alison Pilnick
School of Sociology and Social Policy
University of Nottingham
Nottingham
UK

Anne Warfield Rawls
Department of Sociology
Bentley University
Waltham MA
USA

Marcus Sanchez Svensson
inUse Consulting AB
Malmö
Sweden

Karen Thorpe
School of Psychology and Counselling
Queensland University of Technology
Australia

T. Elizabeth Weathersbee
Department of Sociology
University of Wisconsin, Madison
USA

Helena Webb
Department of Management
King's College London
London
UK

1

Beyond 'doctor and patient': developments in the study of healthcare interactions

Alison Pilnick, Jon Hindmarsh and Virginia Teas Gill

Introduction

Over the last three decades, conversation analytic (CA) studies have illuminated some of the fundamental organisational features and interactional processes in a broad array of medical encounters. Investigations of interactions between physicians and patients have been a cornerstone of this field since the early 1980s. However, conversation analysts have also moved beyond the dyadic doctor-patient encounter to consider interactions between a wider range of healthcare professionals and their clients, and between a variety of healthcare professionals themselves.

Practical motivations spurred some of the earliest CA research on encounters between doctors and patients. Beginning in the late 1970s, a few conversation analysts began videotaping primary care consultations. Among these was Richard Frankel who, as a faculty member in a department of medicine, had a practical interest in improving communication and was exploring how videotapes could be used for physician training. Frankel recognised that CA could be an especially useful tool for understanding the dynamics of medical encounters, given that so much of medical practice consists of real-time conversations between doctors and patients. Recordings of these conversations and detailed written transcripts provide direct and repeated access to the practices the participants use to accomplish actions and activities during medical encounters. This access allows for the systematic study of medical interactions and detailed specification of recurrent interactional processes (Frankel 1983, see also Frankel and Beckman 1982).

The concrete findings CA generates can be used to help doctors (and patients) become more aware of and sensitive to their actions, which ultimately stands to improve health and healthcare. Frankel (1990), along with other pioneers in the field – including Christian Heath, Candace West, and Paul ten Have – took a firm stand that any recommendations for improving communication between doctors and patients must be grounded in the details of actual interaction. As West argues, '…it is only through systematic empirical study of the minutiae of doctor-patient interaction that we can learn what constitutes the alleged communication "gap" between doctors and patients, and how it might be transformed' (West 1983: 103).

The contribution of this work has not been restricted to issues relating to medical communication skills. Through systematic study of the details of medical encounters, conversation analysts have been mining a rich sociological seam for 30 years. Their work shares with other types of observational research in the sociology of medicine (*e.g.* ethnographic studies such as Emerson 1970, Silverman 1987, Byrne and Long 1976, and Strong 1979) a concern to witness and document naturally-occurring social interactions in medical settings. Like ethnomethodological investigations of medicine (Sudnow 1967) and of allied medical fields such as psychiatry and psychotherapy (Coulter 1973, Turner 1972, Wootton 1977, Garfinkel 1967), CA investigations focus on the generation of social order, particularly how participants organise their work routines and engage in (and display) sense-making practices in real time. The CA approach reveals how, turn by turn in conversation, participants produce the social organisation of different types of medical encounters – with their attendant tasks and projects, asymmetries of authority and expertise, and particular interactional dilemmas. This approach enables empirically-grounded, concrete specifications of *what* is done in medical interactions and *how* this is achieved (Halkowski and Gill, forthcoming), findings that can be shown to others and verified by reference to the data (Sacks 1984).

Of particular significance for medical sociology is CA's ability to reveal and unpack the fundamentally collaborative and contingent nature of medical encounters (Maynard and Heritage 2005, Heritage and Maynard 2006a). This is achieved, in part, through its distinctive methodological commitments and concerns. In particular, CA notes that in all interaction, people are ongoingly attentive to the talk and visible conduct of their co-participants. Indeed, they rely on each other to make sense of emergent conduct by virtue of what has happened immediately before; that is, in the light of the sequential context. Because they routinely do so, a speaker can position an utterance in a particular location to give it a particular sense as an action without spelling it out in so many words. A related aspect of the collaborative nature of interaction is that actions are typically accomplished via sequences, where one participant initiates a sequence (*e.g.* asks a question, makes an offer, presents a proposal), making it relevant for the recipient to produce the second part (*e.g.* to answer the question, accept or decline the offer, agree or disagree with the proposal) (Schegloff and Sacks 1973). Whatever is produced after the sequence initiation is likely to be understood as responsive to it, unless marked otherwise. The production of action (the 'what is being done here') is also a contingent matter: in a responsive turn of talk, a recipient might or might not exhibit a particular understanding of a speaker's utterance, and in the ensuing talk, the original speaker might or might not correct this displayed understanding (Schegloff and Sacks 1973). As in ordinary conversation, social actions in medical settings are jointly accomplished over time, as the interaction unfolds (Heritage and Maynard 2006a).

These methodological commitments and concerns have important implications for the investigation of medical encounters and what can be discovered about them. Here we will mention just two of these implications. First, rather than treating aspects of social context (*e.g.* doctors' and patients' respective social statuses, power, knowledge asymmetries, etc.) as exogenous factors that affect participants' behaviour in predictable ways during medical consultations, conversation analysts begin with sequences of talk themselves and show how the participants build consultations with them – *i.e.* how they employ sequences in interactional practices and thereby carry out particular tasks, establish and maintain boundaries of expertise, display knowledge asymmetries, and the like. This approach enables a concrete understanding of how the social reality of medical encounters is accomplished in real time, and how interactional dilemmas (and their solutions) emerge.

A second and related implication is that CA investigations of medical encounters focus as much on *patients'* behaviour as doctors' behaviour. As Heritage and Maynard (2006b: 19) assert, 'It is by acting together that doctor and patient assemble each particular visit with its interactional textures, perceived features, and outcomes'. This approach has generated some significant findings about the nature of patients' participation and agency in medical encounters, findings that would not necessarily be predicted or uncovered if one starts with the assumption that, for example, patients' status precludes the exertion of agency (see Collins *et al.* 2007).

CA research on doctor-patient interaction: key issues

The major themes of the last 30 years of conversation analytic work on medical encounters have, then, emerged from the organisation of the encounters themselves, the tasks that participants accomplish, and the specific interactional issues and dilemmas to which the participants orient. For example, primary care medical consultations (especially acute-care visits, but also some non-acute visits) are typically organised around the twin goals of diagnosing the patient's medical problem and recommending treatment. To do this, the doctor and patient (1) come together and establish a relationship (*opening*), (2) the patient expresses the reason for the visit (*presenting complaint*), (3) the doctor examines the patient (*examination*), (4) the doctor produces an evaluation of the patient's condition (*diagnosis*), (5) the doctor proposes treatment for the condition (*treatment*), and (6) the doctor and patient terminate the visit (*closing*) (Heritage and Maynard 2006b: 14–15, see also Byrne and Long 1976, ten Have 1989, Robinson 2003).

The issues and dilemmas that emerge within these encounters reflect these activities. For example[1]: patients face the issues of how to put their concerns on the floor (Robinson and Heritage 2005); how to show themselves to be properly oriented to their bodies (Halkowski 2006, Heritage and Robinson 2006, Heath 2002); how to direct the doctor's attention toward and away from certain diagnostic possibilities (Gill and Maynard 2006, Gill *et al.* forthcoming, Stivers 2002b); and how to deal with diagnoses and treatment recommendations that may or may not correspond to their own views and preferences (Heath 1992, Stivers 2002a, 2006, Peräkylä 2002).

From the point of view of doctors, issues include eliciting all of a patient's concerns (Heritage *et al.* 2007, Robinson 2001) and designing solicitations that are fitted to the concerns that patients are likely to have (Heath 1981, Robinson 2006); preparing patients for no-problem diagnoses (Heritage and Stivers 1999) as well as difficult diagnostic news (Maynard 2003, Maynard and Frankel 2006); and securing patient agreement in regard to diagnoses (Peräkylä 2006) and treatment recommendations (Stivers 2006, Roberts 1999).

In other genres of medical encounters – *e.g.* those outside doctor-patient interaction – the major tasks may be quite different. Visits may be therapeutic in nature (*e.g.* engaging in physical therapy), administrative (*e.g.* admitting a patient to the hospital), related to instruction (*e.g.* instructing a resident during a surgery), etc. This, in turn, engenders different sets of interactional issues and dilemmas, as we will discuss below.

Beyond the doctor-patient consultation

Over the past ten to fifteen years, we have witnessed an increase in the number of conversation analytic studies that consider settings and activities beyond the doctor-patient consultation. For example, recent studies have explored ante-natal screening and examinations (Büscher and Jensen 2007, Nishisaka 2007, Pilnick 2004), AIDS/HIV counselling (Peräkylä 1995, Silverman 1997), anaesthesia (Hindmarsh and Pilnick 2002), child counselling (Hutchby 2007), health visiting (Heritage and Sefi 1992), dentistry (Anderson 1989, Hindmarsh in press), emergency calls (Whalen *et al.* 1988, Whalen 1995), homeopathy (Ruusuvuori 2005), medical and child helplines (Greatbatch *et al.* 2005, Pooler forthcoming, Potter and Hepburn 2003), pharmacy (Pilnick 1998), physiotherapy (Parry 2004, Martin 2005), psychiatry and psychotherapy (McCabe *et al.* 2002, Antaki *et al.* 2005, Peräkylä *et al.* 2008, Speer and Parsons 2006) and surgery (Koschmann *et al.* 2007, Sanchez Svennson *et al.* 2007, Mondada 2007). Furthermore, there are a range of recent studies relevant to medical sociology that stand outside formal healthcare settings, such as research concerning Alcoholics Anonymous (Arminen 1998) and the family (Beach 1996). Also of note are a set of studies that consider the bodily and vocal skills and competencies of people with communication disorders of various kinds (Goodwin 2003, Wilkinson *et al.* 2007, Beeke *et al.* 2007, Finlay *et al.* 2008, Maynard 2005). In doing so they detail the communicational competence rather than incompetence of people who have difficulties in speech and communication and, as such, have important contributions to make to speech therapy, as well as our understanding of forms of (dis)ability.

It is not simply the breadth of recent conversation analytic work on health and illness that is of value here (although that indeed is of value). More importantly, the consideration of these diverse settings and activities introduces new issues, and allows for the specification of existing issues, of sociological interest that cannot be captured in the study of doctor-patient interactions alone. This range is considerable and we cannot hope to do it justice. However, it may be worth highlighting three particular issues in order to illustrate some of the contributions that these developments are making. These concern: (i) different dilemmas that arise in practitioner-patient interaction beyond encounters between doctors and patients; (ii) interaction between healthcare practitioners, and (iii) how new technologies feature in the course of healthcare delivery. As will become apparent, these three issues have particular relevance for the present collection of studies.

Practical problems in practitioner-patient interaction
The consideration of a wider range of sites for healthcare introduces novel forms of activity and even types of patient. For instance, whereas doctor-patient consultations (especially acute-care consultations) are fundamentally concerned with issues of diagnosis and the discussion of treatment plans, other sites of practitioner-patient encounter relate more centrally to treatment delivery. Examples of such 'hands-on' treatment-based interactions include the work of physiotherapists, dentists, speech therapists and podiatrists. The very involvement of practitioners in physically treating patients raises some distinctive challenges and issues in the interaction. For example, in encounters in physiotherapy and speech therapy, one issue that emerges relates to a patient's performance during therapy sessions. When the patients display forms of physical or verbal 'incompetence' or 'trouble', then this requires correction and management. In their domestic interactions, lapses in competence by the patients tend to be explicitly noted and corrected by partners or relatives. However, studies of institutional encounters (Parry 2004, Lindsay and Wilkinson 1999) find that therapists are less likely to make explicit reference to troubles. Thus, within practitioner-patient encounters, incompetence is produced and oriented to as a sensitive issue. This sensitivity is grounded in the fact that one possible reason for incompetence is a potential lack of effort on the part of the patient, whilst another is the failure (or lack of progress) of the therapy itself. So these findings highlight the ways in which the particular institutional character of the encounter is accomplished in (and through) the forms of talk that feature within the setting.

In other settings, the combination of the tasks that must be performed in the encounter and the specific cohort of patients with whom practitioners interact, produces interactional dilemmas not typically found in doctor-patient encounters – especially those occurring in acute-care visits in primary care settings. For instance, hospital pharmacists in Britain are bound by a code of ethics to ensure that patients know the proper dosage instructions for their medications. However, patients who have chronic illnesses, and their caregivers, may already be well familiar with matters of dosage and administration. When pharmacists interact with these patients and their caregivers, they face the dilemma of how to adhere to ethical codes without treating the recipients as less knowledgeable than they actually are (Pilnick 1998). The move to consider a wider range of healthcare interactions provides opportunities to explore such dilemmas and their interactional solutions, ones which are relatively uncommon in certain types of doctor-patient encounters. Thus, they provide more opportunities to consider how these circumstances are handled as a matter of routine.

These studies also demonstrate the ways in which 'blanket' recommendations for practice struggle in the face of local contingencies. Different types of healthcare place distinct demands on practitioners and patients and there may be different agendas and asymmetries at work. As Peräkylä *et al.* (2007: 140) note with regard to standardised recommendations for patient involvement, 'The relevancy of [different] forms of participation ultimately arises from the overall goal of the encounter, as well as from the theory of healing that guides the interaction'. Indeed, even within a single setting for healthcare delivery, policies and recommendations can raise challenges to practitioners who are dealing with patients with various levels of knowledge, expertise and commitment. To fully understand the impact of these recommendations, therefore, requires analysis of the ways in which they are deployed and treated in a range of practical circumstances of use (see also Collins *et al.* 2007). Moreover, it is valuable to ground the development of policies and recommendations in a solid understanding of actual practice.

Interaction between healthcare practitioners
While much work on communication in healthcare has been concerned with encounters between medical professionals and patients, one strand in the emerging body of conversation analytic work on healthcare considers forms of communication that arise in real time, between members of healthcare teams – in meetings (*e.g.* Housley 2003) or in the very course of treatment (Hindmarsh and Pilnick 2002, Mondada 2007, Sanchez Svensson *et al.* 2007). These investigations, and others, address Atkinson's concern that there is 'far too little research on how medical practitioners from different specialities cooperate or compete in the management of particular conditions' (Atkinson 1995: 34).

Perhaps the most significant body of work on interactions between practitioners concerns an issue of long-standing interest in medical sociology, namely medical (and professional) socialisation and training. A particular dilemma for practitioners in these cases relates to the ways in which medical practice is bound up with medical education. As Bosk (1979: 3) suggests, the superordinate must allow room for the trainee to make what he calls 'the honest errors of the inexperienced' in order to avoid damaging the confidence and the learning experience of the trainee. At the same time supervisors must ensure the quality of the patient's treatment. These can be conflicting concerns.

Some of the most complex and delicate analytic work in this area relates to one of the most complex and delicate medical specialities, surgery. For example, studies by Koschmann and colleagues (2007 and forthcoming) explore the artful practices in and through which surgeons provide instruction while operating. In particular, they consider how surgeons render visible specific features of the anatomy, and stages of the procedure, in the very course of those procedures. These studies are notable as they demand especially close attention to the bodily and material resources brought to bear in the interactional organisation of instruction. As a result, these studies often involve multiple cameras, multiple microphones and live audio-visual mixing in order to capture the action in sufficient detail to support the analysis. Importantly, the studies demonstrate how the surgeon's talk is only understandable (for participant or analyst) by virtue of its association with gestures and visible conduct and the wider 'material' context(s) in which it is produced and seen.

Issues concerning the relationships between medical practice and medical training are further complicated in other settings, for instance general hospital medicine (*e.g.* Pomerantz and Ende 1997, Pomerantz *et al.* 1995). Whereas in many surgical procedures the patient is often (although not always) fully anaesthetised, in general medicine, the patient is fully conscious and aware of the interaction between participants. All parties to the encounter manage the interactional and practical tensions that can arise in balancing teaching and learning with communication with the patient. For instance, Pomerantz and colleagues delineate the practices through which supervisors maintain the junior doctor's role as the primary caregiver while still monitoring their work and advising on the case in hand.

Interaction between healthcare practitioners (and indeed between experts and novices) also introduces more complex and variable forms of participation than are exhibited within general practice doctor-patient encounters. Rather than a straightforward interaction between practitioner and patient, many of these settings involve multiple parties to health-care encounters with variable occupational concerns, specialties and interests. This can have implications for the very ways in which treatment is organised and delivered. Furthermore, it can have an impact upon the quality of communication with patients, as other activities such as training conversations, instructions or even decisions, are managed 'front stage' and are thus hearable (and visible) to the patient.

New technologies and healthcare interaction

Some of the most important developments in healthcare in the past few decades have related to the use of new technologies. Take for example, ultrasound scanners in ante-natal screening, systems to support laparoscopic surgery, telecare monitoring systems, and of course the various scripts and forms, whether on paper or computer, that underpin so many features of healthcare service and delivery today. Given the relevance of technology in modern healthcare, there are numerous recent studies that consider the ways in which anything from inhalers to electronic patient records are changing the organisation and delivery of care (for a review see Heath *et al.* 2003). Most relevant to this collection are a number of studies that consider how participants use technologies in the course of encounters relevant to health and illness. In each case the focus is not on what the technologies are designed to achieve, but rather with how they are put to work, how they feature, and how are they oriented to in sequences of interaction.

One example is the use of expert systems to support medical helplines. In a study of NHS Direct, Greatbatch *et al.* (2005) noted that their clinical assessment system (CAS) was designed to standardise and control interaction between the callers and the nurse call-takers. However, in interactions that emerge in delivering the service, participants work with – and around – features of the technology in artful and unexpected ways. Instead of the system enforcing standardisation, the nurses can be seen to prioritise their own knowledge and expertise and to 'adapt, tailor, qualify and supplement' advice and information for the specifics of the caller's problem' (Greatbatch 2005: 825). The use of the system and the management of the conversation by the nurses are delicately interwoven. This raises fundamental questions about attempts to manage or control healthcare interactions, the tension between abstract procedures and local contingencies, the distributions of expertise between new technologies and professionals and indeed the very nature or purpose of medical helplines.

In these and other ways practitioners need to 'manage' new technologies in the course of communication with patients. The technologies can introduce practical problems for practitioners in ensuring the 'flow' of conversation (Greatbatch *et al.* 1995) and they can also introduce distinctive dilemmas for practitioners in discussing medical issues and concerns. Take, for example, the use of screening technologies in ante-natal care. These new technologies do not lead to definitive diagnoses of potential fetal abnormalities, but rather generate 'risk figures'. Communicating the meaning of these risk figures, such that prospective parents can make informed decisions, is a complex interactional matter (Pilnick 2004). The decisions asked of prospective parents require some understanding of the technology and the associated figures that it generates. So the introduction of the technology poses challenges to practitioners aiming to follow recommendations of shared decision making and the like, as they must not only communicate the figures but the reliability of the tests and technologies involved and their relevance for the pregnancy. These and other studies of healthcare technologies in interaction, therefore, can inform technological developments and indeed training programmes, by emphasising the communicational contexts in which technologies feature, rather than solely their technical operation and functionality.

Introducing the collection

The chapters that we have selected for this book build on the established tradition of applying CA to medical interaction, and many draw heavily on the key themes and findings that we have summarised above. Critically, they advance this work by unpacking some of the distinctive practical problems or institutional dilemmas that arise in different healthcare settings. The authors of these chapters also reflect upon the practical relevance of their work, and the ways in which the understandings they present may be used to address these dilemmas. As the title of the collection suggests, the themes of policy, participation and new technologies are at the forefront of the analyses presented here, just as they are at the forefront of many recent developments in healthcare.

The first chapter in this collection is a groundbreaking study of the solicitation of donated human tissue over the telephone, unpacking how call centre personnel work to solicit donations from the family of the deceased person. Weathersbee and Maynard's analysis shows how solicitation is carried out cautiously, incrementally and tacitly, reflecting both its interactional status as a dispreferred action and its wider delicacy. Their analysis is located within a wider policy context, as they highlight the shortage of donated tissues in the US and a drive to increase donation rates. In this context, the authors show how configurations in the wording of solicitations may operate interactionally but unintentionally to impact on the act of donation, in some cases encouraging it and in others acting to discourage. Solicitation is carried out tacitly, such that callers avoid overtly requesting donations, and instead 'mask' their requests as other actions such as 'ostensible offers', or 'notifications' that the decedent has the potential to donate tissue. However, whilst this orients to the very real sensitivity and delicacy of the situation, it also presents an early opportunity for the call recipient to decline, and Weathersbee and Maynard note that call makers never aggressively strive to convert refusals into consents. It has been argued that donation rates vary as a result of the logistical efforts of procurement organisations, but the analysis presented here shows how examination of actual interaction is critical for understanding this, since aspects of this interaction may exert a very real effect on outcomes. In other words, when policy initiatives do not come to fruition in the way that has been hoped, the authors show how it may be necessary to trace this process back to the fine details of how the involved parties talk to one another. As such, the chapter presents the first step in a crucial programme of research in organ and tissue donation, which until now has focused on who asks for donations or in what context they ask (face to face, over the phone) rather than how they ask.

The relationship between policy and interaction is also a key theme of our second chapter, by Butler, Danby, Emmison and Thorpe. At the same time, the authors address a classic and recurrent theme in the sociology of health and illness: the asymmetrical distribution of knowledge between medical professionals and the lay public. However, here it is applied to a very modern context – calls to a Child Health telephone line. As the authors note, the rising costs of face-to-face primary care have resulted in an increasing provision of broadly defined health services being devolved to telephone contact. The operation of such helplines generally involves clear policies and guidelines regarding appropriate call handling. Such guidelines may relate to professional boundaries and the institutional role of the call taker (for example nurses may not be permitted to diagnose), but they may also relate to the use of a particular paper or computer-based protocol to be followed. The Child Health Line under investigation is intended to offer support and information on children's behaviour, health and development, with guidelines that nurses should not provide specific 'medical advice'. However, callers regularly request medical advice, and assume that the nurses answering their call will be able to offer it. Such an assumption is understandable given the name of the service and a common sense understanding of the term 'health'. The guidelines thus result in multiple constraints, and obvious tensions, to be managed by the call-takers. The authors examine how these nurses manage the apparent paradox of responding to callers' needs by delivering what may be interpreted as medical advice, whilst formally and accountably abiding by service guidelines not to do so. Given the ambiguity and overlap between 'medical' and 'child development' issues, and what counts as advice as opposed to information, it would be virtually impossible for nurses to adhere strictly to the guidelines. The analysis illustrates how they use these ambiguities as a resource, in order to respond to callers' concerns. In this way the chapter shows how institutional guidelines and policies are 'talked into being' in the course of interaction with clients.

Our third chapter also situates itself within a policy context, but this time addresses policies specifically designed to encourage patient participation in healthcare. Talk about the meanings and rationale of procedures and proposals has been identified as a key issue in patient-centred care, shared decision making and patient education (Collins 2005) and is encouraged by official guidelines (*e.g.* NHS 2003). In her chapter, Parry offers an empirical examination of talk about reasons and rationale in healthcare consultations, by focusing on physiotherapists' accounts for the treatment actions they propose, instigate and conduct. Previous work in primary care (*e.g.* Peräkylä 1998, 2006) shows that accounts related to diagnosis do particular kinds of interactional work above and beyond the 'face value' explanations they provide. Critically, in making their reasoning apparent to patients, doctors balance their authority with accountability, and treat patients as individuals who are both interested in and capable of understanding. Accounts tend to occur in circumstances of overt or incipient patient resistance, where proposals run counter to patient expectations, and where the reasoning underlying actions is not obvious. Parry's work builds on this by extending it to a different clinical setting, and by examining accounts for treatment-related actions as opposed to diagnosis. Physiotherapy is a valuable setting for this kind of research because it generally requires visible and effortful co-operation on the part of the patient during treatment, and as such necessitates a particular focus on co-operation, persuasion and motivation. Whilst accounts in this setting are also found in circumstances where patients and therapists do not agree about the best way forward, where patients express concern over physical functions, or there is opacity about the rationale for a treatment proposal, Parry also finds new circumstances which have not been previously documented in the literature. Accounts are associated with removal or adjustment of patients' clothing, and in this sense can be seen to relate to wider issues regarding the body, dignity, and the appropriateness of requests. They are also provided when treatment actions are designed to remediate some locally evident physical failure, and in this context help to build a sense that the problem that has manifested is a solvable matter that can be addressed in partnership. This latter category of accounts is used to persuade, influence and motivate patients, and as such has important implications for practice.

Participation may also come to be treated as a moral matter in healthcare. Obesity has been described as 'the modern epidemic' (WHO 2000) and is a key priority for governments and healthcare systems worldwide. However, there has been a lack of sociological work examining the way in which the condition is managed in the course of weight-loss consultations. This is of particular significance, given that the first line of treatment for obesity is behavioural intervention, achieved through advice giving on diet, exercise and lifestyle. The categorisation of obesity as a lifestyle issue positions the obese individual as normatively responsible for onset of obesity and as responsible to contribute to its management. The chapter by Webb in this volume addresses this gap in the literature through detailed analysis of consultations in two UK NHS obesity clinics. The focus of the analysis presented here is on opening questions, and the way in which patients' answers to these orient to moral issues of responsibility, and perform moral work. Webb shows how, when patients produce their answers to opening questions, they typically imply either 'success' or 'lack of success' in their weight loss programme. Whilst doing this, they construct their personal agency in different ways. Patients enhance their agency when reporting behaviours that would imply success, such as weight loss, continued exercise etc. By contrast, patients whose responses imply lack of success tend to minimise their agency, emphasising instead the role of external or unavoidable factors. As Webb concludes, these different types of response have resonance with the perceived responsibilities of obese patienthood, and highlight the particular moral responsibilities to which patients orient. Like many of the other chapters in this volume, the findings have important implications for healthcare practice, in this case by demonstrating how patients handle the tensions between moral and institutional agendas.

The next chapter considers participation in a more established doctor-patient context, but is distinctive in that it involves more than two participants. Clemente examines how older paediatric patients manage assistance from their parents in chronic pain consultations. In the context of answering questions from clinicians about symptoms, the chapter lays out child-initiated strategies that preclude, solicit or limit parental assistance in situations where the child is having difficulties providing an answer. The wider literature on doctor-patient interaction illustrates that providing clinicians with symptom information is not always an easy task – for example, patients must judge what is relevant and what counts as 'medical' (Heritage and Robinson 2006). This is complicated further in the setting Clemente considers, because in cases of recurrent non-malignant pain there is often a long and complex medical history. Careful analysis shows how information provision is a collaborative process supported in this context by the clinicians' strong commitment to child-centredness. The end result is that children are able to solicit and draw on parental assistance without losing interactional control, or the opportunity to present their own symptom accounts. Ultimately, the success of the children's strategies depends on the fact that they invite specific types of parental support whilst excluding other forms of parental participation. For example, parents' contributions may be framed as temporally limited or as responsive to the child, thereby underlining the role of the child as the primary informant. Through this combination of invitation and exclusion, children manage to assert agency and control. Children's limited participation has been identified as potentially problematic across a range of medical settings, and Clemente concludes by suggesting that clinicians can promote children's participation by being sensitive to the strategies they employ. This chapter makes an important contribution to the wider study of paediatric medicine by illustrating the importance of studying it as a triadic rather than dyadic process. Focusing on doctor-child or doctor-parent communication alone would fail to uncover the delicate inter-relationship between the contributions of all three parties (see Stivers and Majid 2007).

Sanchez-Svensson, Heath, and Luff also consider multi-party encounters, but in a rather different context, where various members of a surgical team manage training episodes within the course of surgical procedures. Indeed, a longstanding interest in the sociology of health and illness has been the way in which healthcare expertise, practice and clinical mentality are established both through formal training and social interaction with peers (e.g. Becker et al. 1961). Less attention has been paid to the way in which forms of training and instruction are managed in moments of social interaction. The authors address this issue by examining the ways in which surgeons, alongside other members of the surgical team, carry out activities of demonstration and instruction. It is widely recognised that surgery requires a mixture of intellectual, technical and manual skills, and as the authors note, these skills can only be acquired through an opportunity to observe and discuss them in situ. Trainees must not only see what is happening, but also know how to make sense of it, and learn how to apply that knowledge contingently. Using video data, Sanchez-Svensson et al. carefully analyse how it is that surgeons make particular phenomena and procedures accessible and intelligible to trainees. What the authors describe as 'momentary revelations of the surgical field' provide the resources for trainees to follow, understand and where appropriate contribute to the production of a complex medical procedure. The intricacy of the tasks at hand make training a particularly complex process in this environment, and this complexity is added to by the fact that throughout the activities of training, the integrity of medical practice must be preserved. The analysis also reveals how instruction and training in this context rely upon the abilities of other professionals who are present, such as nurses and anaesthetists. They must anticipate and remain sensitive to episodes of teaching, to enable these to be interwoven with the surgical task at hand. The findings here have implications for the study of 'situated learning' across healthcare and beyond.

The theme of participation continues into the next chapter, but is explored from a rather different perspective. This chapter also introduces our final theme, that of technology. The need for increased patient participation during interaction with nurses has been foregrounded in a range of recent UK 'best practice' documents (e.g. Royal College of Nursing 2003). Jones's analysis focuses on one particular area of nurse-patient communication, the admissions interview. Specifically, it focuses on the use of the technology of the paper-based admissions document that nurses complete during the interview, and examines how the use of this document affects the interaction that takes place between nurse and patient. The analysis shows how the topics that are discussed, and the way in which they are discussed, are often closely related to the layout of the paper document. Whilst this may be logical in an administrative sense, the juxtaposition of topics on the assessment form (where, for example, the topic 'sleeping' is adjacent to that of 'dying') may make little common sense to patients who are attempting to orient to the discussion as a coherent interactional sequence. If patients' health needs and experiences are discussed as a series of apparently unrelated topic areas, this conflicts both with the ways in which people normally experience illness and the ways in which they normally interact. The end result is that patients' participation is limited both because only one specific and delimited topic is considered relevant at any one time, and because the ordinarily 'messy' talk which is produced by patients must be made to fit into the appropriate topic-limited and space-limited section of the document. These findings are interesting, given that some nurses have resisted the introduction of more traditionally defined technology in the form of electronic patient records, for fear they restrict the patient's voice (Rhodes *et al.* 2006). However, as Jones points out, in order to address these issues and enhance possibilities for patient participation, we must guard against focusing on the templates or technologies, whether they be paper or electronic in form, and examine instead the way in which they are used in practice. Jones concludes by noting that 'best practice' guidelines should be grounded in a better understanding of the interactional dynamics of nurse/patient interaction and the contextual influences of specific nursing tasks.

Our final contribution to this volume continues the theme of the impact of healthcare technologies on medical interaction. However, this chapter examines medical interaction of a rather different kind from the other contributions to this volume: the interaction between doctors' reports of medical treatments, the individuals or systems that formalise them into reports, and the resulting documentation. As Jones's chapter in this volume highlights, medical records of one form or another play a central role in many aspects of healthcare, but little research exists on their creation. Using data from a study of healthcare documentation production, David, Garcia, Rawls and Chand examine the process of medical record creation through the use of speech recognition technology (SRT) and subsequent editing by medical transcriptionists (MTs). Their analysis shows that the work of MTs combines both skilled worksite practices (for example understanding what the normal range of values might be for a particular laboratory investigation) as well as an orientation towards the socially ordered properties of dictated speech. This latter orientation includes an understanding of the way in which spoken language is different from written language, for example the ways in which speakers produce self-corrections, or use voice inflections to indicate punctuation. Medical transcription, then, involves essential knowledge work based on social practices, and since SRTs cannot do this, there are limitations to their use and dangers of over-reliance on them. Through their single case analysis, David and colleagues show how MTs have the ability to create an 'intendedly unified object', and also to recognise and rectify many of the errors that SRT can introduce. The chapter is a timely reminder of the fact that, while new technology often holds the promise of improving healthcare, its application will not automatically result in doing so. As the authors identify, medical records, in common with other forms of socially constructed information, have essential social properties and so need to be considered within the context of their construction and use.

As a collection, the chapters contained in this book address the three themes of policy, participation and new technologies announced in the title, in the ways that we have described above. Taken together, what they also demonstrate is the breadth of medical interaction in which these issues come to the fore. They underline the utility of taking a conversation analytic approach to studying communication in healthcare settings, showing that the smallest details of the way in which the participants talk to one another can have sizeable impacts on the eventual outcomes. The study of doctor-patient interaction has been a cornerstone of the study of healthcare interaction, and CA researchers in this area of the field continue to generate important insights. However, healthcare today is more diverse than ever, and this encompasses not just the range of personnel who deliver care, but the settings in which they do so, the tools and techniques which they employ, the tasks they accomplish, and the dilemmas they confront. CA researchers have already begun to address this diversity, and we mean to add to this endeavour by bringing together the chapters in this collection.

Acknowledgements

We would like to thank all the contributors to the book, and all the reviewers whose timely and generous reviews helped to develop the chapters included here. Special thanks are due to Hannah Bradby and Liz Ackroyd for their efficient and patient assistance in the production of this book.

Note

1   This is an illustrative, and by no means complete, accounting of some issues and dilemmas that emerge in doctor-patient consultations and of the CA publications that explore them. Paul ten Have maintains an online bibliography of CA publications on medical encounters, an excellent resource to discover the range of studies in the field. See http://www2.fmg.uva.nl/emca/medbib.htm

References

Anderson, W.T. (1989) Dentistry as an activity system: sequential properties of the dentist-patient encounter. In Helm, D.T., Anderson, W.T., Meehan, A.J. and Rawls, A.W. (eds) *The Interactional Order: New Directions In The Study Of Social Order*. New York: Irvington.

Antaki, C., Barnes, R. and Leudar, I. (2005) Diagnostic formulations in psychotherapy, *Discourse Studies*, 7, 627–47.

Arminen, I. (1998) Sharing experiences: doing therapy with the help of mutual references in meetings of Alcoholics Anonymous, *The Sociological Quarterly*, 39, 3, 491–515.

Atkinson, P. (1995) *Medical Talk and Medical Work: The Liturgy of the Clinic*. London: Sage.

Beach, W.A. (1996) *Conversations about Illness: Family Preoccupations with Bulimia*. Mahwah, N.J.: Lawrence Erlbaum.

Becker, H., Geer, B., Hughes, E. and Strauss, A. (1961) *Boys in White: Student Culture in Medical School*. Chicago: University of Chicago Press.

Beeke, S., Maxim, J.E. and Wilkinson, R. (2007) Using conversation analysis to assess and treat people with aphasia, *Seminars in Speech and Language*, 28, 2, 136–47.

Bosk, C.L. (1979) *Forgive and Remember: Managing Medical Failure*. Chicago: University of Chicago Press.

Büscher, M. and Jensen, G. (2007) Sound sight: seeing with ultrasound, *Health Informatics Journal*, 13, 1, 23–36.

Byrne, P.S. and Long, B. (1976) *Doctors Talking to Patients: a Study of the Verbal Behaviours of Doctors in the Consultation*. London: Her Majesty's Stationery Office.

Collins, S. (2005) Explanations in consultations: the combined effectiveness of doctors' and nurses' communication with patients, *Medical Education*, 39, 785–96.

Collins, S., Britten, N., Ruusuvuori, J. and Thompson, A. (eds) (2007) *Patient Participation in Health Care Consultations*. Open University Press.

Coulter, J. (1973) *Approaches to Insanity*. Bath, UK: Martin Robertson.

Emerson, J. (1970) Behavior in private places: sustaining definitions of reality in gynaecological examinations. In Dreitzel, H.P. (ed.) *Recent Sociology*. New York: Macmillan.

Finlay, W., Antaki, C. and Walton, C. (2008) Saying no to the staff: an analysis of refusals in a home for people with severe communication difficulties, *Sociology of Health and Illness*, 30, 1, 55–75.

Frankel, R.M. (1983) The laying on of hands: aspects of the organisation of gaze, touch, and talk in a medical encounter. In Fisher, S. and Dundas Todd, A. (eds) *The Social Organisation of Doctor-Patient Communication*. Washington, D.C.: Center for Applied Linguistics.

Frankel, R.M. (1990) Talking in interviews: a dispreference for patient-initiated questions in physician-patient encounters. In Psathas, G. (ed.) *Interaction Competence: Studies in Ethnomethodology and Conversation Analysis (No. 1)*. Lanham, MD: University Press of America.

Frankel, R.M. and Beckman, H.B. (1982) Impact: an interaction-based method for preserving and analyzing clinical transactions. In Pettegrew, L. (ed.) *Explorations in Provider and Patient Interaction*. Louisville, KY: Humana Press.

Garfinkel, H. (1967) *Studies in Ethnomethodology*. Englewood Cliff, NJ: Prentice-Hall.

Gill, V.T. and Maynard, D.W. (2006) Explaining illness: Patients' proposals and physicians' responses. In Heritage, J. and Maynard, D. (eds) *Communication in Medical Care: Interaction Between Primary Care Physicians and Patients*. Cambridge: Cambridge University Press.

Gill, V.T., Pomerantz, A. and Denvir, P. (forthcoming) Preemptive resistance: patients' participation in diagnostic sense-making activities, *Sociology of Health and Illness*.

Goodwin, C. (ed.) (2003) *Conversation and Brain Damage*. New York: Oxford University Press.

Greatbatch, D., Heath, C., Campion, P. and Luff, P. (1995) How do desk-top computers affect the doctor-patient interaction, *Family Practice*, 12, 1, 32–6.

Greatbatch, D., Hanlon, G., Goode, J., O'Caithain, A., Strangleman, T. and Luff, D. (2005) Telephone triage, expert systems and clinical expertise, *Sociology of Health and Illness*, 27, 6, 802–30.

Halkowski, T. (2006) Realising the illness: patients' narratives of symptom discovery. In Heritage, J. and Maynard, D. (eds) *Communication in Medical Care: Interaction Between Primary Care Physicians and Patients*. Cambridge: Cambridge University Press.

Halkowski, T. and Gill, V.T. (forthcoming) Conversation analysis and ethnomethodology: the centrality of interaction. To appear in Bourgeault, I.L., DeVries, R. and Dingwall, R. (eds) *Handbook of Qualitative Health Research*. London: Sage.

ten Have, P. (1989) The consultation as a genre. In Torode, B. (ed.) *Text and Talk as Social Practice*. Dordrecht/Providence, R.I.: Foris Publications.

Heath, C. (1981) The opening sequence in doctor-patient interaction. In Atkinson, P. and Heath, C. (eds) *Medical Work: Realities and Routines*. Farnborough: Gower.

Heath, C. (1992) The delivery and reception of diagnosis in the general practice consultation. In Drew, P. and Heritage, J. (eds) *Talk at Work: Interactional in Institutional Settings*. Cambridge: Cambridge University Press.

Heath, C. (2002) Demonstrative suffering: the gestural (re)embodiment of symptoms, *Journal of Communication*, 52, 3, 597–617.

Heath, C., Luff, P. and Sanchez Svensson, M. (2003) Technology and medical practice, *Sociology of Health and Illness*, 25, 3, 75–96.

Heritage, J. and Robinson, J.D. (2006) Accounting for the visit: giving reasons for seeking medical care. In Heritage, J. and Maynard, D. (eds) *Communication in Medical Care: Interaction between primary care physicians and patients*. Cambridge: Cambridge University Press.

Heritage, J. and Maynard, D.W. (2006a) Problems and prospects in the study of physician-patient interaction: 30 years of research, *Annual Review of Sociology*, 32, 351–74.

Heritage, J. and Maynard, D.W. (2006b) Introduction: Analyzing interaction between doctors and patients in primary care encounters. In Heritage, J. and Maynard, D. (eds) *Communication in Medical Care: Interaction between primary care physicians and patients*. Cambridge: Cambridge University Press.

Heritage, J., Robinson, J.D., Elliott, M.N., Beckett, M. and Wilkes, M. (2007) Reducing patients' unmet concerns in primary care: the difference one word can make, *Journal of General Internal Medicine*, 22, 10, 1429–33.

Heritage, J. and Sefi, S. (1992) Dilemmas of advice: aspects of the delivery and reception of advice in interactions between health visitors and first time mothers. In Drew, P. and Heritage, J. (eds) *Talk at Work*. Cambridge: Cambridge University Press.

Heritage, J. and Stivers, T. (1999) Online Commentary in Acute Medical Visits: A Method of Shaping Patient Expectations, *Social Science and Medicine*, 49, 11, 1501–17.

Hindmarsh, J. and Pilnick, A. (2002) The tacit order of teamwork: collaboration and embodied conduct in anaesthesia, *The Sociological Quarterly*, 43, 2, 139–64.

Hindmarsh, J. (in press) Peripherality, participation and communities of practice: examining the patient in dental training. In Llewellyn, N. and Hindmarsh, J. (eds) *Organisation, Interaction and Practice: Studies in Ethnomethodology and Conversation Analysis*. Cambridge: Cambridge University Press.

Housley, W. (2003) *Interaction in Multidisciplinary Teams*. Aldershot, Ashgate.

Hutchby, I. (2007) *The Discourse of Child Counselling*. Amsterdam and Philadelphia: John Benjamins.

Koschmann, T., LeBaron, C., Goodwin, C., Zemel, A. and Dunnington, G. (2007) Formulating the 'Triangle of Doom', *Gesture*, 7, 1, 97–118.

Koschmann, T., LeBaron, C., Goodwin, C. and Feltovich, P. (forthcoming) 'Can you see the cystic artery yet?': a simple matter of trust, *Journal of Pragmatics*.

Lindsay, J. and Wilkinson, R. (1999) Repair sequences in aphasic talk: a comparison of aphasic-speech and language therapist and aphasic-spouse conversations, *Aphasiology*, 13, 4, 305–25.

Martin, C. (2005) *From Other to Self: learning as interactional change*. PhD Thesis, Uppsala Studies in Education 107, Uppsala University.

Maynard, D.W. (2003) *Bad News, Good News: Conversational Order in Everyday Talk and Clinical Settings*. Chicago, University of Chicago Press.

Maynard, D.W. (2005) Social actions, gestalt coherence, and designations of disability: lessons from and about autism, *Social Problems*, 52, 500–24.

Maynard, D.W. and Frankel, R.M. (2006) On diagnostic rationality: bad news, good news, and the symptom residue. In Heritage, J. and Maynard, D. (eds) *Communication in Medical Care: Interaction Between Primary Care Physicians and Patients*. Cambridge: Cambridge University Press.

Maynard, D.W. and Heritage, J. (2005) Conversation analysis, doctor-patient interaction and medical communication, *Medical Education*, 39, 428–35.

McCabe, R., Heath, C., Burns, T. and Priebe, S. (2002) Engagement of patients with psychosis in the medical consultation: a conversation analytic study, *British Medical Journal*, 325, 1148–51.

Mondada, L. (2007) Operating together through videoconference: members' procedures for accomplishing a common space of action. In Hester, S. and Francis, D. (eds) *Orders of Ordinary Action*. Aldershot: Ashgate.

NHS Modernisation Agency (2003) *Essence of Care: Patient Focused Benchmarks for Clinical Governance*. London: Department of Health.

Nishisaka, A. (2007) Hand touching hand: referential practice at a Japanese midwife house, *Human Studies*, 30, 3, 199–217.

Parry, R. (2004) The interactional management of patients' physical incompetence: a conversation analytic study of physiotherapy interactions, *Sociology of Health and Illness*, 26, 7, 976–1007.

Peräkylä, A. (1995) *AIDS Counselling: Institutional Interaction and Clinical Practice*. Cambridge: Cambridge University Press.

Peräkylä, A. (1998) Authority and accountability: the delivery of diagnosis in primary health care, *Social Psychology Quarterly*, 61, 4, 301–20.

Peräkylä, A. (2002) Agency and authority: extended responses to diagnostic statements in primary care encounters, *Research on Language and Social Interaction*, 35, 219–47.

Peräkylä, A. (2006) Communicating and responding to diagnosis. In Heritage, J. and Maynard, D. (eds) *Communication in Medical Care: Interaction Between Primary Care Physicians and Patients*. Cambridge: Cambridge University Press.

Peräkylä, A., Ruusuvuori, J. and Lindfors, P. (2007) What is patient participation: reflections arising from the study of general practice, homoeopathy and psychoanalysis. In Collins, S. *et al.* (eds) *Patient Participation in Health Care Consultations: Qualitative Perspectives*. Maidenhead: Open University Press.

Peräkylä, A., Antaki, C., Vehviläinen, S. and Leudar, I. (eds) (2008) *Conversation Analysis and Psychotherapy*. Cambridge: Cambridge University Press.

Pilnick, A. (1998) 'Why didn't you just say that?': dealing with issues of asymmetry, knowledge and competence in the pharmacist/client encounter, *Sociology of Health and Illness*, 20, 1, 29–51.

Pilnick, A. (2004) 'It's just one of the best tests that we've got at the moment': the presentation of screening for fetal abnormality in pregnancy, *Discourse and Society*, 15, 4, 451–65.

Pomerantz, A., Ende, J. and Erickson, F. (1995) Precepting in a general medicine clinic: how precep-
tors correct. In Morris, G.H. and Chenail, R.J. (eds) *The Talk of the Clinic*. Mahwah, NJ: Lawrence
Erlbaum.

Pomerantz, A. and Ende, J. (1997) When supervising physicians see patients: strategies used in difficult
situations, *Human Communication Research*, 23, 4, 589–615.

Pooler, J. (forthcoming) Managing the diagnostic space: interactional dilemmas in calls to NHS Direct.
In Buscher, M., Goodwin, D. and Mesman, J. (eds) *Ethnographies of Diagnostic Work*. Basingstoke:
Palgrave.

Potter, J. and Hepburn, A. (2003) 'I'm a bit concerned': early actions and psychological constructions
in a child protection helpline, *Research on Language and Social Interaction*, 36, 197–240.

Rhodes, P., Langdon, M., Rowley, E., *et al.* (2006) What does the use of a computerised checklist
mean for patient centred care? The example of a routine diabetes review, *Qualitative Health Research*,
16, 353–78.

Roberts, F. (1999) *Talking about Treatment: Recommendations for Breast Cancer Adjuvant Therapy*.
New York: Oxford University Press.

Robinson, J.D. (2001) Closing medical encounters: Two physician practices and their implications for
the expression of patients' unstated concerns, *Social Science and Medicine*, 53, 639–56.

Robinson, J.D. (2003) An interactional structure of medical activities during acute visits and its implications for patients' participation, *Health Communication*, 15, 1, 27–59.

Robinson, J.D. (2006) Soliciting patients' presenting concerns. In Heritage, J. and Maynard, D. (eds)
Communication in Medical Care: Interaction Between Primary Care Physicians and Patients. Cambridge: Cambridge University Press.

Robinson, J.D. and Heritage, J. (2005) The structure of patients' presenting concerns: the completion
relevance of current symptoms, *Social Science and Medicine*, 61, 481–93.

Royal College of Nursing (2003) *Defining Nursing*. London: Royal College of Nursing.

Ruusuvuori, J. (2005) Comparing homeopathic and general practice consultations: the case of problem
presentation, *Communication and Medicine*, 2, 2, 123–35.

Sacks, H. (1984) Notes on methodology. In Maxwell Atkinson, J.M. and Heritage, J. (eds) *Structures
of Social Action: Studies in Conversation Analysis*. Cambridge: Cambridge University Press.

Sanchez Svensson, M., Heath, C. and Luff, P. (2007) Instrumental action: the timely exchange of
implements during surgical operations. In Bannon, L., *et al.* (eds) *Proceedings of the 10th European
Conference on Computer Supported Cooperative Work*. London: Springer.

Schegloff, E. and Sacks, H. (1973) Opening up closings, *Semiotica*, 8, 289–327.

Silverman, D. (1987) *Communication and Medical Practice: Social Relations in the Clinic*. London:
Sage.

Silverman, D. (1997) *Discourses of Counselling: HIV Counselling a Social Interaction*. London: Sage.

Speer, S.A. and Parsons, C. (2006) Gatekeeping gender: some features of the use of hypothetical
questions in the psychiatric assessment of transsexual patients, *Discourse and Society*, 17, 6,
785–812.

Stivers, T. (2002a) Participating in decisions about treatment: overt parent pressure for antibiotic
medication in pediatric encounters, *Social Science and Medicine*, 54, 1111–30.

Stivers, T. (2002b) Presenting the problem in pediatric encounters: 'Symptoms only' Versus 'Candidate
diagnosis' presentation, *Health Communication*, 14, 3, 299–338.

Stivers, T. (2006) Treatment decisions: negotiations between doctors and patients in acute care encounters. In Heritage, J. and Maynard, D. (eds) *Communication in Medical Care: Interaction Between
Primary Care Physicians and Patients*. Cambridge: Cambridge University Press.

Stivers, T. and Majid, A. (2007) Questioning children: Interactional evidence of implicit racial bias in
medical interviews, *Social Psychology Quarterly*, 70, 4, 424–41.

Strong, P.M. (1979) *The Ceremonial Order of the Clinic: Patients, Doctors, and Medical Bureaucracies*.
London: Routledge and Kegan Paul.

Sudnow, D. (1967) *Passing On: the Social Organization of Dying*. Englewood Cliffs, N.J.:
Prentice-Hall.

Turner, R. (1972) Some formal properties of therapy talk. In Sudnow, D. (ed.) *Studies in Social Interaction*. New York: Free Press.

West, C. (1983) 'Ask me no questions': an analysis of queries and replies in physician-patient dialogues. In Fisher, S. and Todd, A. (eds) *The Social Organization of Doctor-Patient Communication*. Washington, DC: Center for Applied Linguistics.

Whalen, J. (1995) A technology of order production: computer-aided dispatch in public safety communication. In ten Have, P. and Psathas, G. (eds) *Situated Order: Studies in the Social Organization of Talk and Embodied Activities*. Washington, D.C.: University Press of America.

Whalen, J., Zimmerman, D. and Whalen, M. (1988) When words fail: a single case analysis, *Social Problems*, 35, 4, 335–62.

Wilkinson, R., Gower, M., Beeke, S. and Maxim, J. (2007) Adapting to conversation as a language-impaired speaker: changes in aphasic turn construction over time, *Communication and Medicine*, 4, 1, 79–97.

Wootton, A.J. (1977) Sharing: some notes on the organization of talk in a therapeutic community, *Sociology*, 11, 333–50.

World Health Organisation (2000) *Technical Report Series 894: Obesity: Preventing and Managing the Global Epidemic*. Geneva: World Health Organisation.

2

Dialling for donations: practices and actions in the telephone solicitation of human tissues

T. Elizabeth Weathersbee and Douglas W. Maynard

Introduction

The purpose of this chapter is to demonstrate and analyse how one group of US call centre personnel work to solicit the donation of human tissues such as cornea, heart valves, and bone. With a conversation analytic perspective, we scrutinise audio recordings and transcripts of calls between these 'Family Support Co-ordinators' (FSCs) and the family of the deceased person, and propose that close attention to the talk and social interaction in this healthcare setting can illuminate tissue donation solicitation practices and expand our understanding of the more general practices for facilitating altruistic acts. Our attention to this interaction does not put the family members' donation decision making per se at the forefront of the analysis, but it does highlight that how FSCs approach family members, and how these members deal with solicitations, are *practical* matters that are subject to management on a moment-by-moment or turn-by-turn, contingent basis.

Social psychological and sociological perspectives on donation

Sociologists have contributed important studies in the area of donation particularly as related to altruism and the provision of public goods (Piliavin and Charng 1990) such as blood (Callero 1985, Callero *et al.* 1987, Piliavin and Callero 1991, Healy 2000), time and money (Lee *et al.* 1999), and human organs (Healy 2004). The earliest study of organ donation analysed the 'gift exchange'[1] between the living, related kidney donor and the recipient, focusing on the surgeons who were doing what was then pioneering work in kidney transplantation (Fox and Swazey 1974). However, in an early study that included 'cadaveric' or deceased kidney donors who were not known or related to the recipient, donor families reported that 'altruism and humanitarianism' played a major role in their decision to donate, with some persons noting that they imagined 'what it would be like if their own child were "lying there, waiting for an organ"' (Simmons *et al.* 1977: 351).

The routine, ongoing, institutionalised giving (Healy 2004) of a public good such as blood, time, and money may be predicted by a 'donor role identity' that emerges through repeat giving over time (Callero 1985, Callero *et al.* 1987, Piliavin and Callero 1991, Lee *et al.* 1999). However, this role identity does not necessarily explain variations in socially organised, but typically rare or 'one-shot' events (Healy 2004) such as the donation of bone marrow (Simmons *et al.* 1993), organs (Healy 2004, 2006a, 2006b) or tissues. In fact, Healy (2004) argues that regional, national, and international organ donation rates vary extensively not because of variation in altruistic identities or motives, but rather because of the logistical efforts of organ procurement organisations (OPO) which provide the opportunity for giving. While Healy (2004) recognises that OPOs' 'requesting procedures' (Healy 2004: 395) and the investment in more staff who are better trained in 'the crucial process of requesting consent from families' (Healy 2006b: 1042) may be important factors to consider in any attempt to explain and ultimately increase donation consent rates, his organisational perspective – as well as donor role identity theory – bypasses what happens in the interaction between organisational actors and potential donors. Accordingly, for better understanding of soliciting donations as a collaborative action, but also expanding our understanding of the more general practices for facilitating altruistic acts and how aspects of interaction may influence donation rates, our study proposes that along with individual identity features and organisational factors in relation to altruism, we also must investigate the ordinary conversational practices of soliciting and giving as Family Support Co-ordinators talk with family members directly and in real time.

Other social scientific perspectives on donation

Previous research has regarded the signing of an organ donor card as a 'form of voluntarism' (Piliavin and Charng 1990: 56), but in practice this action may have very little to do with donation. In fact, despite the *US 1968 Uniform Anatomical Gift Act* (UAGA) guaranteeing an individual's right to determine in advance whether or not to donate their organs and tissues upon their death, it is the family member(s) who, after the individual's death, make(s) the final donation decision (Kurtz *et al.* 2007, Healy 2006a, Zink and Wertlieb 2006, Morgan 2004, Rodrigue *et al.* 2003, Siminoff *et al.* 2001, Verble and Worth 2000). Consequently, the exercise of altruism in organ and tissue donation is more complex than the donation of blood, time, or bone marrow because it 'involves the giver in other basic human realities ... death and family relationships' (Prottas 1983: 299). That is, though organ and tissue donation does not involve a physical cost to the person(s) making the donation – as do blood and bone marrow donation – it does involve an intense emotional cost. This begins with the difficulty of reconciling the sight of a loved one's warm body with the diagnosis of brain death. As liver transplant surgeon Pauline Chen[2] notes, given that 'we all harbor [the hope] that our loved one might still be alive ... [since] our life support machines and medications make the brain-dead look as if they are only asleep ... (a)ccepting a loved one's death and then deciding to proceed with organ donation is one of the most emotionally difficult sets of decisions a family member can make.'[3] Despite otherwise positive attitudes towards donation, it can be very difficult to relinquish a loved one's body to be 'cut-up as spare parts' at a time when many believe the body should remain protected, whole and undisturbed (Sque *et al.* 2008: 140).

The stakes are high, however, in terms of increasing organ and tissue donation. Over 100,000 American men, women and children alone currently sit on the national organ waiting list (United Network of Organ Sharing November 2008); while an average of 18 will die each day, waiting for a transplant[4]. The unmet demand for transplantable organs and tissues – what some call a 'profound crisis in US healthcare,' (DeJong *et al.* 1995) – has as yet few sustainable solutions (Koh *et al.* 2007). Despite a plethora of federally-funded initiatives, which include updating UAGA to further protect donors' rights to designate their organs for donation after their death, increasing spending on donor education, and adopting less stringent donor requirements, there has been little increase in the pool of transplantable organs and tissues (Kaserman and Barnett 2002). Consent rates in the United States remain at approximately 50 per cent for organs (Siminoff *et al.* 2001) and 35% for tissues (Rodrigue *et al.* 2003) though the vast majority (95%) of Americans report that they support the donation of organs for transplantation (Gallup 2005).

Economists (Barnett and Kaserman 2000) and other scholars (Epstein 2006, Satel 2006) believe that the current donative system – begun in the early 1980s and codified into law in 1984 through the *National Organ Transplant Act* – by relying on 'altruistic motives to call forth the requisite supply' (Barnett and Kaserman 2000: 336) has clearly and miserably failed. The only remedy for this broken system, they argue, is to create a financial incentive to donate. Others going back to Titmuss's (1971) classic study of blood donation take exception to this perspective, and argue that financial markets may actually *decrease* donations by driving altruists out of the market and replacing them with egoists, or by 'crowding out' various civic virtues that lead the majority of people to donate (Healy 2006b: 10). In the Institute of Medicine's recent report on organ donation (Childress and Liverman 2006), committee members strongly recommended against financial incentives. In short, many scholars agree that we have not yet 'wrung all the supply we can out of the donative system' (Thorne 1998: 247).

Over two decades ago, Perkins (1987) explored what psychologists might do to help alleviate the transplantable organ and tissue shortage, and suggested that the probability of 'obtaining consent from families might be enhanced by the manner in which the request is made' (1987: 925). Yet, more than two decades later, no one has taken '(t)he first step in this research ... detailed examinations of requests as they are made' (Perkins 1987: 928). After their extensive meta-analysis of organ donation studies, Institute of Medicine committee members agreed that, '(c)ommunication and the relational aspects of the donation process are instrumental in creating a positive environment for considering and consenting to donation' (Childress and Liverman 2006: 107). However, studies that illuminate the organ and tissue donation interaction, including those from Scotland (Haddow 2004), Greece (Bellali and Papadatou 2007) and the US (Rodrigue *et al.* 2006) do not look directly at the interaction itself but rather rely on interviews in which family members recollect their organ donation request experience. Additionally, when studies claim to analyse the actual interaction surrounding donation, and even suggest that '(p)roblems with the ways in which families are asked about donation' account for high declination rates (Siminoff *et al.* 1995: 16), they neglect any investigation of how the interaction actually unfolds. That is, they suggest *who* should approach the family about donation, rather than the different issue of the concrete *ways* in which the approaching/asking occurs in the donation interaction. While one French study comparing rates of cornea donation by telephone versus face-to-face interactions approximates actual interaction by describing the components of the 'standardised telephone interview' (Gain *et al.* 2002: 927), they too rely on accounts of observations rather than recordings and transcripts of actual interactions.

While the literature concentrates mostly on organ rather than tissue donation, the issues are the same: to fully understand the donation process, it is necessary to examine actual, real-time interaction between clinic personnel as they solicit the donation from family members who may or may not consent.

Data and methods

These data were collected as part of a wider study on tissue donation practices directed by the second author and initiated by the 'Tissue Center,' a pseudonym for one of the largest organ, eye, and tissue recovery, processing and distribution programs in the nation. From this office, located in a large US city, personnel initiate donation phone calls to families located in multiple – including local and national – geographical regions. These telephone calls are routinely recorded and archived as digital audio files for legal as well as quality control purposes. The overall objective of the wider study was to identify a best practices model that could be used to inform Tissue Center staff training.

Data for this project derive from two sources: digital audio-recordings and transcriptions of the telephone interactions between the Tissue Center's 'Family Support Co-ordinators'

(FSC) and the decedent's family member(s), along with in-depth interviews and observations conducted in the Tissue Center. In the stratified purposive sample of telephone calls (n = 186), the aim was to obtain calls across the range of FSCs, to include racial/ethnic diversity among decedent families, and to incorporate an approximately equal number of donation outcomes, *i.e.* half consents and half declinations. This strategy of oversampling calls to the families of African-American and Latino decedents and consent calls was used to ensure that the final sample would include an adequate number of cases from these subgroups. Accordingly, the final sample includes: 89 (48%) consent and 97 (52%) declination calls placed by eight different Family Support Co-ordinators, the overwhelming majority of whom are White (97%) and female (83%); calls to the families of 135 (73%) White, 24 (13%) African-American, and 27 (14%) Latino decedents.[5] The in-depth interviews, each of which was audio-recorded and lasted approximately two hours, were conducted with five FSCs (four female and one male) and the director of the Tissue Center. These interviews and observations made by the first author were conducted over two three-day periods in 2005 and 2006. Our data collection protocol was approved by the University of Wisconsin (UW) Institutional Review Board (IRB), conditional on preserving confidentiality for all participants, and additionally providing pseudonyms for any geographical references in research reports.

While we suggest that this particular methodological approach to exploring the donation solicitation interaction improves our current analysis, we acknowledge a 'limited affinity' (Maynard 2003: Chapter 3) between ethnography and conversation analysis (CA). Accordingly, the field observations and interviews are used in this chapter to 'describe settings and identities, explicate unfamiliar terms or courses of action, and explain curious sequential patterns' (Maynard 2003: 73-6). Additionally, we follow general analytic procedures for the CA field as outlined, for example, in Clayman and Gill (2004) and ten Have (2007) with the aim of explicating, in a systematic way, the 'machinery' of interaction (Sacks 1984). Although by necessity we are showing a limited number of representative conversational extracts in this chapter, the practices by which participants assemble the interaction are 'methodical occurrences' or 'formal procedures' (Sacks 1984) that generalise in the first place to our entire collection of data but can also, in their generic features, be expected to characterise other settings with possible altruistic actions, *e.g.* interactions wherein participants face related tasks of solicitation and donation.

Institutional setting

The Tissue Center (TC) is staffed 24 hours a day, seven days a week to receive 'referral' calls for tissue donation, initiate calls to families of the deceased, and co-ordinate the procurement of tissues.[6] The referral begins as the triage staff receives the death notification telephone call from the hospital nursing staff or the medical examiner's office, in the case of decedents who did not die in the hospital. Medical staff members are required by federal law to notify the TC and supply information for every deceased patient. During the referral call, the triage staff collects a variety of health and demographic information on the decedent, including the time of death and the name and telephone number of the decedent's next-of-kin. From this information, the triage staff determines exactly which tissues the FSC can 'pursue' in their approach/telephone call to the decedent's next-of-kin. Using the medical information record or 'chart' compiled by the TC triage staff, the FSC determines when and where to telephone the next-of-kin depending on the decedent's time of death and the emotional condition of the family.

Sequential organisation of tissue donation solicitation calls

Identification, epistemic display, and condolence sequences
The vast majority of calls in our collection begin with 'Hello' (as in line 2, Extract 1 below), which in the US is the formal and most common response to a summons, whether that is a ringing phone or one generated by a 'switchboard request', line 3 (*cf.* Schegloff 1979: 30) to reach the targeted recipient (in 41% of our calls, a non-targeted family member or friend answers the phone rather than the targeted, designated next-of-kin.)

Extract 1   D36CJT1[7]

```
 1    ((ringing phone))
 2    A: ↓Hello::,
 3    C: .hh Ye::s > I was < ↑looking for Mister Sierr::a ↑plea:se?
 4    A: This is he:: may I he:lp you,
 5    C: Mister Sierr:a ↑my name is Do::nna and I'm a Family
 6       Support Coordinator with First Regional ↑Donor
 7       ↑Service::s,
 8    A: Ye:s Ma'am-
 9    C: An: Sir the ho:spital informed us of your wife's
10       (p)assing and I wanted ta offer my (.) sis- h (0.1)
11       sincere condolences to you and your fa::mily,
12       (0.4)
13    A: Thank you, =
14    C: = You we::lcome an Sir I'm sorry to be calling you at
15       this difficult ti::me, the reason I need (.) ta speak
16       with you (.) .hh your wi:fe ha:s the ability to
17       donate corneas > to restore vision < ta o::thers hh
18       and I wanna check with ya sir if that might have been
19       in her wi:she::s?
20       (0.2)
```

Although these opening moments may seem inconsequential and routine, they are 'dense' with social actions and interaction, and embody gatekeeping, relationship constitution, and the determination of the reason for the call (Schegloff 1979, 1986: 113, 117). In Extract 1, the FSC asks for the targeted call recipient and receives confirmation that he has been reached (lines 3–4), then identifies herself by first name, occupational title ('Family Support Co-ordinator'), and organisation (First Regional Donor Services) (lines 5–7). We will later examine how the reason for the call is articulated by the FSC, but so far we can see that when at line 8 the call recipient ('Mister Sierra') provides a go-ahead signal by acknowledging his caller's identity, he opens the gate for further interaction and allows for progression of the call (Maynard and Schaeffer 2002a). The relationship between these parties is established as between a person acting in an organisational capacity and an individual with whom the organisational actor is unacquainted (and vice versa).

After the gate is open for further interaction, the FSC produces a stretched 'an' at line 9, proposing the turn as an extension of the previous turn. It suggests further legitimacy for the call beyond the FSC's use of her occupational and organisational identity by referring to the 'hospital' as a source of notification – a 'how-we-know' display that is followed by a formulation of 'what-we-know,' namely that the family member has died – referenced euphemistically as a 'passing' (this turn at lines 9–10 also includes a proposal about the decedent's relationship to the call recipient.) Accordingly, this turn embodies what Whalen and Zimmerman (1990) discuss as 'practical epistemology' – an exhibit of how a party came to know about an event under discussion – and what we refer to as an 'epistemic display' regarding the deceased party (see also Heritage and Raymond 2005).

In our sample of calls, there are no how-are-you exchanges as are typical in ordinary call openings (Schegloff 1986). Instead, given that the FSC has now established that she knows of the family member's death, the initiation of a condolence is made relevant. There is a parallel, however, between condolence and how-are-you sequences, in that just as how-are-you sequences make the current state of the other party a matter of joint concern (Schegloff 1986), a condolence offering *presumes* the current state of the call recipient to be one of grieving and proposes it as a matter of joint concern to be addressed sympathetically by the FSC. Hence, a condolence offering can be called a how-are-you substitute that initiates instead a *how-you-are* sequence. Regularly in our tissue donation calls, the condolence offering (lines 10–11) initiates an adjacency pair whose second part is the recipient's gratuity (line 13) and the exchange is completed with a sequence-closing third turn (Schegloff 2007:120–3) as at line 14 in Extract 1, 'You we::lcome'.

However, in this instance, rather than acknowledging the condolence acceptance and immediately moving to the reason for the call, the FSC (lines 14–15) apologises for the timing of the call, suggesting it to be a 'difficult time' and thereby elaborating and extending the condolence sequence. The recipient withholds acknowledgement or acceptance of this proposal, which may resist it, or at the very least, work to maintain the formal or business nature of the call. This assessment is somewhat more presumptive than the initial and formal condolence by embodying what Labov and Fanshel (1977) call a 'B-statement' about a state of being to which the recipient has primary access and the initiator has only secondary, and in this case, inferential access. The epistemic rights to make such assessments can be very contentious territory (Heritage and Raymond 2005) and, unlike the offering of condolences in conversations between friends and relatives (Maynard and Weathersbee 2006) where condolences can initiate 'troubles talk' (Jefferson 1988), here they do not. Rather, in our sample of calls, the condolence receives either no uptake or a minimal acknowledgement that is regularly followed by a formulation of the reason for the call.[8]

Reason for the call: tacit donation solicitation
The reason for the call is typically the first step in *tacitly soliciting* the tissue donation from the donor family. By suggesting that the solicitation is tacit, we mean that FSCs use various devices that avoid overt requesting, as is demonstrated in other contexts of both ordinary and institutional talk (Maynard and Schaeffer 1997, Curl and Drew 2008). This avoidance is evidence that solicitations, like direct requests more generically speaking, are dispreferred, with offers being preferred over a direct request in both ordinary conversation (Schegloff 2007) and institutional talk (Gill 2005, Maynard et al. 2008).

The preference for offers over requests typically means that one interlocutor may use a device such as a 'pre-request' to elicit an offer from the other party rather than making a direct request of that party and risk rejection of the request, a potentially disaffiliative action (Schegloff 2006). Additionally, parties can avoid making direct requests by 'masking' them as other actions such as 'ostensible offers' (Schegloff 2006: 84–6). For example, FSCs often mask the donation solicitation by formulating the reason for the call as an 'offer' of the 'option ... to donate' (lines 37–38) as seen in Extract 2 below.

Extract 2 DO1CKTR3

```
34    C:  °Yes ma'am° .hh tch an:d (0.1) I know it's a very
35        difficult ↓ti::me for your fa:mily right no:::w,
36        (0.6)
37    C:  .h Just ca:llin ta offer you the option that your
38        >↓hu:sband may be able to donate ↑his < corneas (.) to
39        help restore sight in o:hthe::rs .h
40        (1.0)
41    C:  As well as other tissues for reconstructive surgeries.
42        (1.0)
43    C:  ↑Is that something that you'd ever had a chance to
44        discuss with [him?
45    A:                [.hhu He never had- he never had signed
46        anything like that, so I gue:ss not.
```

The issue of who actually has the agency to make the donation is addressed subtly here as the 'option' is offered to the wife, although it is the husband who would 'be able to donate' (lines 37–39). After indications of resistance at lines 40 and 42, and after the query about whether she had a chance to discuss tissue donation with the husband (lines 43–44), the wife effectively denies the donation by citing the husband's not having 'signed anything like that' as a reason, and declining the 'offer' extended to her with 'so I guess not' (line 46). In addition to showing a tacit way of soliciting donation, this extract also illustrates the subtle ways in which FSCs and family members address this issue of agency, *i.e.* who can or who does make the donation decision.

More regularly than 'offering the option' to donate, FSCs tacitly solicit donation by formulating the reason for the call as notifying the next-of-kin that the decedent has the 'potential to donate' (C55CDG1) or 'would be able to donate' (D04LPH) particular tissues. In some cases, such notifications appear to work something like pre-requests in that, just as they may occasion 'blocking moves' (as in Extract 4, line 19 below), they can generate offers of the desired social object (Schegloff 2007: 90–1). Accordingly, in Extract 3 below, the FSC apologises for the call (line 20), suggests that the 'paperwork at the hospital' is incomplete (lines 21–22), and informs that the decedent 'may be able ta donate' (line 24). In overlap with this latter utterance the call recipient offers to donate the decedent's eye tissues (lines 25–26, 28).

Extract 3 C28CPH

```
20    C:  I apologise again for having ta co::ntact you after she's
21        passed awa::y (0.2) .hh but when it's not kno:::wn (.) what
22        someone's wishes a::re in the pa:perwork at the ho:spital
23        (0.2) .hh about e::ye tissue donation (0.1) that
24        [they may be > able ta < donate
25    A:  [.hh Yea::h (.) u:::h (0.8) u::h (1.1) if the::re's (0.2) if
26        you can use em she had (.) poor eyesight [but if (0.1) > w- =
27    C:                                           [Uh huh
```

```
28    A:  = we: < no have problem with donating.
29    C:  Oka::y .hh uhm (.) I know the hour is la::te (.) and
30         I apologise for havin ta a::sk but (0.1) .hh we have
31         ta do:: what's called a medica::l and social history
32         questionna::ire?
33    A:  Uh huh.
```

The FSC, by initiating the next step in the donation process, the completion of a required medical and social history questionnaire (lines 29–32), displays an understanding that this offer constitutes the call recipient's consent to donation.

Conversely, rather than offering donation in response to a tacit solicitation, call recipients may issue a blocking move that declines the donation solicitation, as in Extract 4 at line 19. This move, especially when coupled with a terminal token such as 'THANK YA' (line 19) and a hanging up of the phone (line 20), represents an early way of declining and works to preempt any further donation solicitation.

Extract 4 D07BDG

```
16    C:  Uh (.) the reason I'm ca::lling you < is that > (.) she
17         do::es have po↓tential (0.4) ta donate corneas
18         [°an- ()
19    A:  [NO MA'AM WE NOT DONATIN ANYTHING HONEY ↑THANK YA
20         ((clicking sound))
21    C:  Tha:t's okay th-
           ((busy signal sound))
```

Otherwise, if the call continues with hesitation (silence) or other responses that do not foreclose further interaction, FSCs are expected to engage practices whereby they can continue their attempts to solicit the donation, but not in so aggressive a manner that they risk damaging public perception of tissue donation. Consequently, FSCs do not aggressively strive, as do survey interviewers, to convert donation declinations into consents (see Maynard and Schaeffer 2002b).

As we see in Extract 5 below, the FSC's initial solicitation formulation receives only minimal uptake in the form of a go-ahead token (line 23). Similar to Extract 1, this FSC masks the solicitation as a kind of offer at line 24. At the completion of her first 'turn constructional unit' (Sacks *et al.* 1974) – *i.e.* at the end of '… as an option your family::' – she produces a sound stretch that would allow for recipient uptake. There is none, and the FSC pursues the matter by inquiring whether the call recipient and her husband had ever discussed 'that,' *i.e.* being a 'cornea and tissue donor.'

Extract 5 C07BKT1

```
20    C:  .hhh there was nothin there on reco::rd indicating your
21         husband's wi:shes (.) regarding the possibility (0.2) hh
22         of being a cornea (.) and tissue dono::r?
23    A:  Uh ~huh
24    C:  We're just extending that as an option to your family:: is
25         that something that you'd ever had a chance ta discuss with
26         hi::m?
27    A:  U::hm (0.5) you know we hadn't discussed it however (0.8)
```

```
28          u::hm (.) I think it would > be a < ↑good thing?
29     C:   Oka::y.
30     A:   .hh If we could ↑do that.
31     C:   Su::re (0.3) .hh uhm (0.1) let me explain to you what we
32          would need to do:: be[fore a donation could ↑take pla::ce.
33     A:   [Okay
```

After hesitation at line 27, the call recipient disconfirms having 'discussed it,' produces a marker of contrast ('however,' line 27), and then volunteers a positive assessment regarding donation (line 28). The rising intonation occasions an acknowledging 'okay' by the FSC at line 29. Next at line 30, the recipient finalises an acceptance that generates an upgraded token – an affirmation – from the FSC (line 31) who pauses before proposing to explain the medical and social history interview that must take place before the tissue recovery team is dispatched.

As noted earlier, FSCs and family members alike demonstrate an artful ability to address the complex issue of exactly who has the agency to consent to donation. As we saw in Extract 1, the FSC suggests that the option to donate is something being offered, and offered first to the targeted recipient, the wife. In Extract 5 above, the option to donate is being 'extended' (line 24) not to the call recipient per se, who is the wife, but to 'your family'. Although, by way of asking about discussion with the husband, his agency is at least obliquely involved in the determination here, the wife claims agency at line 28 as she responds to the FSC's continuing tacit solicitation with an offer that is acknowledged at line 29, re-completed at line 30, and confirmed at line 31.

If consent to donation has still not been given after asking about any discussions with the deceased (Extract 6, lines 6–7), the FSC may use additional practices to solicit the donation. In Extract 6, after the targeted recipient's denial of having a discussion with the deceased (line 9), the FSC first acknowledges that denial (line 10 – in overlap with another negative token at line 11) before proposing the call recipient's relationship to the deceased as 'knowing him the best' and asking for her sense of his wants (lines 12–13) given that she denied having actually discussed it with him.

Extract 6 C40CKT1

```
1      C:   And I apo:logise for the ti::ming of the ca::ll (0.4) .hh
2           u:hm- there was nothing there at the ho::spital
3           indicati::ng Mister Bately's wishe::s regarding the
4           possibility:: (0.3) .hh of being a cornea donor ta help
5           restore sight in someone e::lse (0.3) .hh as well as tissue
6           donatio::n .hh is that something that you'd ever had a
7           chance ta discuss with hi::m,
8           (1.3)
9      A:   U:::h (.) no:: hhhh
10     C:   [°Alright°
11     A:   [Nya
12     C:   An- (.) kno:wing him be::st do you feel like that was
13          something he would have wa::nted,
14          (1.1)
15     C:   Or something that you would be in fa::vor o::f
16     A:   ↑Ye::s:: hh
```

17   C: O::ka::y
18   (1.2)
19   C: A::lright w-

The call recipient withholds answering at line 14, whereupon the FSC asks if it was something the recipient herself would want (line 15). The FSC thereby interprets the recipient's
withholding as due to some inability to formulate the *decedent's* wants regarding 'cornea
and tissue donation.' Upon being asked about her own position, the recipient agrees to
donation strongly and without delay (line 16).

According to TC policy and training, if the interaction is still continuing, but there has
been no donation decision, the FSC should inquire as to whether they can give the call
recipient some 'information about donation' to discuss with the other family members and
possibly then gain consent to the tissue donation. To facilitate this later consent, the FSC
is expected to propose and arrange a return telephone call. Work in progress examines these
other kinds of overtures (Weathersbee, forthcoming).

Discussion

While scholars have recognised the importance of analysing the solicitation of donated
goods such as human organs and tissues, to date none has examined the actual donation
solicitation interaction. Our study is a first attempt at filling this gap by analysing the interaction as it unfolds in real time for its participants. Our close analysis of the sequential
organisation of the tissue donation telephone call shows how solicitation is done cautiously,
incrementally, and – reflecting its status as a dispreferred action – tacitly rather than overtly.
Sometimes immediately in response to the initial formulation of the reason for the call, and
other times after further but still tacit attempts at solicitation, these solicitation practices
can generate offers of donation from family members.

Tacit solicitations, however, are often unsuccessful, as when family members block the
solicitation or, more regularly, meet solicitations with polite denials, as when a family
member suggests they have not discussed donation with the deceased person and use this
– or are taken by the FSC to be using this – as a reason to withhold donation. In any case,
the declination of donation, like the consent to donation, needs to be seen as an interactional
accomplishment. For example, consider how the construction of questions about whether
the family member had discussed the matter with the deceased person may encourage declination. Constructions such as 'is that something that you'd ever had a chance to discuss
with your spouse' (Extracts 2 and 5) have *negative polarity*, structurally preferring an answer
that can operate (or be taken as) a declination to donate. If the targeted recipient of the
phone call is disinclined to donate, such a construction facilitates withholding the donation
(Extract 2).

Conversely, if the recipient is inclined to offer the donation, but there had been no
discussion of donation with the deceased, following structures for dispreferred second-pair
parts may mean effectively acknowledging a failure to do something the FSC has suggested as relevant for the decision, then marking a contrast and producing an affirmative
display as part of an overall disagreement turn, a potentially disaffiliative action. For
example, in Extract 5, after the question about 'ever' discussing donation with the spouse,
the family member says, 'U::hm (0.5) you know we hadn't discussed it.' Then she emits
the contrast marker 'however,' and subsequently a tentative indication that donation is

a 'good thing.' In many cases, then, configurations in the wording of solicitations may operate interactionally but inadvertently to discourage the act of donation that FSCs are attempting to elicit.

Our research has been limited to tissue donation and while the practices of tacit solicitation may be generic and therefore applicable to other settings where altruistic acts are possible, most especially those involving organ donation, we do not yet have the data to verify these claims. However, in this chapter, we have demonstrated that a conversation analytic approach, in analysing the turn-by-turn sequence in telephone interactions involving tissue donation, gains significant ground in understanding the social organisation of such interaction. In future research, the interactional patterns we have identified can be analysed in greater detail to determine where, for example, practices on the part of Family Support Co-ordinators (or other organisational actors in other donation settings) may subtly discourage (or encourage) donation. In the case of organ and tissue donation specifically, if we are to understand why so many initiatives have done so little to increase the pool of transplantable organs and tissues, we must first fully understand the machinery of the donation solicitation interaction.

Acknowledgements

We express our gratitude to Dr. Betty A. Chewning of the University of Wisconsin's School of Pharmacy who connected us to the Tissue Center that supplied us both with the data for this study and the funding to complete it. We are grateful also to its Director, along with several key personnel, who must remain anonymous, but have been extremely helpful in facilitating the research. Additionally, we thank the two anonymous reviewers and the book editors for very helpful comments on earlier versions of this chapter.

Notes

1   See Sque and Payne (1994) for a more recent, modified theory of organ donation as a Maussian gift exchange.
2   See also Chen (2007) pp. 195–203.
3   Read this interview in its entirety at http://www.randomhouse.com/knopf/catalog/display.pperl? isbn=9780307263537&view=qa
4   According to 'Donate Life America' at http://www.donatelife.net/UnderstandingDonation/ Statistics.php
5   The Tissue Center collects demographic information on the decedent during the initial triage call. However, there is no similar information collected on the family members of the deceased.
6   Words in quotation marks reflect vocabularies that staff members use.
7   Pseudonyms are used in transcripts in place of proper names and places. Also note that targeted recipients are denoted 'A' and callers are denoted 'C' in the left margin, at the beginning of each speaker's turn.
8   The regular form for condolences in ordinary conversation is an utterance such as, 'I was sorry to hear X,' rather than 'I want to offer my condolences.' In fact, there are extensive variable features of condolences in both ordinary conversation and in the institutional context of tissue donation phone calls (Maynard and Weathersbee 2006) that are beyond the scope of this chapter.

References

Barnett, A.H. and Kaserman, D.L. (2000) Comment on 'The shortage in market-inalienable human organs': faulty analysis of a failed policy, *American Journal of Economics and Sociology*, 59, 2, 335–49.

Bellali, T. and Papadatou, D. (2007) The decision-making process of parents regarding organ donation of their brain dead child: a Greek study, *Social Science and Medicine*, 64, 439–50.

Brody, J.E. (2007, August 28) The solvable problem of organ shortages, *The New York Times*, p. F.7.

Callero, P.L. (1985) Role-identity salience, *Social Psychology Quarterly*, 48, 3, 203–15.

Callero, P.L., Howard, J.A. and Piliavin, J.A. (1987) Helping behavior as role behavior: disclosing social structure and history in the analysis of prosocial action, *Social Psychology Quarterly*, 50, 3, 247–56.

Chen, P.W. (2007) *Final Exam: a Surgeon's Reflections on Mortality*. New York: Alfred A. Knopf.

Childress, J.F. and Liverman, C.T. (2006) *Organ Donation: Opportunities for Action*. Washington, D.C.: The National Academies Press.

Clayman, S.E. and Gill, V.T. (2004) Conversation analysis. In Hardy, M. and Bryman, A. (eds) *Handbook of Data Analysis*. London: Sage.

Curl, T.S. and Drew, P. (2008) *Contingency and Action: a Comparison of Two forms of Requesting*. Heslington, York: University of York.

DeJong, W., Drachman, J., Gortmaker, S.L., Beasley, C. and Evanisko, M.J. (1995) Options for increasing organ donation: the potential role of financial incentives, standardized hospital procedures, and public education to promote family discussion, *The Milbank Quarterly*, 7, 3, 463–79.

Epstein, R. (2006, May 15). Kidney beancounters, *The Wall Street Journal*, p. A.15.

Fox, R.C. and Swazey, J.P. (1974) *The Courage to Fail: a Social View of Organ Transplants and Dialysis*. Chicago: University of Chicago Press.

Gain, P., Thuret, G., Pugniet, J.L., Riszi, P., Acquart, S., Le Petit, J.C., *et al.* (2002) Obtaining cornea donation consent by telephone, *Transplantation*, 73, 6, 926–9.

Gallup Organisation, The (2005) *National Survey of Organ and Tissue Donation Attitudes and Behaviors*. Rockville, MD: Health Resources and Services Administration.

Gill, V.T. (2005) Patient 'demand' for medical interventions: Exerting pressure for an offer in a primary care clinic visit, *Research on Language and Social Interaction*, 38, 4, 451–79.

Haddow, G. (2004) Donor and nondonor families' accounts of communication and relations with healthcare professionals, *Progress in Transplantation*, 14, 1, 41–8.

ten Have, P. (1999) *Doing Conversation Analysis: a Practical Guide*. London: Sage.

Healy, K. (2000) Embedded altruism: blood collection regimes and the European Union's donor population, *The American Journal of Sociology*, 105, 6, 1633–57.

Healy, K. (2004) Altruism as an organisational problem: the case of organ procurement, *American Sociological Review*, 69, 387–404.

Healy, K. (2006a) Do presumed consent laws raise organ procurement rates? *DePaul Law Review*, 55, 1017–43.

Healy, K. (2006b) *Last Best Gifts: Altruism and the Market for Human Blood and Organs*. Chicago: The University of Chicago Press.

Heritage, J. and Raymond, G. (2005) The terms of agreement: Indexing epistemic authority and subordination in talk-in-interaction, *Social Psychology Quarterly*, 68, 15–38.

Jefferson, G. (1988) On the sequential organization of troubles talk in ordinary conversation, *Social Problems*, 35, 418–41.

Kaserman, D.L. and Barnett, A.H. (2002) *The U.S. Organ Procurement System: a Prescription for Reform*. Washington, D.C.: AEI Press.

Koh, H.K., Jacobson, M.D., Lyddy, A.M., O'Connor, K.J., Fitzpatrick, S.M., Krakow, M., Judge, C.M., *et al.* (2007) A statewide public health approach to improving organ donation: the Massachusetts organ donation initiative, *American Journal of Public Health*, 97, 1.

Kurtz, S.F., Strong, C.W. and Gerasimow, D. (2007) The 2006 revised *Uniform Anatomical Gift Act – A law to save lives, Health Law Analysis*, February, 44–9.

Labov, W. and Fanshel, D. (1977) *Therapeutic Discourse*. New York: Academic Press.

Lee, L., Piliavin, J.A. and Call, V.R.A. (1999) Giving time, money, and blood: similarities and differences, *Social Psychology Quarterly*, 62, 3, 276–90.

Maynard, D.W. (2003) *Bad News, Good News: Conversational Order in Everyday Talk and Clinical Settings*. Chicago: The University of Chicago Press.

Maynard, D.W. and Schaeffer, N.C. (1997) Keeping the gate: declinations of the request to participate in a telephone survey interview, *Sociological Methods and Research*, 26, 1, 34–79.

Maynard, D.W. and Schaeffer, N.C. (2002a) Opening and closing the gate: the work of optimism in recruiting of survey respondents. In Maynard, D.W., Houtkoop-Steenstra, H., Schaeffer, N.C. and van der Zouwen, H. (eds) *Standardization and Tacit Knowledge: Interaction and Practice in the Survey Interview*. New York: Wiley Interscience.

Maynard, D.W. and Schaeffer, N.C. (2002b) Declination conversion and tailoring. In Maynard, D.W., Houtkoop-Steenstra, H., Schaeffer, N.C. and van der Zouwen, H. (eds) *Standardization and Tacit Knowledge: Interaction and Practice in the Survey Interview*. New York: Wiley Interscience.

Maynard, D.W., Freese, J. and Schaeffer, N.C. (2008) *Requesting as a social action: implications for nonresponse and 'Leverage-Saliency' in the survey interview*. American Sociological Association Annual Meeting, Boston.

Maynard, D.W. and Weathersbee, T.E. (2006) *An Initial Investigation on the Use of Condolences in Ordinary Conversation and in Telephone Requests for Tissue Donation*. Presentation at the Annual Meetings of the American Sociological Association, Montreal.

Morgan, S.E. (2004) The power of talk: African Americans' communication with family members about organ donation and its impact on the willingness to donate organs, *Journal of Social and Personal Relationships*, 21, 1, 112–24.

Organdonor.gov (2007 January 25) Organ and Tissue Donation, http://www.organdonor.gov/default.htm.

Perkins, K. (1987) The shortage of cadaver donor organs for transplantation: can psychology help? *American Psychologist*, 42, 10, 921–30.

Piliavin, J.A. and Charng, H. (1990) Altruism: A review of recent theory and research, *Annual Review of Sociology*, 16, 27–65.

Piliavin, J.A. and Callero, P.L. (1991) *Giving blood: The Development of an Altruistic Identity*. Baltimore, MD: Johns Hopkins University Press.

Prottas, J.M. (1983) Encouraging altruism: public attitudes and the marketing of organ donation, *The Milbank Memorial Fund Quarterly/Health and Society*, 61, 2, 278–306.

Rodrigue, J.R., Scott, M.P. and Oppenheim, A.R. (2003) The tissue donation experience: a comparison of donor and nondonor families, *Progress in Transplantation*, 13, 4, 258–64.

Rodrigue, J.R., Cornell, D.L. and Howard, R.J. (2006) Organ donation decision: comparison of donor and nondonor families, *American Journal of Transplantation*, 6, 1, 190–98.

Sacks, H. (1984) Notes on methodology. In Atkinson, J.M. and Heritage, J. (eds) *Structures of Social Action: Studies in Conversation Analysis*. Cambridge: Cambridge University Press.

Sacks, H., Schegloff, E. and Jefferson, G. (1974) A simplest systematics for the organisation of turn-taking for conversation, *Language*, 50, 696–735.

Satel, S. (2006, 15 May) Death's waiting list, *The New York Times*, p. A.21.

Schegloff, E.A. (1979) Identification and recognition in telephone conversation openings. In Psathas, G. (ed.) *Everyday Language: Studies in Ethnomethodology*. New York: Irvington Publishers, Inc.

Schegloff, E.A. (1986) The routine as achievement, *Human Studies*, 9, 111–51.

Schegloff, E.A. (2007) *Sequence Organisation in Interaction: a Primer in Conversation Analysis*. Cambridge: Cambridge University Press.

Simmons, R.G., Klein, S.D. and Simmons, R.L. (1977) *Gift of Life: the Social and Psychological Impact of Organ Transplantation*. New York: John Wiley and Sons.

Simmons, R.G., Schimmel, M. and Butterworth, V.A. (1993) The self-image of unrelated bone marrow donors, *Journal of Health and Social Behavior*, 34, 4, 285–301.

Siminoff, L.A., Gordon, N., Hewlett, J. and Arnold, R.M. (2001) Factors influencing families' consent for donation of solid organs for transplantation, *Journal of the American Medical Association*, 286, 71–7.

Sque, M. and Payne, S. (1994) Gift exchange theory: a critique in relation to organ transplantation, *Journal of Advanced Nursing*, 19, 45–51.

Sque, M., Long, T., Payne, S. and Allardyce, D. (2008) Why relatives do not donate organs for transplants: 'sacrifice' or 'gift of life'? *Journal of Advanced Nursing*, 61, 2, 134–44.

Thorne, E.D. (1998) The shortage in market-inalienable human organs: a consideration of 'nonmarket' failures, *American Journal of Economics and Sociology*, 57, 3, 247–60.

Titmuss, R. (1971) *The Gift Relationship: from Human Blood to Social Policy*. New York: Vintage.

Verble, M. and Worth, J. (2000) Fears and concerns expressed by families in the donation discussion, *Progress in Transplantation*, 10, 48–55.

Weathersbee, T.E. (forthcoming) Requesting, altruism, and the case of human tissue donation. University of Wisconsin-Madison: Dissertation.

Whalen, M.R. and Zimmerman, D.H. (1990) Describing trouble: Practical epistemology in citizen calls to the police, *Language in Society*, 19, 465–92.

Zink, S. and Wertlieb, S. (2006) A study of the presumptive approach to consent for organ donation: a new solution to an old problem, *Critical Care Nurse*, 26, 129–36.

3

Managing medical advice seeking in calls to Child Health Line

Carly W. Butler, Susan Danby, Michael Emmison and Karen Thorpe

Introduction

A central theme in medical sociology, first introduced by Parsons nearly sixty years ago, has been the asymmetrical distribution of power and knowledge between medical professionals and the lay public. As Parsons (1951) argued:

> The physician is a technically competent person whose competence and specific measures cannot be competently judged by the layman [sic]. The latter must therefore take these judgments and measures 'on authority' (1951:463).

Consistent with his overall sociological vision, Parsons' depiction of the medical relationship was almost entirely theoretically derived. Subsequently, research has demonstrated how medical authority is produced and oriented to in the course of actual medical consultations (e.g. Heath 1992, Heritage 2005, Maynard 1991, Peräkylä 1998, Gill 1998, West 1984). However, little has been written about how displays of authority and accountability in medical interactions relate to institutional policies and guidelines within which medical professionals operate.

The rising cost of direct face-to-face primary care has resulted in the provision of medical services being increasingly devolved to telephone contact via medical and health helplines. The operation of such helplines often involves clear policies and guidelines regarding what knowledge health professionals are entitled to display. These guidelines can relate to both the institutional role of the call-taker (for instance, nurses cannot offer diagnosis, see Pooler 2007), and in terms of institutional practices (such as the use of computer software packages to undertake medical assessments, see Greatbatch *et al.* 2005).

In this chapter we examine how nurses on a Child Health Line manage the apparent paradox of delivering medical advice when they are bound by service guidelines not to offer such advice. As we show, there are recurring practices through which these policies are 'talked into being' by nurses, whilst still meeting the demands of callers who seek medical advice regarding their ill children. In addition to showing how medical authority is enacted in actual health interactions, the chapter contributes more broadly to the growing body of research on helpline interactions (Baker, Emmison and Firth 2005, Edwards 2007), and in particular, on the role of institutional guidelines in shaping the nature of the help the call-taker is able to provide (see Danby, Baker and Emmison 2005, Emmison and Danby 2007). Help lines are crucial sites where knowledge claims and entitlements by the parties to the call (e.g. Potter and Hepburn 2003), and their attendant rights and responsibilities (e.g. Raymond and Zimmerman 2007), are particularly salient. Epistemic considerations are shown to play an important part in both the framing of the problem by the caller and the concomitant advice by the expert call-taker. These themes are also found in the limited literature on medical helpline interaction (*e.g.* Drew 2006, Greatbatch *et al.* 2005, Pooler 2007).

Calls to health lines embody an assumption that the call-taker is able to offer advice on medical matters, using knowledge to which the caller may not have access or entitlement. An asymmetrical distribution of specialised knowledge and authority is, of course, central to the medical encounter. However, doctors' authority and entitlement to know about medical issues is balanced by accountability in the delivery of diagnosis – showing 'how they know' and communicating this to the patient (Peräkylä 1998). Whilst research has focused largely on primary care interactions, a growing number of studies have examined how expertise, knowledge and skills are occasioned in interactions between clients and other health professionals, including pharmacists (Pilnick 1998, 1999), HIV counsellors (Silverman 1997), genetic counsellors (Sarangi and Clarke 2002), health visitors (Heritage and Sefi 1992) and nurses (Greatbatch *et al.* 2005, Leppanen 1998, Pooler 2007).

How knowledge and authority is displayed and oriented to in interactions with clients amongst various health professions is often bounded in terms of what medical advice or information can be offered. For instance, Sarangi and Clarke (2002) show how genetic counsellors invoke such boundaries by engaging in hedging, or by contrasting their expertise with other medical professionals to formulate uncertainty in their responses to clients' requests for information and advice. Through invoking their professional knowledge and institutional roles, the counsellors construct their 'zones of expertise'.

Pooler (2007) discusses how nurse advisors in the National Health Service Direct (NHSD, a UK-based telephone helpline) are constrained by institutional requirements that they do not offer diagnostic assessments. The nurse advisors engage in what Pooler describes as 'boundary setting' in the initial stages of a call by advising callers that they cannot diagnose a problem. Following the use of a computer-assisted clinical assessment system, nurses produce problem formulations in ways that display caution and uncertainty, and which downgrade their epistemic authority. Greatbatch *et al.* (2005) show how NHSD nurse call-takers depart from the institutionally mandated use of an 'expert system' aimed at standardising nurse-caller interactions. Nurses privilege their own expertise in their delivery of the system's algorithmic questions and dispositions, and in their recommendations – both overriding and underriding the assessments given by the system.

In this chapter, we examine how nurses on an Australian Child Health Line manage their boundaries of expertise and institutional remit in response to callers' requests for medical advice. Child Health Line offers support and information on children's behaviour, health and development, operating under guidelines that nurses should not provide specifically 'medical advice'. Parents, however, regularly request medical advice on the assumption that the nurses have the professional authority and institutional warrant to offer such advice. Such an assumption is not surprising, given the name of the service and a common-sense understanding of the mutual relevance of health and illness. The boundary between wellness and illness is far from clear cut and there can be ambiguity as to where a child's behaviour or symptoms may sit on the health continuum – particularly when the nurse is unable to see the child. The problem is further complicated by the blurred line between what constitutes 'medical' or 'non-medical' advice.

The institutional guidelines thus result in multiple constraints and tensions to be managed in the course of the calls. The practical dilemma facing the nurses involves discerning whether the problem falls within their realm of expertise, and managing this discriminatory work within the bounds of the institutional guidelines and the local contingencies of the interaction. In this sense, calls seeking medical advice are managed on institutional, practical, and interactional levels. We show that while Child Health Line nurses do indeed offer medical advice and information, they do so in ways that reveal the tensions between the service guidelines and the practicalities of responding to parents' requests for medical advice.

Child Health Line

Child Health Line is an Australian 24-hour telephone service funded by Queensland Health. Established in 2000, the service answers approximately 50,000 calls per year (Ferguson 2005), and is advertised through Child Health clinics, in the information section of the phone book and in the parent-held child health record booklet. Local call costs apply for metropolitan users and a toll-free number is available to callers outside Brisbane. The call centre operates from a residential parenting clinic. On each shift, calls are taken by two experienced paid nurses with general nursing qualifications and midwifery and/or child health postgraduate certificates. Staff participate in professional development workshops, such as parenting programmes (Ferguson 2005). A clinical nurse consultant oversees the provision of the service and staff performance.

Unlike many tele-health services (such as the NHSD in the UK), Child Health Line does not use a clinical assessment system. Nurses enter demographic details of the caller and child, and the main reason for the call into a database. Calls are not routinely recorded and monitored, and documented only if an emergency or child protection matter is reported (Ferguson 2005).

A quantitative analysis of 300 calls within the corpus collected for this project indicates that most calls are about infants (mean 7 months). A small proportion of calls (4%) seek service information, 48 per cent exclusively seek parenting advice, 22 per cent exclusively seek medical advice, and a further 26 per cent present combined medical and parenting problems. Overall, 48 per cent of calls present an issue with some medical content.

Data and method

This study draws from a corpus of over 700 calls to Child Health Line recorded over four weeks during the 2005–2006 Christmas and New Year period. Twelve nurses gave written consent to participate in the study, and callers were advised that calls would be recorded for research purposes. Callers and nurses could opt out of having a call included in the corpus.

A preliminary analysis identified a subset of calls in which callers solicited medical advice or assessments (for instance, seeking a diagnosis or asking whether it was necessary to seek medical attention for their child) and in which there appeared to be an orientation to the practical, epistemic and institutional boundaries around advising on medical matters. These extracts were transcribed using Jeffersonian conventions (Jefferson 2004). The analysis draws on ethnomethodological conversation analytic methods, entailing detailed examination of members' descriptions and the sequential organisation of turns at talk (Hutchby and Wooffitt 1998, Schegloff 2007). Turns at talk are understood as being responsive to just prior talk and consequential for a next turn; that is, utterances are both *context sensitive* and *context renewing* (Heritage 1984). By looking at how turns at talk are designed, their sequential placement and their interactional relevance, analysts can demonstrate how people produce and make sense of social action.

Analysis

The analysis focuses on cases where nurses' epistemic and institutional entitlement and authority are occasioned in relation to calls seeking diagnostic assessment, advice about seeking medical attention and information about ostensibly medical conditions. We describe three ways in which the child health nurses manage medical advice and information seeking: by using membership as a nurse to establish boundaries of expertise, by privileging parental authority regarding decision making about seeking treatment for their child, and by respecifying a 'medical' problem as a child development issue.

Establishing boundaries of expertise
One way nurses manage calls seeking medical assessment or advice is by making reference to the limits of their knowledge and institutional role, and offering explicit descriptions of what advice or information they can or cannot offer. Nurses suggest that the caller obtain the information, advice or assessment they seek from somebody better qualified to offer it, such as a doctor or pharmacist.

The first example is from a caller asking about giving medication to her son for his high temperature. The nurse had earlier advised the caller to take the child to the hospital if he got worse, and the caller sought clarification as to when this should happen (lines 1 and 3 below). Of particular interest here is the sequence in lines 20–43 where the caller appears to be seeking an assessment of her son's welts.

[NB: C = Caller; CT = Nurse]

Extract 1

ZC5CNJ41P

1	C:	<u>A</u>nd is [it ri::ght that once he hits like that thirty ni:ne=
2	CT:	[°Yeh°
3	C:	=degrees he should go to the hospi↑tal is that right?
4	CT:	k.hhh ↑Oh:-↑ (0.3) we:ll if he's got °i-° o:other °e-° ah
5		sy:mptoms as well if y:ihn: not getting it do:wn an:d ah
6		.hhhh (0.2) yih know he's a- (0.2) unusual ↑ra:sh:↑ or he's
7		got any °e-° (0.3) sort'v. hhh (0.4) you know neck ↑stiffness↑
8		or vo:miting: or .hhhhh
9	C:	Ye:a[h
10	CT:	[You kno:w °he° seems (.) tih (.) di:slike bri:ght ↑li:ghts
11		or has a ↑hea:da:che↑↓or (1.1) you kno:w,
12		(0.3)
13	C:	Yeap=
14	CT:	=Unusual cry:ing,
15		(0.3)
16	CT:	°Um:::°
17	C:	g.HHH Yea:h well see out of those, like cos he's got a <u>c</u>ough,
18		(.)
19	CT:	[Yeh
20	C:	[.hh B't u:m my <u>dau:gh</u>ter (.) for a:ges,
21	CT:	Yep=
22	C:	=And a doctor sa:w this and jist said it's an

```
23                 allergic reaction has been getting like hi:ves
24                 like welts coming up on her? .HHH
25    CT:          °↑Ye[ah.↑°
26    C:               [And then (0.2) tida:y_like she's had this since
27                 the start of Dece:mbe:r, .hhhh (.) an'- (0.2) tida:y he
28                 actually got a couple on his back and then on his ha:nds
29                 but they've just gone away ag↑ain?
30    C:           .hhhhhh An'-
31    CT:          °↑Mm::↑°
32    C:           Both of them seem to be complaining about being a bit
33                 itchy?
34                 (0.6)
35    CT:          °↑O:h ri:ght,↑°
36    C:           Ye[:ah.
37    CT:            [Ye:ah.
38                 (0.3)
39    CT: ->       .h ↑W'll↑ i- um (1.3) well I don't know wha:t that is but
40         ->      it could- ye:ah as you say the doctor said it could
41         ->      be a reaction to something and I'm- I'm just a nu:rse
42         ->      =So I just have to depend on the .hhhhhhh (0.3) the- what
43         ->      the doctor (0.4) diagnoses?
44                 (.)
45    CT:          Y[eah.
46    C:            [Yep. B't-=
47    CT:          =<Yeh I wou:ld- (.) ah me:ntion to the doctor as well.
48    C:           Okay an' [(.) b't (.) we:lts (.) are the:y ah like in=
49    CT:                   [°And ah°
50    C:           =a different category to: (0.4) like (0.3) rashes aren't
51                 they? ...
```

After the caller proposes a candidate reason for taking her son to the hospital (a temperature of 39°C (102.2°F)), the nurse qualifies this with a list of possible co-occurring symptoms that would warrant taking the child to hospital – an unusual rash, neck stiffness, vomiting, dislike of bright lights, headache, and unusual crying (lines 6–14). In describing these symptoms the nurse can be seen to be offering medical information. The caller then begins an assessment of her child's current condition using the list of symptoms offered by the nurse with 'see out of those' (line 17). She initially offers 'a cough' as a current symptom, which was not in the nurse's list and downgrades the seriousness of the child's state, and then continues with a description of her son's welts (lines 20–33). The relevance of the welts appears to tie back to the nurse's mention of a rash in line 6, and the caller appears to be seeking an assessment of the welts.

The caller alludes to the possibility that the welts appearing on her son are related to her daughter's, which had been diagnosed by the doctor as an allergic reaction (lines 20, 22–24). However, an element of uncertainty is raised by the report of the timing of the son's welts; whereas the daughter's had been evident since 'the start of December' (four weeks previously), the son's welts appeared only that day and had since 'gone away again'. The more recent and temporary nature of the son's welts might suggest a relationship with his current illness, and the possibility that the welts may be a rash requiring urgent medical attention. The ambiguity alluded to, the proffer of a speculative explanation (Gill 1998), and the caller's questioning intonation, make assessment a relevant next action for the nurse (Gill and Maynard 2006, Stivers 2002).

The nurse responds initially with a high-pitched newsmarker, 'oh right' (line 35), which registers the information but does not project a forthcoming assessment. In lines 39–43 she responds to the caller's description, with the restart, 'wells', delays, and perturbations marking this response as dispreferred (Pomerantz 1984). While orienting to the relevance of an assessment of the child's symptoms as a next action, the nurse claims insufficient knowledge to offer an explanation for the welts (line 39–41) and whether these might be considered a rash. Recycling the caller's report about what the doctor said ('as you say the doctor said', line 40) about the daughter's welts, the nurse accounts for her lack of entitlement to make an assessment by identifying herself as 'just a nurse' who has to 'depend on what the doctor diagnoses'. In this way, the nurse makes relevant her institutional category membership to downgrade her epistemic authority and defer to the doctors' entitlement to undertake medical assessment. In line 48 the caller acknowledges receipt of the advice to ask the doctor about the welts (at line 47), but then asks explicitly whether welts are in a 'different category' from a rash. In doing so, she can be heard to reformulate the gist of her initial problem presentation, and orients to the absence of an assessment by the nurse.

Thus, while the nurse offered medical information regarding the kinds of symptoms that warrant taking the child to the hospital, she avoids proffering a 'diagnosis'. On the one hand, making such a diagnosis over the telephone is problematic due to the absence of visual information – but of interest here is the way that the nurse invokes her institutional role in accounting for her inability to suggest what the welts may be (*i.e.* whether they are a rash or not). Although a tentative suggestion is made, this draws on the report of what a doctor had said and the nurse displays her lack of entitlement to undertake diagnosis.

When nurses did allude to medical diagnoses, they displayed caution in their diagnostic activities in ways similar to those identified by Pooler (2007). In the following example, the caller rang regarding his six-weeks-old son whose belly button was 'bulging up hugely' (data not shown here). After a series of questions regarding the bulging, the nurse proposes an assessment of the problem (lines 56–58):

Extract 2

ZC5CRB21J

```
56   CT:   I- I mean I can't see him so I don't know but it
57          sounds like he's got you know a little .h (.)like a
58          little h↑ernia there [maybe?
59   C:                         [Yeah th-
60   CT:   >Yeah<>.h we're not allowed to give medical advice
61          so .h obviously. h you hav- .h see the doctor t- to
62          confirm (0.2) to confirm thi:s,
63   C:    Yeah.
```

A possible diagnosis – that the child may have a 'little hernia' (line 58) – is prefaced with a disclaimer 'I mean I can't see him so I don't know', which attends to the practical constraints on doing diagnostic activity over the telephone, in that nurses do not have visual information. The diagnosis is strongly hedged, with the evidential verb 'sounds like' (Peräkylä 1998) and the 'maybe' at the end of the turn establishing the assessment as speculative and cautious (see Pooler 2007). The caller comes in quickly with an agreement and, while more is projected to follow, the nurse begins a new turn (line 60). With the collective proterm 'we', the nurse draws on her membership as a Child Health Line nurse, and explicitly states the rules by which the service operates whereby nurses are 'not allowed to give medical advice'. The suggestion that the bulge is a hernia may be understood as a breach of this rule in that a diagnosis is proffered, but by invoking the institutional rules immediately after offering 'medical advice', the nurse hedges the strength of her assessment.

In Extracts 1 and 2, we see the nurses offering medical advice and information – but they do so in a way that makes visible their institutional membership and associated rights and entitlements. In each case, after engaging in diagnostic activity, the nurses invoke their membership as a nurse and use this to both account for and display their professional boundaries. In Extract 1 the nurse claims a lack of knowledge and defers to the greater epistemic authority of the doctor to identify the nature and cause of the welts on the caller's child. In Extract 2, the doctor is referred to as the proper person to confirm a strongly hedged candidate diagnosis. The nurse's identity as a nurse is thus invoked not in terms of a state of knowledge, but in terms of the institutional mandate under which they operate. Furthermore, the fact that the nurse cannot see the child is made relevant – thus, there is an orientation to both practical and institutional epistemic entitlements, which make diagnostic activity problematic.

Privileging parental authority

A number of calls to Child Health Line invite the nurses to engage in triaging – assessing whether a problem requires medical attention. Nurses, while not supposed to offer medical advice, have professional, legal, and moral obligations to advise the caller to seek medical assessment when it appears necessary. In a number of cases there is ambiguity as to whether medical attention is warranted, and practical and institutional constraints further complicate the provision of advice in such instances. In the extracts presented here, triaging activities were managed by the nurse privileging the right of parents to make their own decisions about seeking further medical advice or treatment, and thereby downgrading their authority.

In the following example, the caller's baby had fallen off the bed and had a lump on her head. Prior to this extract the nurse had asked about the child's symptoms and it was established that the child appeared calm and happy, and was not displaying any signs of injury.

Extract 3

ZC618820J

```
1    CT:   ↑Because I↑ am not there with you I can't
2          see her, [I can't (0.3) °ng° sort'v say .h
3    C:              [Yeih
4    CT:   oh she's oka:y no she's no:t okay, [.hh I =
5    C:                                        [Ye:ah
6    CT:   =haf tuh say tuh you you should go (.)
7          and get her checked out.=Okay?
8    C:    Ye:s
9    CT:   .h U::m (.) but it's you:r choice. It's your
10         decision?
11   C:    Yeah=
12   CT:   =On (.) o-on um: her (.) signs and symptoms of what
13         she's doing at the moment.
```

While all indications are that the child is 'okay' other than the lump on her head, the nurse avoids making an explicit assessment and appeals to the practical constraints on her ability to make an assessment (as in Extract 2). Then, by framing her advice as something she 'has to say', the nurse invokes the institutional constraints on the nature of her advice (lines 4, 6–7). In lines 9–10, the nurse orients to the caller's authority to decide whether or not to get the baby checked out and, in doing so, withholds her own authority. In this way she appears to disalign with the institutional mandate to tell callers to have their children seen by a doctor, and downgrades the directiveness of her advice by orienting to the caller's right to make a decision about the course of action to take, based on his own observations of the child's condition.

In this case, institutional policy can be heard explicitly as requiring the nurse to offer what could be considered 'medical advice' in the sense that taking the child to be checked out is recommended. However, by drawing on her lack of visual access, the nurse indirectly alludes to the possibility of underriding this advice (Greatbatch *et al.* 2005) – and puts the onus on the parent to make this decision.

The caller in Extract 4 has asked whether they should be concerned about their child's temperature (37.4C/99.3F) following immunisation shots given earlier that day. In data not shown here, the nurse assures the caller that 37 is 'normal' and at '37.4 she's probably feeling a little bit uncomfortable but that's okay'. The nurse suggests making the child more comfortable by wiping her with a wet cloth and dressing her in comfortable clothing, advice that can be understood as ways of treating an essentially well (albeit uncomfortable) child and addresses the caller's query regarding whether they should be concerned. The caller then asks the first of several queries regarding the 'warning signs' to 'look for in case she gets a reaction'. The nurse describes some symptoms – a temperature, localised pain, crying and being 'miserable' – and suggests extra fluids, comforting the child and, 'according to what the doctor said, panadol'. Thus, the nurse relates only mild reactions to immunisations that may be treated by parents at home, and defers to the advice of the doctor in relation to administering panadol.

Perhaps in response to the absence of symptoms that might be considered to raise concern, or be understood as 'warning signs' (as the advice offered so far relates to 'at-home' care), the caller pursues this line of questioning by asking (line 3) when he should 'start to get concerned':

Extract 4

ZC617GO6T

```
1    C:    .hh Wha- if the temperature continues to ri:se,
2    CT:   Yeh=
3    C:    =When do I start to get conce:rned.
4          (0.7)
5    CT:   Tch .hh Okay, thirty seven fi:ve she's prob'ly
6          feeling (.) you know like uncomfortable,
7    C:    Yih
8    CT:   An:- (.) bit hot, .h thirty ↑eight I'd say she's
9          got a ↑temperature .h so I'd be (.) you know
10         like doing what I sai:d wiping 'er over with a wet
11         cloth, or[: .h u:m and pushing the extra fluids=
12   C:              [Yih
13   CT:   an' [that, .h u:m and if she was really *a-*=
14   C:        [Mhm,
```

```
15   CT:   =miserable, [u:m you could (.) um consider giving=
16   C:              [°Yeah,°
17   CT:   =her some pa:nadol if that's whatcha doctor
18          [recommended, .h we- we don't pu:sh the panadol=
19   C:     [↓Yea:h
20   CT:   =these days because it's .h it can mask (.)
21          symptoms?=
22   C:     =No: well that' [s right- .hhh [wha-
23   CT:                    [Okay.        [So: um an'
24          then anything above that, um: (.) sort of
25          she- (.) she is (0.4) feeling (.) unwell.
26          Yeah. She's got a fe:ver.
27   C:     Okay and then: .hh if it's above thirty
28          eight, then I: I- ° m° I:'d prob'ly need tuh
29          maybe consider (.) calling a doctor or going
30          to a doctor or:: is that- .hh
31          (1.5)
32   CT:   .hh Ah:::m well it's ↑up↑ to you:,
```

The nurse begins her response (lines 5–21) by essentially repeating information already given about comforting a child with a mild temperature and discomfort. At lines 23–26 she suggests that a temperature above 38° (100.4°F) means the child has a fever. The caller acknowledges this and then proffers a candidate course of action if the temperature goes above 38° (calling or going to a doctor, lines 28–30). The proposed course of action is constructed so as to continue the nurse's turn with the connector 'and then' proposing a completion. This works to invite the nurse to confirm 'going to the doctor' as an appropriate action. The caller qualifies his assertion with the hedging 'probably' and 'maybe' and the open-ended alternative at line 30. The nurse's response is delayed and withholds a recommendation by telling the caller that 'it's up to you' (line 32). The apparent ambiguity as to when further medical help should be sought appears to be treated as problematic by the caller, who then repeats his request a few turns later:

Extract 5

ZC617GO6T

```
1    C:     =.hh [bud- (0.6) I jist wanted to make sure .hh=
2    CT:         [>Yeh<
3    C:     =wha:t are thee warning signs where we need to
4           suddenly rush 'er off to a doctor or to: the-
5           the children's ho:spital
6           (0.7)
7    CT:    Well I gue:ss u:m: °i- eh° i's sort'v °i-°
8           yee- (0.4) agai:n y:ou'd have tuh go on h- you:r
9           gut i:nstinct there or watch (.) the signs and
10          symptoms that she's showing you,
```

The caller's question (lines 3–5) is designed as seeking information (about the 'warning signs'), but strongly implicates a proposed course of action ('rushing off to the hospital) that is hearable as a request for advice. The nurse's response is delayed, as in Extract 4, and has a troubled beginning with a number of false starts. The nurse avoids offering either information or advice and, as before, leaves the decision to seek further help to the caller, suggesting he 'rely on his gut instinct'. While earlier the nurse had provided both information and advice in terms of managing mild temperatures and discomfort, in response to the caller's repeated queries regarding when the child might be considered unwell enough to warrant further medical attention, the nurse withholds advice. Thus while medical information is provided (*i.e.* a temperature above 38 degrees indicates that the child is unwell), decisions about medical treatment are deferred to the caller. In this way, it may be possible to suggest that a distinction is made between the delivery of medical *advice* as compared to medical *information*. While the nurse provides facts about children's temperatures, the nurse refrains from making a recommendation when it comes to what this particular caller should do about the specific symptoms of their child. As in Extract 3, the decision as to what to do is left up to the caller.

Drawing on expertise to re-specify a 'medical' problem
When callers ring with concerns about what they consider to be a medical issue, nurses at times draw on their authority in the domain of parenting and child development to offer information and advice that address the problem, without giving medical advice. In these cases, nurses address the problem within the bounds of their area of expertise and institutional remit by respecifying a medical issue as either a parenting or child development matter.

In Extract 6, the caller initially asks if the help line is 'medical health for babies' (lines 3–4). In this sense, the nature of the caller's request is framed as a medical matter. The nurse states that Child Health line is not a medical help line, but gives a go-ahead for the caller to ask her something.

Extract 6

ZC5CSG59M

1	CT:	Child Health Line may I help you Kerry A:nne
2		speaking?
3	C:	Yeah is this u:m (0.3) medical health for
4		ba:bies?
5		(0.3)
6	CT:	No this is the Child Health Line = So it's
7		not a medical help line.
8		(0.4)
9	C:	O::h=(I j-)
10		(0.4)
11	CT:	But I ca:n y- I mean if you wa:nna ask me something?
12		(0.2)
13	C:	A::h I'm jist I'm wo:ndering about projectile
14		vo:miting.
15		(0.2)
16	CT:	Sorry?
17		(0.5)
18	C:	I was wondering about projectile vo:miting?
19	CT:	How old is the ba:by.
		((34 lines omitted in which nurse asks about timing and frequency of the vomiting))

```
53   C:    U:::m (0.8) tch .h we:ll be was burping like I burp
54         him after the [f- during the fee[d so yea:h he had=
55   CT:              [Yeah           [yeah
56   C:    =wi:nd.
57   CT:   Alrigh'=.h ↑what can happen with small babies is
58         they've go:t (.) imm:aturity at thee .h the bowel=at
59         the gut there?
60         (.)
61   C:    Yep.
62   CT:   And the milk will just pop up and down all
63         the time.=So sometimes different position[ns? .hh
64   C:                                             [((cough))
65         [>Yep<
66   CT:   [Like if you'd fed a baby one side and then you
67         lay them down?,
68   C:    Mm=
69   CT:   =and try to change the nappy so whilst you're lifting-
70         lifting their little le:gs up?,
71         (.)
72   C:    Ye::ah=
73   CT:   =You're lifting their .h tummy hi:gher >you know< you're
74         lifting [(         [              ) bring it out?
75   C:            [Ye::ah (0.8)   [ye:ah.
76         (0.4)
77   C:    Ye:ah=
78   CT:   >wil' jus'< come back (.) out through the mouth agai:n.
```

By indicating that she is seeking information, the caller presents projectile vomiting as a topic rather than as a symptom of her child – possibly orienting to the opening turns where it was established that Child Health Line did not give medical help. In asking the child's age immediately after the caller's turn (line 19), the nurse displays her understanding of the call as not simply a request for information, but relating to a symptom or condition of the caller's child. In lines not shown, she asks a series of questions relating to the frequency and timing of the vomiting. After the caller confirms that the baby had wind (lines 53–53/56), the nurse offers an explanation for the child's vomiting.

The nurse's explanation draws on her knowledge of children's physical development, and describes what is effectively normal in 'small babies' – 'immaturity of (…) the bowel (…) the gut', which means that milk 'will just pop up and down all the time' (lines 62–63). The nurse's description of the milk just coming 'back out through the mouth again' (line 78) is a much milder version of what the caller had described initially as 'projectile vomit-ing', and establishes the problem as something that occurs in the everyday activities of child care. Use of non-personalised information (Silverman 1997) through generic descriptors ('small babies', 'if you fed a baby', 'you're lifting their little legs up') serve as normalising devices. The generalised account of babies vomiting is heard to account for this baby vomit-ing. Thus, while the caller had initially presented her problem as a medical issue, the nurse draws on her expertise in the area of child development and parenting to re-specify the problem as non-medical and as an expected and normal occurrence.

Whilst the symptoms are re-specified as non-medical, the nurse engages in work that can be understood as diagnostic activity. After the caller identifies her child's problem, the nurse's questioning serves as the basis for the production of a differential diagnosis, *i.e.* not projectile vomiting in the clinical sense. The hedging and caution evident in the diagnostic work suggested or alluded to in Extracts 1 and 2 are noticeably absent in this call. Rather, the nurse appears to speak with authority, and without any allusions to her institutional membership and entitlements. Thus, the 'medical work' undertaken in this call appears less problematic as it falls within the realm of expertise of the Child Health nurse.

Extract 7 offers a clear example of a nurse displaying authority with respect to child health and wellness. The caller had rung regarding her eight-week-old child's lack of bowel motions, and reported having previously taken her child to the doctor (not shown) who prescribed medication leading to a bowel movement four days prior to the call. The reason for the call is concern about the absence of any movement since then, and indications that the baby is in some discomfort.

Extract 7

ZC5CV01R

13	C:	.hh but um ↑he hasn't been to the toilet since
14		and he's passing like a lot of wi::nd an- .hh
15		[(0.2) gets upset during the feeding¿
16	CT:	[H:m.
17		(0.3)
18	C:	t.hhhh[h [like he has got a pai::n:- (0.2) there?
19	CT:	[Ye:[ah.
20	CT:	.h (0.3) Um:: and he- he's passing urine?=an' he's:
21		and he's gaining weight?=↑Your baby?
22		(.)
23	CT:	<E[v'rything like that's going well?
24	C:	[Yea:h.
25	C:	Yeah
26	CT:	.hh And- the doctor didn't talk about the- normal
27		behaviour where- °m° breastfed babies (.) at this
28		age don't poo for up to a coupla weeks?
29		(0.3)
30	C:	.h Well I said that to him, 'cos one of the um (.)
31		child (0.5) h:ealth: nurses at the ((hospital name))
32		had said that tuh me:.
33	CT:	Yea:p.
34	C:	.hh And he said no no that's not ri:ght.
35	CT:	Oh it i:s.
36		(0.4)
37	C:	.h Oh:. [hihihi .hhhh
38	CT:	[hihihi haheh very right;
39	C:	[O:h. = 'Co]s then I'm thinking ↑o:h no=he's goin'=
40	CT:	[(Well-) we-]
41	C:	=oh no he should be going every day he should have
42		[three or four poops a da:y=an' I'm thinking ↑o:h=
43	CT:	[°M:m m:m.°
44	C:	=go:sh h .h
45	CT:	↓No. .hh breastfed babie- I mean we deal with

46   breastfed babies all the time an' a norm↑al
47   baby¿=I s'pose¿=as child health nu(h)rses (…)

After describing the history and treatment of the problem, the caller presents her child's symptoms (lines 13–15, 18). The problem presentation invokes the relevance of an assessment of these symptoms by the nurse. The nurse responds by asking about further symptoms (lines 20–21, 23) with three questions that anticipate – and receive – optimised, or 'no-problem' responses (Boyd and Heritage 2006). The nurse continues with a detailed interrogative regarding what the doctor 'didn't say' about the 'normal behaviour for breast-fed babies' (line 26–28) that sets up a preference for a 'no' response. While on the surface the question appears to seek information, it carries an assumption that the doctor did not provide the caller with this information. There is also a possible evaluative component to the interrogative in that the doctor's presumed lack of information provision, and the pre-scription of medicine, is criticised.

The caller reveals that a child health nurse at a hospital had given her this information and that she had raised it with the doctor, who disagreed (line 34). The nurse's response, 'oh it is' (line 35), comes quickly and is said firmly and authoritatively, suggesting an independent epistemic position which is then upgraded by 'very right' at line 38. After the caller continues with an account of her reaction to the doctor's assertion, the nurse does a disagreement (line 45), countering both the doctor's assessment/diagnosis, and the reported concern of the caller. Demonstrating her institutional alignment with the nurse from the hospital with 'we' (line 45) and the category mapping 'as child health nurses' who 'deal with' breastfed and 'normal' babies 'all the time' (lines 45–47), the nurse's knowledge and experience is used to establish her epistemic authority in this matter. In contrast it is suggested that the doctor lacks experience and access to this specialised body of knowledge.

Over the next two minutes the nurse describes in detail the normal behaviour of breastfed babies. The end of this informing sequence is shown below:

Extract 8

ZC5CV01R

89   CT: But they're not constipated constipation is a hard
90   dry pebbly poo and that's the definition of it,=not
91   how often they go¿ but what the consistency of the
92   poo is when they do: go.
93   C: Oh:ka:y
94   CT: .h (0.2) So: ahm: I'll have to disagree:e [*er:* um=
95   C: [Yeah
96   CT: =(0.4) with the doctor, there's a lot of evidence
97   (0.3) er:m th't- (0.2) this is a no:rmal phenomenon in
98   breastfed babies and we see it a:ll the time.
99   C: Oh okay, .h

Over these turns, the nurse establishes the factual basis of her knowledge of constipation – referring to the 'definition' of constipation, and the 'evidence' that supports this understanding of lack of bowel motions as a 'normal phenomenon' (lines 89–92), and explicitly formulates her disagreement with the doctor (lines 94, 96). Referring to her collective membership in closing this extended turn, the nurse again invokes the epistemic authority of Child Health Nurses. The nurse orients to both authority and accountability in her assessment of the problem by describing *how she knows* what she knows (Peräkylä 1998), and explicitly contrasts her domain of expertise with that of the doctor's. In so doing, a problem initially presented as a medical matter on the basis of the doctor's treatment of the problem is re-specified as an aspect of normal child development.

As noted in relation to Extract 6, by making an assessment of the child's symptoms, the nurse could be seen to be engaging in medical work – even though the diagnosis itself is not a 'medical' one. Also similar to Extract 6 is the absence of hedging or disclaimers evident in the earlier examples where the nurses deferred to the authority of the doctor. On the contrary, the nurse appears to privilege her epistemic authority and entitlement in Extracts 7 and 8. Institutional membership as a child health nurse is used to override the 'medical advice' of the doctor (*cf.* Greatbatch *et al.* 2005), contrasting with Extracts 1–3 where this membership was invoked to downgrade and account for the nature of the advice provided.

Conclusions

The contributions of this chapter are threefold. First, the chapter contributes to the body of literature on the interactional organisation of medical authority, and, more specifically, to the limited literature on how nurse authority is displayed (Greatbatch *et al.* 2005, Pooler 2007). Secondly, it demonstrates how institutional guidelines and policies impact upon displays of authority and are talked into being in the course of interactions with clients. Finally, the chapter contributes more generally to research on telehealth services in revealing some practical dilemmas facing nurses who staff such services. These findings have implications for policy, training and practice in relation to telephone health lines, and telenursing, by demonstrating how service guidelines are relevant for the in situ organisation and classification of healthcare interactions.

The chapter builds on studies of the interactional production of authority in medical interactions, to demonstrate how specific institutional roles and mandates intersect with the practical management of the underlying asymmetry between health professionals and clients. In line with Peräkylä's (1998) finding that doctors attend to their obligations to reveal the grounds on which medical assessments are made, we observe in Child Health Line calls a strong orientation to the accountability of nurses' assessments, information and advice in relation to their epistemic entitlements. The downgrading, and upgrading, of epistemic entitlements in these calls demonstrates how states of knowledge are treated as distinct from having rights to use that knowledge (Drew 1991, Gill 1998). As Drew (1991: 45) suggests, 'when speakers orient to their asymmetrical position as regards some knowledge, they orient to the normatively organized social distributions of authoritative access to bodies or types of knowledge'.

Epistemic and institutional boundaries were used not only to qualify and downgrade the strength of nurses' assessments, but were also invoked when the nurses' professional expertise in the domain of child development and health (or wellness) was made relevant. The bounded nature of authority and expertise was displayed when nurses invoked their membership as a nurse in cases where an assessment of a child was requested – whether or not this assessment resulted in a 'medical diagnosis'. Displays of epistemic entitlement, however, were differentiated in terms of whether symptoms could be considered to relate to a 'medical' or 'child health' matter. Whilst epistemic downgrading was evident in relation to 'medical problems' (Pooler 2007, Sarangi and Clarke 2002), where a problem could be understood in terms of child development rather than medical problems, categorisations and epistemic upgrading were used to display the Child Health nurses' authority in regard to such matters.

The management of epistemic access and entitlement was both facilitated and complicated through the use of institutionally determined guidelines and practices. We have demonstrated how institutional roles and policies can be 'talked into being' by medical professionals in the course of their interactions with clients. The Child Health Line guideline, promoting the view that 'the service does not offer medical advice', seems at the outset a straightforward regulation for implementation. However, this analysis shows how the guideline poses interactional tensions for the nurses in responding to parental requests for support and advice about their child's health and illness. By necessity, the nurses engage in medical work in order to identity whether 'medical advice' is sought and/or necessary. Medical advice and information (diagnosis, triaging and so on) is delivered in ways that display the boundaries around nurses' institutional obligations as well as their medical expertise. Even when nurses appear to be able to identify an explanation for a child's symptoms, they are institutionally bound to be cautious in delivering such explanations (*e.g.* Extract 2).

It would be next to impossible for the Child Health Line nurses to adhere strictly to the service guidelines, given the nature of the calls that they receive, and the ambiguity and overlap between matters of 'normal' child development and parenting, and medical matters. Many parents call the service precisely because they are concerned that their child's symptoms may indicate a medical issue, and the nurses are expected to be able to advise on this. What we observe, then, is the nurses' management of the fuzzy boundaries around health versus illness, and between advice and information. For example, in Extract 4, the nurse provided information in relation to dealing with a child's temperature, which could be heard as medical advice. However, this sort of advice (cooling the child down, providing lots of fluids and so on) falls on the boundaries between matters of 'health' and 'illness', and between information and advice (see Pilnick 1999, Silverman 1997). A slight rise in temperature following immunisation is 'normal' and can be dealt with by the parent, so such advice may not necessarily be considered as 'medical'. However, when the caller persisted with requests for advice about seeking further medical attention, there was a marked lack of epistemic entitlement and authority displayed by the nurse. The boundary had been reached and the nurse maintained her position on one side of that boundary.

The findings presented here have implications for the operation of the Child Health Line service and for telehealth more generally. The detailed analysis may be useful for training purposes to demonstrate how nurses reconcile the tensions arising in adhering to service guidelines whilst meeting callers' requests for help. It also illustrates the value of recording and examining actual calls as part of the development of institutional guidelines and policies to see how such tensions arise. On a more specific level, the remit that nurses should not offer medical advice appears to be at odds with the name of the service. The name, 'Child Health Line', clearly suggests that the helpline is equipped to handle calls of a medical nature, and so it is no surprise that the service receives numerous requests for medical advice and information. Changing the name to one that more accurately reflects the aims of the service might help reduce the frequency with which such calls are received.

Whilst at the time of writing, Child Health Line did not use standardised assessment protocols or software packages, the service has since merged with a statewide telehealth service. Callers now speak first with a registered nurse on the general health line and an algorithm is used to determine if the call is best handled by a Child Health Line nurse, or by general nursing staff. Consequently, it is likely that the incidence of medical-related calls forwarded to Child Health Line nurses will be reduced. However, this chapter has shown that the question of whether a problem is a medical one is not always clear-cut, and nurses can draw on their expertise in child development and parenting to respecify ostensibly medical problems as wellness matters. Nurses triaging the calls to the general health line may not have the necessary expertise to distinguish between problems presented by callers as medical from ones better understood as child development issues. Furthermore, as discussed by Greatbatch *et al.* (2005), the use of an expert system to standardise service delivery may have limited value as nurse expertise is regularly privileged over computer software to offer an individualised service. As shown here, institutional practices and guidelines can be understood in terms of the limitations they pose for nurses, and also in terms of the opportunities they provide for nurses to display their unique experience and expertise.

Acknowledgements

We acknowledge the support of our funding bodies, the Royal Brisbane Children's Hospital Foundation, Perpetual Trustees, and Queensland University of Technology. We thank those who made the study possible, the management of Riverton Early Parenting Centre and participating Child Health Line nurses and parents. We also thank Alison Pilnick, Jon Hindmarsh and Virginia Teas Gill and the anonymous reviewers for their insightful comments, and Toni Dowd and Fairlie McIlwraith who contributed to early work on this project.

References

Baker, C.D., Emmison, M. and Firth, A. (eds) (2005) *Calling for Help: Language and Social Interaction in Telephone Helplines*. Amsterdam: John Benjamins.

Boyd, E. and Heritage, J. (2006) Taking the history: questioning during comprehensive history taking. In Heritage, J. and Maynard, D.W. (eds) *Communication in Medical Care: Interaction between Primary Care Physicians and Patients*. Cambridge: Cambridge University Press.

Danby, S., Baker, C.D. and Emmison, M. (2005) Four observations on openings in calls to Kids Help Line. In Baker, C., Emmison, M. and Firth, A. (eds) *Calling for Help: Language and Social Interaction in Telephone Helplines*. Amsterdam: John Benjamins.

Drew, P. (1991) Asymmetries of knowledge in conversational interactions. In Markovà, I. and Foppa, K. (eds) *Asymmetries in Dialogue*. Hemel Hempstead: Harvester Wheatsheaf.

Drew, P. (2006) Mis-alignments in 'after-hours' calls to a British GP's practice: a study in telephone medicine'. In Heritage, J. and Maynard, D.W. (eds) *Communication in Medical Care: Interaction between Primary Care Physicians and Patients*. Cambridge: Cambridge University Press.

Edwards, D. (2007) Calling for help: Introduction to the special issue, *Research on Language and Social Interaction*, 40, 1, 1–8.

Emmison, M. and Danby, S. (2007) Avoiding giving advice in calls to Kids Help Line. *Paper presented at the International Pragmatics Association Conference*, Sweden, July 2007.

Ferguson, R. (2005) Telephone helplines for parents. In Wootton, R. and Batch, J. (eds) *Telepediatrics: Telemedicine and Child Health*. London: Royal Society of Medicine Press.

Gill, V.T. (1998) Doing attributions in medical interaction: patients' explanations for illness and doctors' responses, *Social Psychology Quarterly*, 61, 322–60.

Gill, V. and Maynard, D.W. (2006) Explaining illness: patients' proposals and physicians' responses. In Heritage, J. and Maynard, D.W. (eds) *Communication in Medical Care: Interaction between Primary Care Physicians and Patients*. Cambridge: Cambridge University Press.

Greatbatch, D., Hanlon, G., Goode, J., O'Caithain, A., Strangleman, T. and Luff, D. (2005) Telephone triage, expert systems and clinical expertise, *Sociology of Health and Illness*, 27, 6, 802–30.

Heath, C. (1992) The delivery and reception of diagnosis in the general practice consultation. In Drew, P. and Heritage, J. (eds) *Talk at Work*. Cambridge: Cambridge University Press.

Heritage, J. (1984) *Garfinkel and Ethnomethodology*. Cambridge: Polity Press.

Heritage, J. (2005) Revisiting authority in physician-patient interaction. In Duchan, J. and Kovarsky, D. (eds) *Diagnosis as Cultural Practice*. New York, Mouton De Gruyter.

Heritage, J. and Sefi, S. (1992) Dilemmas of advice: aspects of the delivery and reception of advice in interactions between Health Visitors and first-time mothers. In Drew, P. and Heritage, J. (eds) *Talk at work: Interaction in Institutional Settings*. Cambridge: Cambridge University Press.

Hutchby, I. and Wooffitt, R. (1998) *Conversation Analysis: Principles, Practices and Applications*. Cambridge: Polity Press (UK and Europe).

Jefferson, G. (2004) Glossary of transcript symbols with an introduction. In Lerner, G.H. (ed.) *Conversation Analysis: Studies from the First Generation*. Amsterdam: John Benjamins.

Leppanen, V. (1998) The straightforwardness of advice: advice-giving in interactions between Swedish district nurses and patients, *Research on Language and Social Interaction*, 31, 209–39.

Maynard, D.W. (1991) On the interactional and institutional bases of asymmetry in clinical discourse, *American Journal of Sociology*, 97, 448–95.

Parsons, T. (1951) *The Social System*. New York: Free Press.

Peräkylä, A. (1998) Authority and intersubjectivity: the delivery of diagnosis in primary health care, *Social Psychology Quarterly*, 61, 301–20.

Pilnick, A. (1998) 'Why didn't you just say that?': dealing with issues of asymmetry, knowledge and competence in the pharmacist/client encounter, *Sociology of Health and Illness*, 20, 1, 29–51.

Pilnick, A. (1999) Patient counselling by pharmacists: Advice, Information or Instruction? *The Sociological Quarterly*, 40, 4, 613–22.

Pomerantz, A. (1984) Agreeing and disagreeing with assessments: some features of preferred/dispreferred turn shapes. In Atkinson, J.M. and Heritage, J. (eds) *Structures of Social Action: Studies in Conversation Analysis*. Cambridge: Cambridge University Press.

Pooler, J. (2007) Managing the diagnostic space: interactional dilemmas in calls to a telephone health help line. *Working paper submitted for Ethnographies of Diagnostic Work, Lancaster, April 2007*.

Potter, J. and Hepburn, A. (2003) 'I'm a bit concerned' – early actions and psychological constructions in a child protection helpline, *Research on Language and Social Interaction*, 36, 197–240.

Raymond, G. and Zimmerman, D.H. (2007) Rights and responsibilities in calls for help: the case of the Mountain Glade Fire, *Research on Language and Social Interaction*, 40, 1, 33–61.

Sarangi, S. and Clarke, A. (2002) Zones of expertise and the management of uncertainty in genetics risk communication, *Research on Language and Social Interaction*, 35, 2, 139–71.

Schegloff, E.A. (2007) *Sequence Organization in Interaction: a Primer in Conversation Analysis*, Vol 1. Cambridge: Cambridge University Press.

Silverman, D. (1997) *Discourses of Counselling: HIV Counselling as Social Interaction*. London: Sage Publications.

Stivers, T. (2002) 'Symptoms only' and 'candidate diagnoses': presenting the problem in pediatric encounters, *Health Communication*, 14, 299–338.

West, C. (1984) *Routine Complications: Trouble with Talk between Doctors and Patients*. Bloomington: Indiana University Press.

4

Practitioners' accounts for treatment actions and recommendations in physiotherapy: when do they occur, how are they structured, what do they do?

Ruth Parry

Introduction

Most of the time, we do not overtly talk about the meanings, reasons and rationales of our actions. In certain circumstances we raise these matters, in particular where actions are somehow transgressive, or potentially understandable as such (Heritage 1984, Antaki 1994). Therefore, this kind of talk occurs where sensitive matters are addressed or enacted. People also refer to meanings, reasons and rationales when attempting to encourage, influence and persuade others to change their behaviour (Johnson 2008).

Given this, it is unsurprising that talk about the meanings and rationales of procedures and proposals is thought to play a pivotal role in healthcare consultations and to be important in patient-centred care, shared decision making and patient education (Collins 2005). Official guidance encourages clinicians to communicate the rationale for treatment to patients and carers (*e.g.* NHS 2003). Nevertheless, healthcare recipients express dissatisfaction about this aspect of communication (Partridge 1994, West and Frankel 1991) and some observations suggest it is an area in which professionals underperform (Talvitie and Reunanen 2002, Campion *et al.* 2002).

In this chapter, I empirically examine talk about meanings, reasons and rationale in healthcare consultations. I do so by focusing on practitioners' verbal accounts for the treatment actions they instigate and conduct, and the proposals they make.

Accounts

When people verbally account for their actions, they express some kind of reason and explanation (Buttny and Morris 2001). Accounts display events and activities as interpretable in particular ways – for instance as rational, sensible and justifiable (Potter 2003). Ranging from single words to lengthy sequences (Buttny and Morris 2001), accounts are sometimes explicitly worded as accounting, via formats like: 'X because Y'; 'X in order to Y', but can also be produced through other formats such as descriptions, reports and versions of events (Buttny and Morris 2001). These implicit accounts are hearable as accounting because of local contextual and sequential features (Antaki 1988).

Accounts may follow interlocutors' 'why' questions or be volunteered under certain circumstances (Antaki 1994). As noted, these circumstances tend to entail some irregularity of conduct and social practice: 'where projected or required behaviour does not occur' (Heritage 1988: 133), so accounts play a role in actions such as apologising, excusing and justifying. Accounts also play a part in making sense of unusual events and actions; promoting interactional alignment (Buttny and Morris 2001); and influencing or persuading others to change their conduct or accept someone else's conduct (Johnson 2008). Accounts for

Who	instigates, delivers, receives, and responds to the account?
What	is accounted for? - what is the 'referent' of the account?
What	does the account invoke? - opinions, 'facts', events or actions? - local or more global matters? - because or in-order-to reasoning?
How	is the account structured? - what is the turn and sequence design? - how is it worded? - is it an explicit or implicit account (in terms of wording, sequential context and response)? - what response is projected and produced?
When	is the account produced? - what activities precede, accompany and follow it? - does it follow, precede or replace the accounted for action?

Why	what can the account be seen to do, how does it function?
	- how does it function with regard to the accounted for
	    action or event?
	- how does it function with regard to broader activity and
	    institutional contexts?

Figure 1 *Components and features of verbal accounts for actions*

actions can be considered as falling into two types: because-accounts and in-order-to-accounts (drawing on Schutz's (1967) concept of because and in-order-to motivations). Because-accounts invoke causes, precipitating factors, needs, *i.e.* existing or prior matters which are either present or absent. In-order-to-accounts invoke aims, aspirations, purposes: things that will be achieved or avoided as a result of the action. Figure 1 summarises components and features of accounting turns and sequences.

Accounts in healthcare interactions have been empirically researched, though in a rather narrow range of settings and clinical activities. Patients' accounts for their symptoms (Gill and Maynard 2006) and their decisions to consult (Heritage and Robinson 2006) have been examined in primary care. Other research has examined doctors' accounts, specifically primary care and outpatient-clinic doctors' accounts for their diagnostic pronouncements (Peräkylä 1998, 2006, Maynard 2004). Peräkylä shows that doctors produce accounts where there is 'extended inferential distance' between examination and diagnosis; where diagnosis is uncertain; and where it involves explicit rejection or correction of diagnostic suggestions expressed by the patient during the examination (1998: 314).

Peräkylä's seminal analyses (1998, 2006) show that accounts do interactional work above and beyond what we might call their *straightforward* functions of justifying, clarifying or explaining specific local procedures or proposals. In accounting for their diagnostic pronouncements and making their reasoning apparent for patients, doctors balance their medical authority with their accountability to patients. Accounting also works to treat patients as individuals who are – at least potentially – interested in and capable of understanding such matters. Maynard (2004) finds that where doctors offer a predecessor account by citing the evidence prior to stating the diagnosis, this can accomplish a sense of mutuality, understanding and agreement' (2004: 71), contributing both to reducing patient resistance and building medical authority.

There has been less research on accounts for treatment actions and recommendations. Stivers' (2005a, 2006) shows that in primary care consultations involving children with upper respiratory tract infections, doctors sometimes produce accounts when recommending against antibiotic prescription – particularly where parents resist their recommendation. Some of Greatbatch's primary care data (2005) show doctors producing accounts alongside recommendations of a 'do not do X' format, though his analytic focus is elsewhere. Stivers notes accounts' role in patient education (2005a) and demonstrates their role in encouraging acceptance of treatment recommendations (2005b).

These understandings about when accounts arise and how they function have been established in a narrow range of settings and for a narrow range of actions. Very little attention has been paid to the structure of practitioners' accounts or to patients' responses. In this chapter I extend previous work through examining accounts in a different setting – inpatient physiotherapy rehabilitation – and through analysing the occurrence, structure and functions of practitioners' accounts for a range of treatment-related actions and proposals.

Although a specialist setting, physiotherapy features topics, tasks, and challenges relevant to many forms of healthcare. A defining feature is that physiotherapists apply specialist and complex knowledge about human movement, movement problems and their physical remedies through interventions that include physical exercises, teaching and learning activities. These often require considerable and effortful co-operation both within and beyond the consultation. This mandates attention to co-operation, persuasion and motivation – matters relevant to many areas of healthcare. Physiotherapy interactions are rich in communication about bodily matters, topics clearly central to many healthcare interactions.

Data and methods

The data comprised 41 video-recordings of neurological physiotherapy sessions in two rehabilitation units in England. Twelve therapists were recorded; all had some specialist clinical experience in neurology. The 21 patients recorded were undergoing rehabilitation for stroke or brain injury. Images were recorded using a Sony MiniDV camcorder on a tall tripod placed behind screens in a corner of the treatment area. A tie-pin microphone and transmitter were worn by the therapist with a receiver connected to the camera. The researcher avoided looking through the camera except for necessary camera adjustments (Heath and Luff 1993).

Data were digitised, watched through, and brief descriptive notes written. Extracts, observations and collected episodes were managed using Transana software (Woods and Fassnacht 2009). For the purposes of this study, it was taken that accounts ranged from those explicitly formulated as such to those where their production and hearability as accounting was ambiguous (Buttny and Morris 2001). I therefore searched for any actions by a clinician, in interaction with a patient, whereby they referred overtly or obliquely to 'in-order-to' and 'because' aspects of treatment actions, proposals and recommendations. Patients also produced such accounts. I do not however examine these here.

During overview of the data, an initial collection of 60 relevant episodes was made and transcribed using Jeffersonian conventions (Jefferson 2004). These were analysed using the perspectives and methods of conversation analysis (Clayman and Gill 2004, Heritage 2005). Preliminary analyses were tested and extended by examining five treatment sessions selected to include patients with a variety of clinical presentations and lengths of 'rehabilitation career', and therapists with a range of experience levels. These sessions were transcribed from start to finish, and closely examined for any overt, implicit and/or fragmented accounts. Data sessions with other researchers and with participating clinicians contributed to the

- Following a patient's expression of concern about some aspect
  of physical state or performance
- Subsequent to a patient's report of performance of an activity,
  or expression of preference or expectation about treatment,
  where therapist recommends otherwise
- When requesting and conducting adjustment or removal of
  clothing items preparatory to treatment
- When treatment actions or recommendations remediate some
  locally evident physical failure
- When there is interactional evidence for likely differences in
  patient's and therapist's perspectives about underlying rationale

Figure 2 *The five broad circumstances in which accounts arose in the data*

analysis. The framework shown in Figure 1 provided a guide for the analysis of individual account sequences. Thus, each collected sequence was examined in terms of when it occurred, what was accounted for, what the account invoked, its sequential, lexical and morphological format; and its functions.

Analysis

Therapists' accounts were either (1) responsive to certain interactional contributions from patients, or (2) occasioned by the instigation and performance of certain treatment-related activities. Overall, five circumstances in which accounts arose were identified. These are summarised in Figure 2 and examined in detail below.

   In the following section I report my analysis of the location, structure and functioning of accounts by examining a series of cases which exemplify each location. One point to make before moving to these individual extracts is that in the data as a whole the majority of instructions, actions and proposals are actually conducted without accompanying accounts; I consider later how my analysis sheds light on this observation.

Accounts occasioned by patients' expressions of concern
In the first extract, a therapist produces an account in response to a patient's comment about a local physical trouble. During a break within a series of aim movements assisted by the therapist, the patient remarks that he is not managing to move his left (most badly affected) arm as far as his right arm.

Extract 1 ParryPDExp:KT3~18.25

```
1    P      .hh I can't get as far as my right one=
2    T      =.pth. no I know, ((sympathetic tone)) but
3           we- we're >gunna work on it together >I'm
4           gonna (ginu) little bi =<help. .h even if
```

5		you ca:n't get as far Andrew, =you- you a:re
6		getting .h some (of) the moo- muscle moving
7		there, .pth and I think it's .h it's good-
8		(.) practice >I mean even if you don't get
9		a:ll the way, .h we're strengthening up- (.)
10		the bit that you a:re able to work an- .hh
11		an it's thinking about the the next little
12		bit, =.h >right, go on let's bring yer elbows
13		in together

((*Further repetition of the arm movement, with
instructions and positive evaluations by the
therapist*))

19	T	a::ll the way back down onto the pillow
20		(1.0)
21	T	Even-even if you're ima:gining a movement?
22		(1.2)
23	T	It's trying to fi:n:d and fi:re up the right
24		area of the bra:in .hh okay? >so even though
25		you might not- .pthh feel that you're not getting
26		very >far if you're thinking about the
27		movement, = that's .h sending the right
28		signals
29		(0.3)
30	T	Okay let's go again

((*Further instructions and physical response*))

On the video, subsequent to line 1, the patient appears attentive in terms of his gaze, but produces neither gestural (*e.g.* nodding) nor verbal responses to the actual account(s) through the course of this extract. After sympathetically acknowledging the patient's remark and making a general proposal for dealing with the problem mentioned (lines 2–4), the therapist produces a series of interlinked accounts.

The first account is: 'even if you ca:n't get as far Andrew, =you- you a:re getting .h some (of) the moo- muscle moving there'. This accounts for the current arm exercise, conveying it as worthwhile in the face of and despite the problem the patient has pointed out. Its format is a compound turn construction unit (Lerner 1991) of the form 'Even if X, Y'. The first part references and responds to the patient's comment, recycling and prefacing his words: 'even if you ca:n't get as far'. The accounted-for matter could be glossed as 'the arm exercise even if performed incompletely', and the account invokes a physical and, in this context, positive consequence of performing this (incomplete) exercise.

The therapist's subsequent 'and I think it's .h it's good practice' is perhaps hearable as an account invoking her clinical opinion as a reason for the action. If it is indeed an account, then it rests on the authoritative status of her opinion. However, she treats her assertion as needing justification: 'I mean even if you don't get a:ll the way, .h we're strengthening up- (.) the bit that you a:re able to work on' ... it's thinking about the ... next little bit'. The initial 'I mean' conveys that what comes next thoughtfully adjusts the preceding talk in such a way as to justify it (Fox Tree and Schrock 2002). The account once again takes an 'even if X, Y' form, the first part referencing the patient's initial comment and its import. It is an in-order-to account which invokes two consequences of the arm activity. The first: 'strength-ening up- (.) the bit that you a:re able to work an-' is precisely tailored to the patient's assertion of incomplete performance. The second: 'an it's thinking about the ... next little bit' introduces the idea that 'thinking about the movement' is beneficial. Noticeably, this part of the account implicitly rests on an assumption that thinking will translate into move-ment – a notion the therapist addresses more directly subsequently.

Another arm movement is instigated, the patient promptly co-operates, and the therapist then embarks on a further account: 'even if you're ima:gining a movement? ... It's trying to fi:n:d and fi:re up the right area of the bra:in .hh okay?'. This constitutes a shift from accounting for the arm activity to accounting for the activity of thinking about or 'imagin-ing' movement. That is, the therapist incrementally unpacks her account, with a matter previously invoked as an account now itself accounted for. By referring to 'a movement' rather than 'the movement', the therapist makes this account hearable as possibly applying beyond the current movement to past, current and future activities. She thereby moves to accounting for a broader range of activities. The rationale is also broadened: finding and firing up 'the right area of the bra:in' suggests a generic or in-principle consequence of thinking about movements. This sense is enhanced by referring to the brain rather than your brain because using 'the' rather than 'your' for body parts which are singular (e.g. trunk, head, neck) can convey a sense of generic, 'in principle' reference (Parry 2007).

The therapist produces yet another account, this time so-prefaced, thereby implying some form of conclusion or upshot (Raymond 2004): '>so even though you might not- . pthh feel that you're not getting very >far, if you're thinking about the movement, =that's .h sending the right signals'. Once again, the first part of the 'even though X, Y' construc-tion lexically references the patient's initial 'can't get as far' comment. The account leaves some ambivalence about just what is being accounted for. It could be heard as referring back to the specific arm exercise, or as referring to exercises and movements in a more general sense, thereby building on the just prior account. In summary, in these final two accounts within the sequence, the therapist closely tailors her accounting to the patient's initial comment about a specific action whilst nevertheless expanding the range of activities referred to in the account and the reasoning and rationale conveyed.

The arm exercise is again repeated, and then (beyond the transcript) the patient overtly questions the premise that thinking about, or imagining a movement is beneficial: 'If that's true, I should be walking now, or running'. Its verity or otherwise is not pursued further because both parties collaboratively move into talk about the technical terminology for the recommended activity (mental imagery), and its sporting applications. Patient resist-ance or rejection of accounts is not unusual, and a transcribed example will be considered shortly.

Patient conveys a preference, and therapist recommends against
Accounts sometimes occur where a patient has conveyed an expectation or preference about some activity or indeed reports performing that activity already, and the therapist subse-quently recommends otherwise. The next extract illustrates. It is quite lengthy because it spans previous patient contributions that occasion the account, as well as the account itself. Also, this episode entails an account for an activity to be conducted remotely to the current consultation, whereas Extract 1 entailed accounting – at least initially – for an immediate, within-session activity. Shortly before Extract 2 begins, the therapist has asked about between-session activities: 'How's the walking been over the weekend d'you think?' In response, the patient reports practising walking and conveys that limping is a problem. Line 1 is the therapist's response.

Extract 2 Parry:PDEx:MT1~3.30

```
 1   T    Is there anything thut you can sor' of sa::y: well-
 2        this feels like it's wrong or this feels like
 3        it's wron[g.
 4   P                 [tch no not rea:lly.
 5   P    =[>I mean i]t di- u- when I take the: splint off .h
 6   T     [okay.    ]
 7   P    it just feels weak.
```

*((They talk about weakness, sensation and balance
problems. Patient proposes that sensation is coming
back in her knee))*

```
13   P    Yeah uh- it ↑is co:ming back definitely. >und um:
14        (.) every time I take thee splint ↓off I wu- s- (.)
15        fiddle with me toe:s. te see if the(h)y're(h)
16        [still worki(h)ng a little bi]t. Ye[s
17   T    [Are they getting any be- ]    [Are you
18   T    getting any more of tha[t-  (.)   pulling ]out?
19   P                           [Bi- a ↑little bit]
20   T    [En toe move]men[t
21   P    [Little    bit.]   [Yeah =sometimes, .h I mean it's-
22   P    it va:ries depending how tired I am I think
23        but-.hh thee um-
24        (0.6)
25   P    The little toe: ↑quite often comes out quite
26        a lo(n)g way. (.) So tha's good? eh heh
27   T    ↑Okay. .h[hhh
28   P             [An I ↑try to think when I haven't got
29        the splint on to- to remember to-
30        (0.6)
31   P    Lift it up?
32        (0.2)
33   P    You know thee-
34   T    Ho:w much walking are you doing without the splint
35   P    =Not a lot. j[ust m-]
36   T                 [°kay° ]
37   P    just first- thing in the morning and when I'm
38   P    getting °h [(°into the) ↑bed    ]
39   T               [What so you're out] to the loo or::
40        (.)
41   P    Yes to the °loo. [n that] sort of thing°
42   T                     [okay ]
43   T    And you're no[t- ]
44   P                 [Sh]ould I try and do a bit mo:re?
45        >What do you [think?]
46   T                 [ tch ] well
47        (1.0)
```

48	P	No[t. e̲uh]
49	T	[I̲'m a >li]ddle bit concerned about h[ow:]
50	P	[Yes,]
51		(0.6)
52	T	If::
53		(1.1)
54	T	(You/yknow)= your toes were to c̲atch.
55		(0.2)
56	P	Y̲eah.
57	T	Thu:t
58		(0.7)
59	T	You would go flying¿
60	P	Y̲e̲s, ((gestures: her arm mimics a body falling
61		over))
62	T	And I uh-
63		(1.2)
64	T	M̲y̲::
65		(0.3)
66	T	>sort of feeling is that your, .hhh (.) the am̲o̲unt
67	T	of movement that you've got in your a̲nkle, i̲sn't (.)
68		umm
69		(1.2)
70	T	Re:ally consistent enough:.
71	P	No̲((nodding))
72	T	Yuh know the a̲ctual pulling yer ankle u̲p?
73	P	No ((nodding))
74		(0.6)
75	T	Isn't consistent enough at this sta:ge, to (.) um:
76		ptch .hh (>walk up/on-) – I mean there are
77		different-
78		(0.6)
79	T	>Y'know different perspe̲ctives on it.
80	P	[M
81	T	[And on:e o̲ne perspective is that- (.) unless you
82		↑have to use it you won't [(.) learn] to use it
83	P	[ptch .hh]
84	P	Y̲e::ah I know::
85	T	So I think to do a liddle bit- isn't a bad idea.
86	P	[Mm.
87	T	[.hh Bu' also just to sor' of ↑s̲it (in the)
88		↑practice.
89	P	=Y̲e:s
90	T	Yo[u know so when you're] n̲ot up on yer feet. [.hh]
91	P	[yes I (could) do that] [m]

((Further discussion of this, including a more
forthright commitment to doing so by patient. The
therapist then proposes 'having a look at' this
exercise))

The splint in question fits behind the patient's calf and under her foot, keeping her foot at right-angles to her lower leg. It stops her toes catching on the floor when she walks. Early in the extract, the patient refers several times to not wearing it (Lines 5, 14, 28–9). The therapist asks a related question at Line 34: 'How much walking are you doing without the splint', following up with further probes (lines 39 and 43). The patient minimises how much she is doing 'Not a lot'. This suggests some recognition that the therapist's question may imply a view that too much is being done without the splint. Nevertheless, she goes on to ask 'Should I try and do a bit mo:re?' (line 44). Initially formatted to project agreement, this is immediately revised: 'What do you think?'. The ensuing 'tch well' and pause indicate some sort of trouble in the therapist's upcoming response (Pomerantz 1984, Heritage 1984), and the patient pre-empts with a compressed negative reply to her own question: 'Not. euh'.

An account sequence then commences. The first part is: 'I'm a >liddle bit concerned about how: ... If:: (1.1) you/y know) = your toes were to catch thut you would go flying;'. Thus, rather than directly voicing a recommendation against activities without the splint, the therapist produces an account that invokes a possible negative consequence of doing so. The patient agrees, and gesturally signals her understanding. A further account follows. Like its predecessor, it is tentatively worded and hesitantly produced: 'your, .hhh(.) the amount of movement that you've got in your ankle, isn't (.) umm ... Re:ally consistent enough: ... Yuh know the actual pulling yer ankle up? ... Isn't consistent enough at this stage, to (.) um .hh (>walk up/on-)'. This hesitancy and tentativeness, alongside subsequent reference to different perspectives at Line 79, convey that her (implied) recommendation against the patient's apparent preference is done with deliberation and sensitivity. Both the act of producing an account and the way it is formatted allow the therapist to avoid overtly and starkly producing a disaffiliative recommendation, whilst nevertheless conveying it. The reference to different perspectives (lines 79–82) also acts both to pre-empt any potential counter by the patient, and to imply that what the patient has been doing was reasonable.

As is common in accounts, the account in Extract 2 necessitates reference to the patient's performance shortcomings. Nevertheless, the therapist uses forms of talk that reduce the seriousness of the shortcoming: the ankle movement is not consistent *enough*. In line with this, she also incorporates an implicit anticipation of improvement: the movement is not consistent enough *at this stage*.

At the end of the sequence, the therapist makes an alternative recommendation: to do activities without the splint in a sitting position. Although the patient shows some signs of agreeing and accepting at this point, later on, when the session is drawing to a close, the patient returns to her concerns:

Extract 2b Parry:PDEx:MT1~36.42

```
1    P    what I worries me (that/a bit)
2         if I'm wearing the splint? (.) um- is
3         that not- (.) encouraging me to use my
4         own tendons and muscles and things a bit?
5    T    Wear- uh will will wearing the splint stop
6         you do you mean?
7    P    Ye [s
8    T        [Yes. d'jyou mean will it hold you back
9    P    Yes I wondered
         ((A further lengthy therapist account follows,
         revisiting matters raised in Extract two)).
```

As noted, it is not atypical for patients to more or less directly reject accounts and/or the recommendations these account for. Thus, accounts are produced, repeated, recycled, and referred back to within what is often a lengthy process of clinicians' attempts to harmonise patients' expressed views towards their own clinical perspectives and treatment recommendations. Particularly in this circumstance, where patients' expectations or preferences and therapist's recommendations are misaligned, accounts are regularly delivered through long, indirect, fragmented and repetitive sequences.

Alongside adjusting or removing items of clothing

Accounts are sometimes occasioned by certain preparatory treatment activities. Such preparations include arranging the environment by fetching and positioning pieces of equipment. At this point, therapists often describe what they were doing – particularly when this involves leaving the patients' visual field or having some physical impact upon the patient, for instance raising the treatment bed. Extract 3 includes an example at lines 1–3. Whilst therapists regularly explain *what is* being done in arranging the environment, they do not at this point account for *why* it is being done. However, there is one form of preparatory activity that does receive such accounts: where there is adjustment or removal of items of the patient's clothing.

Extract 3 Parry:PDExp:GT4~7.26

```
 1   T      .hhh >Let's -have a little look at yer
 2             <balance. and just grab a
 3             (0.7)
 4   T      A stoo: l
 5             (1.3) ((therapist leaves treatment area and returns
 6                 with a stool))
 7   T      Do you mind taking yer sho:es off?
 8             (0.3) ((sound of stool scraping on floor))
 9                 ((patient immediately bends down))
10   P      Yes ((starts to raise left foot))
11             (0.2)
12   T      'Cause I'd li:ke to see what yer feet do.
13             (4.5) ((patient removing her shoe))
14   P      >It's the only my <pur:pose is err go on my
15             legs. that's it?
```

Following the therapist's question at Line 7, the patient makes an immediate physical response, making the first moves towards taking her shoes off, and she also responds verbally with a 'yes' although not until the noise of the stool on the floor stops. The patient's combined verbal and physical responses indicate that she treats the therapist's 'do you mind' as a straightforward request to take her shoes off. The therapist's account (line 12) comes when the patient has already started to remove her shoes. Thus, it does not appear to be produced in an effort to resolve problems of response or co-operation. Rather it works to convey the therapist's request as an accountable matter in itself. The patient's next spoken turn does not address the account. Instead, it returns to a distinct topic which was first raised a few minutes earlier.

In invoking the therapist's wish to see the patient's feet, the account conveys and trades on an assumption that it is reasonable and conventional for a therapist to inspect unclothed body parts. By actually producing an account though, the therapist conveys doing so as something that should nevertheless be subject to some explanation. In turn, this builds a sense of what is appropriate in therapy. Accounts at this juncture can also work to rule out alternative, possibly inappropriate, reasons for undressing (this is more obvious in other examples where items of clothing such as shirts rather than footwear are removed).

In general, those accounts that accompany adjustment and removal of clothing in the data are not associated with compliance problems; are brief and invoke a single therapeutic reason; rule out alternative less respectable reasons; and neither project nor receive direct verbal response from the patient.

Accounts accompanying actions and proposals that remediate locally evident problems
All therapy activities could, of course, be characterised as remediating – in that they all somehow address physical troubles and failures. However, I use the term here in connection with treatment actions and proposals that address, that attempt to remediate, troubles and failures that are evident and salient locally, at that moment. Some of these were accompanied by accounts, and Extract 4 is an example. When it begins, the patient and therapist are preparing for the patient to move from wheelchair to bed (lines 1–4).

Extract 4 ParryPDExp: JT2~2.20

```
 1   T    Now .hmm >when you gun- before you gunna
 2        stand up? what d'you need to think about
 3   P    =Feet on the ground.
 4   T    Bo:th feet on the ground. that's it? ((patient
 5        stands up and starts to pivot round) )
 6        (0.2)
 7   T    [>Hang on]
 8   P    [They    a] :: re (n)
 9        (0.4) ((by end of pause, patient has completed the
10        move from wheelchair to sitting on treatment bed) )
11   T    Was both feet on the floor?
12        (1.1)
13   P    £I d(h)on' t ↑think so,
14   T    I: don't think it was either, >so
15        we really need to think about .h when
16        you're standing,
17   P    Yeah
18   T    That you take your weight- (.) down through
19        that leg as well.
20   P    Mm.
21   T    'Cause otherwise only this side.
22   P    Yeah
23   T    Helps with the movement.
24        (1.0)
25   T    ptch °and we want both sides helping with
26        the movement°
27        (0.3)
28   T    Kay?
          ((Patient nods repeatedly and action moves to
          removing the patient's cardigan and talking about
          the agenda for the session)))
```

Despite references to both feet on the ground before the movement (lines 3–4), the video shows the patient hopping round, *i.e.* exclusively relying on her non-affected leg. This contrasts with what has been collaboratively proposed, and also with the rehabilitation approach used in this setting, which aims to persuade and teach the patient actively to use the affected side again rather than compensate by relying on unaffected limbs. By asking 'Was both feet on the floor?' the therapist ensures joint attention to and voicing of the problem. The therapist then makes a recommendation: '>so we really need to think about ...', which is swiftly followed by an account: 'Cause otherwise only this side ... helps with the movement. ... °and we want both sides helping with the movement°'. The first part of this account invokes negative future consequences of not doing as recommended[1]. The second part invokes an aspiration, produced as purportedly mutually desired and agreed upon via an 'institutional we' (Drew and Heritage 1992).

Accounts for remediating actions and recommendations can also occur before treatment activities actually commence. Specifically, when therapists in the data propose an overall plan or agenda for the day's session they sometimes account for these proposals by pinpointing particular problems or concerns raised during foregoing history-taking and examination.

Whatever the treatment phase in which therapists accounted for remediating actions and proposals, they initially worked to ensure collaborative attention and agreement with regard to both the existence and nature of the problem addressed. This allows the recommendation and account to be produced on a foundation of mutual attention to, and agreement about, the problem addressed. As I discuss at more length after a final extract, making clear the connection between the evident problem and the corrective action or instruction also builds a sense of the problem being a matter that can be resolved or reduced.

Accounts occasioned by possible differences in perspective regarding ongoing treatment actions

The final overall circumstance in which accounts arise is where there are some interactional grounds for anticipating differences in perspectives about the rationale of activities. The final extract illustrates this. For several minutes before it begins, both parties have been engaged in discussing and examining weakness in the patient's toes. As it starts, the patient is bringing his legs to rest on the treatment bed so as to demonstrate the toe movement. It is relevant that an ongoing theme in this session has been the patient's gloom at his slow progress and the therapist's countering – building a case that good progression is being made.

Extract 5 Parry: PDExp: LT1~7.44[2]

1	P	Just gonna put ↑foot up THERE? (.)
2	P	because I ↑thi:nk
3		(0.4)
4	P	Easier,
5	T	Okay
6	P	To show you how the- (.) toes are mo[ving.
7	T	[fi::ne alright

((*Therapist briefly leaves treatment area, tidying away the patient's splint. Patient then shows the therapist his toe movement and remarks on his previous inability to move them*))

```
12   P    I can actually move ↑this joint now. which is-
13        (1.7)
14   T    So la::st week when we checked that d'you- were you
15        able to do that?
16   P    N[o (way)
17   T     [N^o:: [::?
18   P           [Well a tiny fract[ion]
19   T                            [TI ]ny,
20   P    °But° nothing in the to[es, I mean (bu/n-) now]
21   T                           [.hhmm tch ay-        ]
22   P    the toes are b- really beginning to move, >I can't
23   P    wriggle them.
24   T    >Yep
25        (0.2)
26   P    [my u- ]
27   T    [.hh So] ju- (.) so how many times can you go up and
28   T    down with yer toes. >so if we do t^en. =so ready,
29        o::ne
30        (1.5)
31   T    Two::
32        (0.6)
33   T    When do they ti:re that's >whad ay >wanna wanna
34        know, Three
         ((Exercise continues, therapist counting
         each repetition)
37   T    ↑Te:n good. .h so z'this one have to help does it?
         ((They go on to talk about how his other foot is
         moving at the same time))
```

Until line 33, an ongoing shared topic has been the patient's ability to move his toes *at all*.
At line 33 the therapist raises a different element – tiring, *i.e. endurance* rather than *ability*
to move. The hearability of this utterance as an account is not absolutely clear. As earlier
noted, it is well recognised that various kinds of turns can be hearable as accounts (Buttny
and Morris 2001, Antaki 1994). However, where they are not explicitly marked as accounts
through their sequential location and/or lexical marking, limited evidence is currently available to ground a definitive analysis of whether or not particular utterances constitute
implicit accounts. Thus, in this case one hearing is that at lines 33–34 the therapist is speci-
fying her instruction by implicitly telling the patient to let her know when he feels tiredness.
On the other hand, her talk is produced in a place where an account is fitting because the
perspective and rationale regarding the therapist's instructions is unavailable and divergent
from the perspectives expressed beforehand. If lines 33–34 constitute an account, then this
is an account that attends to achieving mutual perspectives on the treatment activity and
its rationale.

Conclusion

Practitioners' accounts for their clinical actions are seen as important components of
healthcare communication. Prior research has shown they can foster mutuality and reduce

patients' resistance; build medical authority; balance authority with accountability; and construe patients as individuals who can engage with reasoning about and understanding of clinical processes and actions (as opposed to merely performing and complying with them). Previous work has noted that accounts arise in circumstances of overt or incipient patient resistance; where clinicians' proposals run counter to patients expectations; and where the reasoning underlying actions is likely to be opaque. These prior findings on when accounts arise and what they do have derived from a fairly narrow range of settings, mainly primary care medicine. They have also derived from analyses of a fairly narrow range of accounted-for activities, these being diagnostic pronouncements and prescription/non-prescription of pharmaceutical interventions.

My analysis complements and extends knowledge about when accounts arise. I have shown that practitioners sometimes produce accounts when patients express concern about bodily state or performance. This has resonance with previous findings: Buttny (1993) describes how accounts follow emotional state descriptions – in the physiotherapy data they may follow avowals of *physical* states and performances. I also showed accounts arising when patients had reported performing, or expressed preferences or expectations regarding particular activities that did not match therapists' subsequent recommendations, and also when therapists instigated treatment actions in contexts of likely misalignment about their underlying rationale. These locations again accord with prior findings about medical inter-actions (Stivers 2005a, Peräkylä 1998). However, some of the circumstances that I identified have not been previously described: these being where accounts were associated with removal or adjustment of patients' clothing, and where they were provided in association with actions and recommendations addressing local and evident shortcomings or failures.

My analysis also complements and extends understandings about the functioning of clinicians' accounts. Whilst reflecting prior findings that they contribute to minimising patient resistance (Maynard 2004, Stivers 2005b) and to providing education (Stivers 2005a), my analysis goes further by showing *how* accounts do so, and it also identifies previously undocumented aspects of their functioning. My analysis suggests that accounts' well-recognised role in dealing with resistance should be seen as overlapping with their contribution to persuading, influencing and motivating patients. Various aspects of the structure and timing of accounts contribute to this. By producing accounts when patients express concern about their difficulties and when their recommendations run counter to expressed preferences or expectations, practitioners ensure that patients' concerns are addressed there and then within the interaction – even where these concerns are indirectly expressed or incipient. Timely production of accounts at this juncture is likely to increase their persuasive force. The persuasiveness of account sequences is also increased where they are overtly linked back – through overt verbal referencing – to the original patient contribution that prompted them. Another feature that can increase persuasiveness is where the account subtly incorporates an assumption that the patient's problems will lessen and their capability will progress. Accounts that have an 'in-order-to' format lend themselves to conveying this kind of assumption. Persuasiveness is also built through incrementally expanding accounts so that they move from accounting for individual and specific actions towards conveying fundamental or broad rationales for multiple activities.

My analysis also illustrated some of the specific mechanisms by which accounts contribute to patient education. For instance, producing accounts in close conjunction with patients' expressed concerns allows provision of timely information, thus enhancing learning. Also, expanding their specific accounts for local activities towards more far-reaching and fundamental matters allows practitioners to provide extensive education and information.

Functions of accounts highlighted in this analysis that have not been explored before include their contribution to managing the challenges inherent in addressing people's physical shortcomings and failures. Though central to many healthcare activities, addressing people's shortcomings and failures is nevertheless a socially delicate and interactionally demanding enterprise because it carries negative connotations for both patient and therapy (Parry 2004). Even though accounts commonly focus attention on patients' shortcomings, their production, timing and format can nevertheless work to manage sensitively these shortcomings and imbue them with some positive slant or meaning. For instance, accounts can convey that physical failures constitute reasons for further efforts, rather than for giving up. Accounts can treat failures as solvable matters rather than irredeemable obstacles, particularly where the account predicates expectations of progress, improvement or resolution. A further element of accounts' functioning that has received little previous attention was highlighted by identifying and analysing accounts produced in contexts of undressing. Therapists' accounts in this context can work to provide a sense that the consultation is a place where undressing is not presumed to be merely routine and unquestioned, but rather is treated as a potentially sensitive or imposing activity (Houtkoop-Steenstra 1990). In general, accounts convey the accounted-for treatment actions as needing special sensitivity and attention in terms of explanation and justification.

This analysis also reveals features that may explain why observational studies in physiotherapy and elsewhere have found that clinicians' accounts are rather infrequent. First there were no clear cases in the physiotherapy data where patients asked 'why' questions about reasons for treatment actions, and thus there were no clear cases of clinicians' accounts being occasioned by such enquiries. It is well recognised that during consultations, patients preserve a differential status between themselves and clinicians by making contributions that are qualified, indirect or limited in various ways, and that doing otherwise would undermine the underpinning logic of the consultation and the rationale of expert healthcare (ten Have 1991, Heath 1992). Applying these understandings to the matter in hand, if a patient attempted to elicit reasons for actions or recommendations from a therapist, this would risk implying questioning or distrust, which in turn could threaten the underlying rationale of therapy. As a result, a circumstance in which accounts commonly arise during everyday interactions very rarely arises in clinical interactions. A second factor that may explain accounts' scarcity concerns how accounts often entail alluding to or attending to some bodily trouble. Doing so is regularly avoided in therapy consultations because of potential connotations for patients' personal competence and for therapy's success (Parry 2004). Finally, analysis showed that accounting sequences can be lengthy; since treatment sessions are time-limited, such accounts unavoidably reduce time available for physical activities. This might make therapists less likely to embark on accounting, particularly given that physical activities are often thought of (by both therapists and patients) as the mainstay of therapy. Before leaving this topic, it is worth noting some 'ways around' these various factors that work against the production of accounts. In the face of a lack of direct patient enquiries prompting accounts, therapists can instead treat certain patient comments as providing *opportunities* for accounting. With regard to a possible tendency to avoid accounts because they refer to physical shortcomings, analysis showed that accounts can be produced and shaped so as to sensitively and constructively manage such troubles. Finally, although some account sequences are indeed lengthy, it is also possible for therapists to produce very brief accounts and to incorporate these within physical activity sequences (*e.g.* Extract 6).

Understanding why professionals may avoid referring to the reasons and rationale of their actions has some bearing on debates within medical sociology about why practitioners do and do not raise and discuss certain matters with their patients. In contrast to notions that professionals avoid explaining things to patients because of an overriding orientation to maintaining knowledge and power differentials, I have shown how professionals' limited references to the rationale and reasoning underlying treatment reflect practical, interactional and social constraints on accounting. Practical constraints include the time that accounting takes; interactional ones include an absence of direct patient enquiries about reasons; social constraints include the sensitivities of verbally attending to patients' physical shortcomings and the fact that accounting often requires such attention.

My analysis could be used in building practical recommendations for practitioners about how to employ accounts reflectively and purposefully within treatment sessions in order to manage or pre-empt patient resistance, foster agreement, deal sensitively with patients' shortcomings, encourage motivation and efforts, and so on. Such recommendations would incorporate the findings about how accounts can be timed and worded so as to help accomplish particular functions.

Several lines of future investigation are suggested by this analysis. As noted, the kinds of circumstances I have examined are by no means always accompanied by accounts. There is thus room for further specification of precisely when and why practitioners do and do not produce accounts. This would require comparative analysis of ostensibly similar treatment activities and circumstances wherein accounts did and did not arise. It would also require some consideration of external factors that might play a part – particularly practitioners' level of experience and expertise, which prior research has suggested is associated with the range and frequency of explanations clinicians produce (Jensen *et al.* 1992, Heritage and Stivers 1999: Footnote 11). Another relevant line of investigation would be the various kinds of reasons and rationales invoked within accounts. In the extracts I examined, clinicians sometimes invoked their own perspectives and concerns and at other times they invoked those of patients. They sometimes invoked very local physical features and sometimes invoked broader functional achievements and aspirations. Also, accounts may invoke 'because matters' or 'in-order-to matters' and consequences. There is room for further exploration of when and why clinicians invoke particular matters within accounts. As noted, there is also room for refining the analytic and evidential bases for identifying whether particular utterances are or are not hearable as accounting. A final important but as yet unanswered question is whether clinicians' accounts actually affect patients' views, knowledge and conduct in the long term, and hence their health outcomes.

Clinicians' accounts for treatment actions and proposals can be produced at various junctures within consultations, although there are practical, interactional and social constraints on their production. Their accounts contribute in a number of ways to therapeutic interactions, for instance by persuading and motivating patients, providing education, discouraging resistance, and by communicating sensitively and informatively about difficult and demanding activities and topics.

Acknowledgements

I would like to thank the patients and physiotherapists who allowed me to record and analyse their interactions, and the conversation analytic communities at Loughborough University and the University of Nottingham for comments on various parts of the data. Tanya Stivers provided important support and advice on analysis. Editors' and reviewers' comments on earlier manuscripts were very helpful in developing this chapter. Data collection and the bulk of analysis was conducted as part of a programme of research funded by a postdoctoral fellowship awarded by the National Coordinating Centre for Research Capacity Development (National Institute for Health Research) UK, fellowship number NCCRCD PDA/N&AHP/PD02/038. Analysis was refined during research visits funded by the British Council Partnership Programme in Science (British Council and Platform Beta Techniek), reference number PPS RV07, to the Max Planck Institute for Psycholinguistics in Nijmegen.

Notes

1   The overt account in this case is an in-order-to account, however a because-account has been conveyed as a predecessor account (Maynard 2004) via the earlier talk about the failure to move from bed to chair with two feet on the ground.
2   As in previously published extracts of these physiotherapy data (Parry 2004), I use the sigma sign Σ to encapsulate effortful sounding vocalisation and exhalations.

References

Antaki, C. (1988) Explanations, communication and social cognition. In Antaki, C. (ed.) *Analysing Everyday Explanation*. London: Sage.

Antaki, C. (1994) *Explaining and Arguing: The Social Organization of Accounts*. London: Sage.

Buttny, R. (1993) *Social Accountability in Communication*. London: Sage.

Buttny, R. and Morris, G. (2001) Accounting. In Robinson, W. and Giles, H. (eds) *The New Handbook of Language and Social Psychology*. Chichester: Wiley and Sons.

Campion, P., Foulkes, J., Neighbour, R. and Tate, P. (2002) Patient centredness in the MRCGP video examination: analysis of large cohort, *British Medical Journal*, 325, 691–2.

Clayman, S. and Gill, V. (2004) Conversation analysis. In Hardy, M. and Bryman, A. (eds) *Handbook of Data Analysis*. Beverly Hills: Sage.

Collins, S. (2005) Explanations in consultations: the combined effectiveness of doctors' and nurses' communication with patients, *Medical Education*, 39, 785–96.

Collins, S., Drew, P., Watt, I. and Entwistle, V. (2005) 'Unilateral' and 'bilateral' practitioner approaches in decision-making about treatment, *Social Science and Medicine*, 61, 2611–27.

Drew, P. and Heritage, J. (1992) Analyzing talk at work: an introduction. In Drew, P. and Heritage, J. (eds) *Talk At Work: Interaction in Institutional Settings*. Cambridge: Cambridge University Press.

Fox Tree, J. and Schrock, J. (2002) Basic meanings of *you know* and *I mean*, *Journal of Pragmatics*, 34, 727–47.

Gill, V. and Maynard, D. (2006) Patients' explanations for health problems and physicians' responsiveness in the medical interview. In Heritage, J. and Maynard, D. (eds) *Communication in Medical Care: Interaction between Primary Care Physicians and Patients*. Cambridge: Cambridge University Press.

Greatbatch, D. (2006) Prescriptions and prescribing: coordinating talk and text-based activities. In Heritage, J. and Maynard, D. (eds) *Communication in Medical Care: Interaction between Primary Care Physicians and Patients*. Cambridge: Cambridge University Press.

ten Have, P. (1991) Talk and institution: a reconsideration of the 'Asymmetry' of doctor-patient interaction. In Boden, D. and Zimmerman, D.H. (eds) *Talk and Social Structure*. Cambridge: Polity Press.

Heath, C. (1992) The delivery and reception of diagnosis in the general-practice consultation. In Drew, P. and Heritage, J. (eds.) *Talk at Work: Interaction in Institutional Settings*. Cambridge: Cambridge University Press.

Heath, C. and Luff, P. (1993) Explicating face-to-face interaction. In Gilbert, N. (ed.) *Researching Social Life*. London: Sage.

Heritage, J. (1984) *Garfinkel and Ethnomethodology*. Cambridge: Polity.

Heritage, J. (1988) Explanations as accounts: a conversation analytic perspective. In Antaki, C. (ed.) *Analysing Everyday Explanation*. London: Sage.

Heritage, J. (2005) Conversation analysis and institutional talk. In Fitch, K. and Sanders, R. (eds) *Handbook of Language and Social Interaction*. Mahwah NJ: Lawrence Erlbaum.

Heritage, J. and Robinson, J. (2006) Accounting for the visit: giving reasons for seeking medical care. In Heritage, J. and Maynard, D. (eds) *Communication in Medical Care: Interactions between Primary Care Physicians and Patients*. Cambridge: Cambridge University Press.

Heritage, J. and Stivers, T. (1999) Online commentary in acute medical visits: a method of shaping patient expectations, *Social Science and Medicine*, 49, 1501–17.

Houtkoop-Steenstra, H. (1990) Accounting for proposals, *Journal of Pragmatics*, 14, 111–24.

Jefferson, G. (2004) Glossary of transcript symbols with an introduction. In Lerner, G.H. (ed.) *Conversation Analysis: Studies from the First Generation*. Amsterdam: John Benjamins.

Jensen, G.M., Shepard, K.F., Gwyer, J. and Hack, L.H. (1992) Attribute dimensions that distinguish master and novice physical therapy clinicians in orthopedic settings, *Physical Therapy*, 72, 10, 711–22.

Johnson, D. (2008) *Contemporary Sociological Theory: an Integrated Multi-level Approach*. New York: Springer.

Lerner, G. (1991) On the syntax of sentences-in-progress, *Language in Society*, 20, 441–58.

Maynard, D. (2004) On predicating a diagnosis as an attribute of a person, *Discourse Studies*, 6, 53–76.

NHS Modernisation Agency (2003) Essence of Care – Patient-focused benchmarks for clinical governance: NHS Modernisation Agency. http://www.dh.gov.uk/en/Publicationsandstatistics/Publications/PublicationsPolicyAndGuidance/DH_4005475

Parry, R. (2004) The interactional management of patients' physical incompetence: a conversation analytic study of physiotherapy interactions, *Sociology of Health and Illness*, 26, 7, 976–1007.

Parry, R. (2007) *Referring to body parts: when is 'your' arm 'the' arm?* Paper presented at the 10th International Pragmatics Association, Goteborg, Sweden.

Partridge, C. (1994) *Evaluation of Physiotherapy for People with Stroke: Report of a Workshop on Appropriate Outcomes of Physiotherapy for People with Stroke*. London: Kings Fund.

Peräkylä, A. (1998) Authority and accountability: the delivery of diagnosis in primary health care, *Social Psychology Quarterly*, 61, 4, 301–20.

Peräkylä, A. (2006) Communicating and responding to diagnosis. In Heritage, J. and Maynard, D. (eds) *Communication in Medical Care: Interaction between Primary Care Physicians and Patients*. Cambridge: Cambridge University Press.

Pomerantz, A. (1984) Agreeing and disagreeing with assessments: some features of preferred/dispreferred turn shapes. In Atkinson, J.M. and Heritage, J. (eds) *Structures of Social Action*. Cambridge: Cambridge University Press.

Potter, J. (2003) Discourse analysis. In Hardy, M. and Bryman, A. (eds) *Handbook of Data Analysis*. Beverly Hills: Sage.

Raymond, G. (2004) Prompting action: the stand-alone 'so' in ordinary conversation, *Research on Language and Social Interaction*, 37, 185–218.

Schutz, A. (1967) [Translated by Walsh, G. and Lehnert, F. (1980)] *The Phenomenology of the Social World*. London: Heinemann Educational.

Stivers, T. (2005a) Non-antibiotic treatment recommendations: delivery formats and implications for patient resistance, *Social Science and Medicine*, 60, 949–64.

Stivers, T. (2005b) Parent resistance to physicians' treatment recommendations: one resource for initiating a negotiation of the treatment decision, *Health Communication*, 18, 41–74.

Stivers, T. (2006) Treatment decisions: negotations between doctors and patients in acute care encounters. In Heritage, J. and Maynard, D. (eds) *Communication in Medical Care: Interaction between Primary Care Physicians and Patients*. Cambridge: Cambridge University Press.

Talvitie, U. and Reunanen, M. (2002) Interaction between physiotherapists and patients in stroke treatment, *Physiotherapy*, 88, 2, 77–88.

West, C. and Frankel, R. (1991) Miscommunication in medicine. In Coupland, N., Giles, H. and Wieman, J. (eds) *'Miscommunication' and Problematic Talk*. Newbury Park, CA: Sage.

Woods, D. and Fassnacht, C. (2009). Transana v2.230 http://www.transana.org. Madison, WI: The Board of Regents of the University of Wisconsin.

5

'I've put weight on cos I've bin inactive, cos I've 'ad me knee done': moral work in the obesity clinic

Helena Webb

Introduction

The title of this chapter quotes a patient responding to a doctor's question at the start of a specialist consultation about obesity. As a medical term, 'obesity' describes a condition of excess bodyweight, predominantly caused by an imbalance between the amount of energy entering the body through food and drink and the amount leaving it through physical activity. Obesity is regarded as a health problem since it is associated with numerous co-morbidities, including type-2 diabetes, stroke, heart disease and some cancers (Department of Health 2004). In recent years, statistics have suggested the existence of a global obesity 'epidemic' (WHO 2000), posing a significant challenge to healthcare systems and governments over how to 'cure' and 'manage' the condition. In the UK, National Health Service (NHS) treatments begin with diet and exercise modifications promoting weight loss, which may be combined with pharmaceutical and surgical interventions. NHS guidance (NICE 2006) acknowledges that diet and exercise regimes require significant lifestyle changes, and emphasises the need for supportive communication in medical encounters, recommending that practitioners should praise, listen to and negotiate with their obese patients. The same policy advice states that to receive care patients must display a commitment to change (NICE 2006) and that obesity is a 'lifestyle issue which the Department of Health cannot by itself be expected to cure' (NAO 2001: 1). This positions the individual as normatively responsible for the onset of obesity and, in part, its management.

This chapter describes how moral issues become visible when doctors and patients discuss obesity. I use conversation analysis (CA) to discuss opening questions and responses in obesity-related medical consultations. Opening questions function to solicit information from the patient that enables the consultation to begin. In my data, patients answer with information relevant to the medical context. Typically, they report and/or assess their treatment status and behaviours between appointments. A key difference emerges in these answers according to whether or not the patients report information that can be heard as implying 'success' or 'lack of success' in weight-loss progress. For example, reports of continued exercise, weight loss and improved health can all be heard in the medical context to imply success. Significantly, patients producing these kinds of responses tend to enhance their own agency when reporting their behaviours. By contrast, patients who respond to opening questions with reports of weight gain (which imply lack of success) tend to minimise their agency by emphasising the role of unavoidable or external factors. By constructing their agency in these different ways, patients orient to obesity and weight loss as moral issues. The moral issues invoked in their responses have resonances with the perceived responsibilities of patienthood and certain dynamics identified in existing analyses of the modern obesity 'crisis'. My analysis demonstrates that normative issues of obesity are constructed collaboratively through talk in this medical setting. As such, it makes a valuable addition to the sociology of obesity and indicates that policy guidelines on how practitioners should talk to obese patients need to recognise the complexity of the interactions that occur.

Background: obesity and medicine – the central role of interaction

As concerns about the prevalence of obesity have grown, sociological interest in the condition has also increased. Existing literature intersects with fields such as academic feminism, gender studies, the sociology of the body and size-acceptance activism to highlight the status of obesity as a social and moral problem. However, there is also space to consider the central role of interaction when the 'problem' of obesity is dealt with in a medical setting.

Literature in the sociology of obesity includes discussions of how the organisation of modern societies can cause collective weight gain (*e.g.* Crossley 2004), including gains that are unevenly distributed according to class, ethnicity and gender (*e.g.* Crossley 2004, Boardman *et al.* 2005, Batnitzky 2008). The obese body can be seen to have become medicalised over time (Sobal 1995), with its definition subject to change (Chang and Christakis 2002). Obesity science itself is characterised by uncertainties, for example regarding the persuasiveness of the dominant energy imbalance model (Gard and Wright 2005, Monaghan 2005) and the supposed connections between weight loss and improved health (Aphramor 2005). Critics of the obesity 'crisis' argue that these uncertainties are glossed over as facts, enabling an ethically questionable 'war on fat' that is partly underpinned by moral attitudes favouring thin bodies over large ones (Monaghan 2005, Rich and Evans 2005).

The obese body as a moral problem is a major theme within the literature. Modern societies can be seen to idealise thin bodies, associating them with the characteristics necessary for capitalist success: hard work and self-control. By contrast, obese bodies represent laziness and greed, symbols of individual moral failure (Bordo 1993, Sobal 1995). Since we culturally assume that bodies mirror an individual's 'real' self, an obese body becomes a marker of a discredited self as well as a visual indicator of ill-health (Jutel 2005). This 'moral model' of the body is argued to remain prevalent (Bordo 1993), mediating certain claims made in obesity science and policy (see above) and inspiring an alternative, 'political model' that promotes size acceptance (Sobal 2003). These medical, moral and political arguments are the basis for framing contests over how obesity is perceived in modern life (Saguy and Riley 2005) and can also be found in individuals' descriptions of their own obese bodies. Whilst individuals may demonstrate awareness of obesity measures or accept their obesity as problematic, they also explain and experience their weight via their personal histories rather than clinical categories (Warin *et al.* 2008), presenting their own, often morally defined, understandings of what constitutes a healthy weight (Monaghan 2007) and resisting constructions of their obesity as due to individual moral failure (Throsby 2007).

The sociological literature indicates that, despite some interweaving and competition between models, obesity has become dominantly positioned as a medical condition. Consequently, individuals categorised as obese are likely to experience medical attention. Interview studies have included obese people's accounts of their patient histories and treatment decisions (Sarlio-Lahteenkorva 2000, Throsby 2007) whilst surveys have revealed how infrequently patients report that they have been advised about their weight in primary care (Loureiro and Nagya Jr 2006). However, there is a lack of research investigating what actually occurs in obesity-related medicine, in particular the interactions that occur during consultations about the condition. This kind of analysis has the potential to make a significant contribution to sociological understanding of the obesity phenomenon, for example by observing how alternative medical, moral and political understandings of obesity become visible in consultations. Furthermore, the particular medical tasks taking place provide relevant themes for analysis. As noted above, obesity treatments prioritise diet and exercise regimes. These take place away from the medical gaze, so patients are required to produce verbal reports of them. Much of the consultation may involve discussions of diet and exercise behaviours, including the provision of advice-giving from the medical practitioner. Talk is therefore a medium for treatment and a form of treatment in itself. Existing work on medical interactions demonstrates the analytic utility of studying talk between practitioners and patients and indicates the benefits of this approach for the study of obesity. In particular, it demonstrates how themes of responsibility for illness and commitment to change – found in the policy literature above – may be constructed as moral issues in the medical encounter.

Talk is a central feature of medical practice and certain types of talk occur in different types of consultation. In his classic observational study, Strong (1979) describes interactions in NHS consultations as following a 'bureaucratic format' in which medicine is assumed to deal exclusively with natural phenomena, leaving moral character assessment absent. Silverman (1987), observing diabetes consultations, adds that this polite form of interaction is at times breached when the condition being discussed is one that emphasises the active commitment of the patient. In these cases the consultation can become 'a kind of trial for the patient in which [he/she] is to be held accountable for [his/her] actions' (1987: 215), leading to tensions in the interaction. Similarly, discussions about smoking in General Practice consultations (Pilnick and Coleman 2003) can lead to interactional difficulties when a patient's health status is connected to his/her own lifestyle behaviour. As with diabetes and smoking, obesity treatment requires the active involvement of the patient as well as frequent discussion of lifestyle behaviours. It is possible that similar forms of tension may be observed when talk involves reference to normative issues of commitment and responsibility for condition and cure. These types of study highlight the value of conducting detailed analyses of medical interactions and identifying how talk between practitioners and patients can construct a particular topic being discussed as a morally 'sensitive' one. The analysis reported in this chapter adds to this body of work by describing how moral issues concerning 'success' and 'lack of success' in weight loss become visible during interactions at the start of medical consultations about obesity.

Methodology

This chapter draws on data from my doctoral research on doctor-patient interactions in obesity-related medical consultations (Webb 2009). Fieldwork took place in the UK in two NHS clinics specialising in treating obese patients. Patients at the clinics attended routine appointments to receive support in losing weight. All were advised to modify their diet and exercise behaviours and some also received pharmaceutical and surgical treatments. Fieldwork involved the video-recording of consultations. A group of 18 patients and one doctor (a diabetes consultant with a specialist interest in obesity) gave formal consent to have their consultations video-recorded over a period of nine months, resulting in 39 recordings and approximately 20 hours of data.

The recordings were transcribed and analysed using conversation analysis (CA). CA identifies and analyses recurrent patterns of interaction. Taking an ethnomethodological approach (Garfinkel 1967), it treats interaction as accomplished collaboratively by those present (Sacks 1992). Verbal utterances and non-verbal phenomena such as gesture, body movements etc are treated as forms of social action and analysed in terms of what actions they perform and how they construct social encounters. We use interaction to present our selves and our behaviours to others as creditable; as such, interactions always have a moral element. This moral element may be connected to the particular context in which interaction occurs. In this chapter I highlight the distinctive moral work occurring during the opening phases of medical consultations about obesity.

This chapter discusses the doctor's opening questions and patients' responses in the data. Medical consultations typically begin with general greetings followed by a question from the practitioner (Byrne and Long 1976, ten Have 1989). This question is an opening question which functions to solicit information from the patient about his/her condition and therefore start the medical 'business' of the encounter. Opening questions take different forms. If the consultation is about a new problem (as in many primary/acute care visits) it may be 'What can I do for you today?', a question that functions to solicit the patient's new concern (Robinson 2006). Alternatively, where patients are attending follow-up or routine consultations, as in these data, opening questions may solicit a progress report on the existing problem. The question may refer to the problem specifically, for example 'How is your hand?' or may be more general, for example 'How have you been?' (Robinson 2006). The production of an opening question projects that the patient will produce an answer to the question in response. Lexical choice may also project what type of information the answer will contain. A question such as 'How is your hand?' pre-selects the topic of the patient's answer, whereas 'How have you been?' selects no topic and is therefore less constraining.

In producing a response that fits (or otherwise) the opening question, the practitioner and patient jointly accomplish the start of the consultation. Although their answers may be constrained by the wording of the opening question asked, patients often have an opportunity to produce an extended response. In this way, opening question and answer sequences are 'the only phase of medical visits in which patients are systematically given institutional licence to describe their illness in their own terms and in pursuit of their own agenda' (Heritage and Robinson 2006: 90). They therefore represent a particularly fruitful area for analysis. In routine appointments, patients tend to answer opening questions with reports of treatment-related behaviours between consultations (Heritage and Robinson 2006). This provides an opportunity to analyse how they represent themselves and their behaviours in their talk. Drew (1998) writes that a constant feature of social life is that in describing our own (or others') behaviours we design our talk to display the appropriateness or inappropriateness of that behaviour. We select from a range of possible modes of description and our talk 'may always ... be understood as doing moral work – as providing a basis for evaluating the 'rightness' or 'wrongness' of whatever is being reported' (1998: 295). Patients' answers to opening questions can therefore be analysed as performing moral work.

Four extracts are presented for discussion. They have been chosen as they represent typical sequences in the dataset in terms of the structure and wording of questions asked; the range of response lengths and topics referred to; and, in particular, the interactional devices employed by patients in their answers. The extracts have been transcribed using the CA system devised by Jefferson (reproduced in Atkinson and Heritage 1984) which marks interactional features such as word stress, intonation and pause length. Analysis discusses how the opening questions are formed and responded to. The data show that the doctor's opening questions tend to take a relatively open, non-constraining form. In response, patients provide information relevant to the medical context through reports and assessments. They also provide information that hearably implies 'success' or 'lack of success' in terms of weight loss progress. Whilst doing so, they invoke agency in relation to their own behaviours in ways that perform particular types of moral work.

Analysis

The analysis describes the systematic interactional practices observed in the data that: (1) accomplish the start of the consultation and (2) can be heard to imply 'success' or 'lack of success' regarding each patient's weight-loss progress. In connection with this second point, the analysis further describes how patients construct their own agency in different ways according to whether they imply success or lack of success, and highlights these alternate constructions as forms of moral work. These interactional practices occur as part of the doctor's opening questions and the patients' responses to them. The key phenomena analysed are the structure, wording and timing of the doctor's questions; the structure and wording of patients' answers, as well as the topics patients choose to address and the order in which they produce them; and the doctor's subsequent utterances after the patients' responses.

Implying 'success'

Extracts 1 and 2 demonstrate typical features of opening questions and responses in the data. Furthermore, they show the type of responses that can be heard as implying 'successful' progress in weight loss. In these answers patients enhance their own agency with regard to their treatment actions and efforts.

After opening greetings the doctor and patient are sitting facing one another. In response to the doctor's opening question the patient produces a positive assessment and report of his exercise behaviours.

Extract 1

1	Doc:	How're you <u>feeling</u>?
2	Pat:	<u>Br</u>illiant. <u>Br</u>illiant.
3		(0.4)
4	Pat:	<u>Ex</u>cellent hh I'm I'm
5		still going to the <u>gy</u>m, un
6	Doc:	You've lost <u>weight</u> <u>ha</u>ven't you?

In line 1 the doctor asks 'How're you <u>feeling</u>?' This wording and the grammatical structure are similar to general enquiries, such as 'how are you?', that we often ask at the start of social encounters. However, several features of its delivery suggest that here it can be heard as a medical opening question. It is delivered about 30 seconds into the consultation, once the doctor and patient have already exchanged initial greetings and are in physical, sitting positions that indicate they are ready to start 'business' (Heath 1986). Additionally, the verb form 'feeling' can express an interest in bio-medical status (Robinson 2006), suggesting that, in this context, the question is a medically relevant one. In this way, 'How're you <u>feeling</u>?' appears designed to start the consultation. Although it is asked in an obesity consultation, this opening question does not refer specifically to weight. This is the case in all four extracts presented here and the vast majority of consultations in the data. The reference to 'feeling' does not propose that the patient should refer to weight – or any other topic – in his response. As an opening question, 'How're you <u>feeling</u>?' is therefore relatively non-constraining.

In line 2 the patient begins his answer with '<u>Br</u>illiant. <u>Br</u>illiant.' followed by '<u>Ex</u>cellent' in line 4. These strongly positive assessments can be heard to provide information about how the patient is feeling. The assessments are outside the neutral range of responses that normally follow a general enquiry (Jefferson 1980) and this suggests that they refer to the specific biomedical sense of 'feeling'. The patient's utterance can be heard as assessing his health status in a way that may be relevant to the clinic setting. This sense is enhanced by his continued response in lines 4–5 which reports that he is still going to the gym. This information implies efforts to become fit and to lose weight through exercise, so is directly relevant to the goals of the consultation. It also provides an update of his treatment behaviours between consultations. It is noticeable that the patient reports information relevant to a medical obesity encounter, even though the doctor's question did not mention this specifically. The patient appears to draw on the context of the current interaction to interpret the doctor's question and produce an opening question response relevant to the consultation.

The structure of the patient's answer implies that he has been successful in his weight loss behaviours. By answering the opening question with strongly positive assessments and combining these with a report about his activities, the patient implies that he is doing well in addition to feeling well. By extension, this suggests that his weight-loss efforts have been successful. The patient's answer also emphasises that this implied success is the result of his own activity. This is achieved through the 'I'm' in line 4 and in particular the use of 'still', in line 5, which displays that the gym work has been continuing for some time. This suggests that the effort of going to the gym is not temporary but a continued effort. In line 6 the doctor asks 'You've lost weight haven't you?'. This directly topicalises weight and suggests that the doctor is treating the patient's previous response as relating to his weight status. The utterance is constructed as an observation, 'you've lost weight' followed by a confirmation-soliciting tag question, 'haven't you?' In this context the observation about weight loss is hearable as a positive comment. It draws out the implications of the patient's answer and implicitly affiliates with the positive slant of his report.

Extract 2 further illustrates the ways in which patients enhance their agency when implying success in weight-loss progress.

Extract 2

The patient is sitting down facing the doctor after exchanging opening greetings and making 'small talk' about waiting times.

```
 1   Doc:   So:::. (1.3) How uh you?
 2   Pat:   .hhh
 3          (1.3)
 4   Pat:   OKay, (.) my knee is no:w (1.5) ninety five
 5          per cent be:tter
 6          (0.3)
 7   Doc:   Okay.
 8   Pat:   °er° I've avoided having any operations on it,
 9          so suh .hh that's good
10   Doc:   Ptch °yes°
11   Pat:   um .hh I sta:rted the swimming
12          (0.4)
13   Doc:   Grea:t
14   Pat:   .hh I went twice, (0.3) and then
15          I was told by: .hh er °um° the guy
16          at thuh City to stop because both
17          times my knee (0.6) swelled u:p
```

```
18   Doc:   Right. You set off your knee.
19   Pat:   Yeah a:nd he said =
20   Doc:   = °OK°
21   Pat:   thut what's proble:y (0.6) happening wuz it
22          wuz actually over extending,
23   Doc:   °Right.°
24   Pat:   °Right.° .hhh So: I've stopped that, but I've
25          been goi:ng to the gy:m,
26   Doc:   ↑Oh grea:t
```

The 'How uh you?' in line 1 is the doctor's opening question. As in Extract 1, it shares the wording of a general enquiry, but is delivered after greetings and once the doctor and patient are in physical positions that suggest they are ready for the consultation to start. The question is also prefaced with a sound-stretched and emphasised 'So:::.'. This has the effect of connecting the 'How uh you?' to some unfinished business that has gone on previously (such as the patient's prior consultations). It marks it as relating to a matter of on-going concern and invites an expanded response from the patient (Bolden 2006).

The patient produces an in-breath, suggesting some oncoming talk, in line 2 and shifts his body position during the silence in line 3. At the start of line 4, he says 'OKay,' with an enhanced volume and continuing intonation which suggests it may announce the onset of some further talk. The patient goes on to say that his knee is now 'ninety five per cent be:tter' (lines 4–5). This information implies that the knee has been a problem in the past but is now much improved. It forms a positive report, displaying that progress has been made. The topic is medically relevant. Although the patient does not explicitly relate his knee problem to his weight, his reference to improvement could be heard to imply that improved mobility enabled increased exertion or even that the improvement in the knee was a result of weight loss. Once again, the patient draws on the context of the talk to answer the doctor's generally worded opening question with information relevant to the consultation.

In line 7 the doctor says 'Okay.', which as a short, acknowledging utterance enables the patient to continue with his response. In line 8 the patient continues about his knee: 'I've avoided having any operations on it,'. The verb 'avoided' generally conveys that the action it is connected to – e.g. having an operation – is less than favourable, so here the patient is implying more success. By stating 'I've avoided' he positions himself as the grammatical subject of the talk and credits himself for this success. An operation is usually something that is medically necessary and caused by a serious problem, so by suggesting that he has been able to avoid it, the patient makes strong claims about his medical progress and his own agency. In line 9 he assesses this news: 'that's good'. This makes explicit that he is treating his news about the knee, and his efforts in connection with it, as positive. It positions him as aware of what is medically 'good' for him and as capable of assessing his own illness experience (Gill 1998).

In line 10 the doctor produces a quiet and minimal agreement, 'yes', and in line 11 the patient begins to talk about swimming. This topic can also be heard as relevant to weight loss as it refers to exercise and provides a continuation of the opening question response. The patient says 'I sta:rted the swimming'. Referring to it as 'the' swimming, rather than just 'swimming', implies that this activity has been discussed by the doctor and patient previously. By reporting that he started swimming after it had been discussed, the patient displays that he has listened and responded to medical advice. He therefore presents himself as compliant and willing to make an effort. However, the use of 'sta:rted' in the past simple (compared, for example, to 'I have started') implies that the activity has since been stopped. After a positive comment from the doctor in line 13, the patient explains why he stopped swimming from lines 14 to 22. He reports it as something he was told rather than chose to do (line 15), positioning stopping as beyond his control. Furthermore, he reports that he was told this by 'the guy at thuh City' (lines 15–16), meaning a practitioner at a local hospital and a medically legitimate source of advice. The addition of that practitioner's observation about the knee over-extending (line 22) justifies the stopping as medically necessary and again displays that the patient listens to medical advice.

After a doctor acknowledgement (line 23) the patient reports the upshot of the situation, 'So I've stopped that,' and continues 'but I've been goi:ng to the gy:m,' (lines 24–25). The report of the 'failure' – stopping swimming – is immediately offset by positive news about gym visits and further evidence that the patient is making an effort to lose weight. In fact, by reporting the failed difficulties caused by swimming first, the patient indicates that his efforts include overcoming obstacles. In line 26 the doctor responds '↑Oh grea:t'. The 'Oh' functions as a change of state token, acknowledging new information (Heritage 1984) and the 'grea:t' provides a positive comment on it. As it follows the patient's report about going to the gym, the 'grea:t' is hearable as displaying a positive orientation to the patient's efforts to continue exercising despite having to stop the swimming. In this way the patient's answer is jointly constructed as implying successful progress at weight loss.

These two extracts demonstrate typical features of the opening questions and responses in my data. The doctor's opening questions appear to be non-constraining, with some similarities to general enquiries. In response, patients draw on the context of the interaction to produce answers that report information relevant to the start of the consultation. This information typically refers to or assesses patients' treatment status and behaviours. Extracts 1 and 2 also demonstrate the ways in which patients respond to opening questions with answers that imply success in weight-loss progress. Here the patients imply success through reports of exercise and improved health. In other cases in the data, patients report additional treatment behaviours, including diet regimes, and sometimes connect them to weight-loss amounts or reduced clothes sizes. Extracts 1 and 2 also show that patients attribute this implied success to their own efforts and activities. In Extract 1 the patient indicates that his gym visits are an ongoing effort and in Extract 2 the patient displays his willingness to overcome obstacles. This is typical across the data. Patients emphasise their own role in undertaking exercise, improving their health, following diets etc and in doing so present the implied successes as their own accomplishment (Maynard 2003). With these references patients perform moral work. They present what can normatively be understood in the context as 'good' – exercise, avoiding operations, making an effort, overcoming difficulties – as personal achievements. Patients' responses implying lack of success are very different, as shown in Extracts 3 and 4.

Implying 'lack of success'
Extract 3

This patient reports weight gain and connects it to external factors that have prevented him from being active.

```
1   Doc:   So how uv things bin since (.) last time
2          you came?
3   Pat:   U::m (.) I've put weight on, cos I've bin
4          inactive
```

```
 5              (.)
 6   Pat:    cos I've 'ad [me knee] done.
 7   Doc:               [the knee]
 8              (0.7)
 9   Doc:    Ri:ght
10              (0.5)
11   Pat:    But u:mm ho:pefully: (0.8) I shoul- I might
12              be getting a gastric band in February, (.)
13   Doc:    Grea:t
14   Pat:    that's what I'm working towards.
```

As the extract begins, the doctor and patient are sitting down and the patient has just commented that 'it's been a long time' since his last visit. The doctor's question in lines 1–2 takes up this topic and asks 'So how uv things bin since (.) last time you came?' As an opening question this is slightly more constraining than the other questions discussed here since it explicitly references the medical setting and selects a time frame for the patient. The patient begins his response in line 3 with 'U::m' and then states 'I've put weight on'. By mentioning weight he takes up the doctor's reference to the setting and produces an opening question response relevant to the consultation. The use of the present perfect, 'I've put', corresponds to the time frame in the doctor's question.

In the context of the obesity clinic, the patient's report of putting on weight is hearable as implying lack of success in his treatment progress. The patient immediately links his weight gain to being inactive (lines 3–4), suggesting the absence of exercise, a key feature in obesity treatment. This is then connected to having a knee operation (line 6). The repeated 'cos' that links these statements constructs the connection between the weight gain, inactivity and the operation as causal and logical. It also conveys that the patient is knowledgeable about his own weight status and what influences it. The placing of 'I've 'ad me knee done' at the end of the patient's answer positions the operation as causing the other two factors: it meant he could not exercise and therefore gained weight. As noted in Extract 2, an operation is generally a medically necessary procedure. So the operation, and its associated consequence of weight gain, can be heard as an unavoidable, understandable course of action undertaken by the patient rather than something he can be blamed for doing. It is noticeable that although 'I've 'ad me knee done' is a grammatically active structure, it also carries a passive sense which conveys that the operation was done to the patient. This can be heard to reduce the patient's agency to some extent in relation to his implied lack of success. For example, it may be hearable as suggesting that the patient had the operation because he needed it rather than because he wanted it.

After a doctor acknowledgement in line 9, the patient continues in lines 11–12: 'But u:mm (0.2) ho:pefully: (0.7) I shoul- I might be getting a gastric band in February,'. The word 'ho:pefully:' displays that the patient regards the operation – which promotes weight loss – as a positive development. It also displays that he has knowledge of what is medically 'good' for him. The inclusion of a specific month for the operation, 'February', indicates that he is taking an active interest in his treatment by keeping track of what might happen to him and when. In line 13 the doctor assesses this news with 'Grea:t' and in line 14 the patient continues 'that's what I'm working towards'. The 'that's' refers back to the gastric band operation so here the patient suggests he is working towards having the operation in February. With the 'I'm working towards' the patient changes back to a more clearly active structure. In combination with the sense of effort and purpose implied by the verb form 'working', this has the effect of emphasising that this operation

– in contrast to the knee one – is something he is actively pursuing and having an influence over.

As in the previous extracts, the patient answers the doctor's opening question with information relevant to his weight-loss status and behaviours. However, his response implies lack of success rather than success. He reports putting on weight and being inactive. In contrast to Extracts 1 and 2 the patient reduces, rather than emphasises, his agency in relation to these behaviours. He connects his weight gain and inactivity to having an operation. This provides a medically and morally acceptable reason for his subsequent weight gain and so limits the extent to which he can be held responsible for it. In this way, lack of success is connected with a mitigating factor. The patient then emphasises his own effort and activity in relation to future treatment that might lead to success: a gastric band operation. The minimisation of agency through reports of mitigating factors occurs consistently across the data when patients' answers imply lack of success. This can be seen in Extract 4.

Extract 4

This patient attends with her mother and speaks with a relatively strong local accent. She produces a long opening question response that initially hints at lack of success. She reports difficulties taking a prescribed drug and, ultimately, weight gain.

```
 1    Doc:    [> but any]way < (.) doesn't matter. How are
 2    Pat:    [   Ri::ght.]
 3    Doc:    you?
 4            (0.6)
 5    Pat:    I'm alri:gh, I tri:ed the Xenical
 6    Doc:    hmmm?
 7    Pat:    .hh But me docto::r thought differently
 8            to yo:u,
 9    Doc:    Okay.
10    Pat:    An he seh and he did it (0.5) gradulee
11            (1.0)
12    Doc:    hmm.
13    Pat:    Which at fi:rst there was no effect,
14    Doc:    °kay° =
15    Pat:    = but then when I 'it three: (0.7)
16            I couldn't 'ave gone to werk.
17            (.)
18    Doc:    Oh really.
19            (0.3)
20    Doc:    Right. [ S   o ] what did you do?
21    Pat:           [Not un]
22            (0.8)
23    Pat:    I wuz always on the loo:: wun't [ a  h? ]
24    Mum:                                    [°yeah°]
25    Pat:    > WEll I'd got me mum, < (.) that [when it] hit
26    Mum:                                      [Y e a h]
27    Pat:    that [time, my] mum ud ad a new knee:
28    Mum:         [y e a h]
29            (0.3)
30    Pat:    .hh so I was off werk so I was lucky, (0.3)
```

31		but I've I I <u>ad</u> to come <u>off</u> them.
32	Doc:	Ptch Did you go <u>back</u> down to <u>two</u> or did you
33		just [stop them entirely?]
34	Pat:	[.hh No I'm jusuh] I've? not had <u>any</u>.
35		Because [.hhh] once I'd took the <u>three</u>,
36	Doc:	[Right]
37	Doc:	mm[h m ?] =
38	Pat:	[= when] I went do:wn, (0.3) I was still
39		going a lo:t [wasn't ah?] But they <u>ma</u>de me
40	Mum:	[(m m m)]
41	Pat:	<u>really</u> <u>ungrey</u>
42	Doc:	mhm. mm
43	Pat:	I was <u>starvin</u>, so I've <u>et</u> a lot [mo:re] =
44	Mum:	[y u -]
45	Pat:	= .hh I've <u>definitely</u> put <u>weight</u> on

This extract starts two minutes into the consultation. The doctor, patient and her mother are all sitting down and there has been some preceding talk about the patient's notes before the '<u>Ho</u>w are you?' in lines 1 and 3. After a slight delay (line 4) the patient begins her response in line 5 with 'I'm alri:gh' and continues: 'I tri:ed the <u>Xenical</u>'. Xenical is an anti-obesity drug available on the NHS. It is therefore a relevant topic for the consultation. As in Extract 2, reference to 'the' drug displays that Xenical has been discussed previously and that the patient has listened to medical advice. Her use of 'tried' indicates that she has followed advice and taken the drug. It also implies that she has made an effort with regard to a treatment behaviour encouraging weight loss. However, 'tried' in the past simple tense suggests that the drug-taking has now been stopped and that, despite the patient's personal effort, it proved unsuccessful. This provides a hint that the patient's answer will imply lack of success in her weight-loss efforts.

The patient then reports her (negative) experiences with Xenical. She says that at first there was no effect but when she reached the full dose she couldn't have gone to work (lines 13–16). The doctor then prompts further patient talk on the topic, first with a news marker (Heritage 1985), 'Oh really.', in line 18 then a question in line 20: 'So <u>what</u> did you do?' The patient reports that she was on the toilet all the time. Her use of the extreme form '<u>always</u> on the <u>loo</u>::' combines with the previous definite assertion '<u>couldn't</u> ave gone to <u>werk</u>' to underscore the negative effects of the drug. Going to the toilet frequently is a common consequence of taking Xenical, as the drug stops the body absorbing some fat from food. The unabsorbed fat then leaves the body in the form of involuntary diarrhoea. The patient's references to being on the toilet reports what happened to her rather than what she did and as such does not 'fit' the doctor's question. By focusing on what happened to her, the patient presents herself as passive rather than active in this report. She then says that she was off work anyway to look after her mother but that she had to come off the drug. The 'when it hit that time,' (lines 25 and 27) once again positions the negative drug experience as something that happened to her. In line 31 she finally reports her actions in response to the drug, and produces an answer that fits more with the doctor's question. She reports coming off the drug and presents this as a necessity rather than a choice: 'but I've I I 'ad to come <u>off</u> them'. The patient has delayed reporting her actions until she has completed the report of what happened to her. This enables her to convey her extreme, negative experience before stating that she has stopped taking the drug. In this way, the action of no longer taking the drug can be heard as a logical outcome of her negative experiences and not something she can be blamed for choosing to do.

In lines 32–33 the doctor asks the patient whether she went down to two doses a day or stopped taking the drug entirely. This seeks clarification of the patient's reference to 'coming off' the drug. Unlike continuers, such as 'okay' (line 9), this question projects a specific way for the patient to go on with her answer. It is possible to hear the question as hinting at the 'correct' response to Xenical's effects: lowering the dose rather than 'just' stopping it 'entirely'. This hinting may connect to the complicated and apparently contradictory response the patient produces in lines 34–39. She begins her answer with 'No I'm jusuh' then cuts off and restarts to state that she hasn't had any of the drug. She then says that after taking three a day she went down but was still going to the toilet a lot. It is possible that the switch from appearing to say she had not taken any to saying that she had gone down and then stopped orients to the implicit normative response implied in the doctor's question. This normative element remains implicit and the doctor does not pursue a definitive response, instead acknowledging the patient's talk with tokens such as 'Right' (line 36) and 'mmhm?' (line 37).

Following a confirmation-soliciting 'wasn't ah?' ['wasn't I?'] directed towards her mother, the patient reports another problem with Xenical: 'But they made me really ungrey' ['hungry'] (lines 39 and 41). Using 'they' – the drugs – as the grammatical subject again emphasises her passive role in this experience. The problem of the drugs making her hungry is reinforced by upgrading 'ungrey' ['hungry'] to 'starvin' ['starving']) in line 43. The patient then says 'so I've et a lot mo:re', ['so I've eaten a lot more'] (line 43). The connector 'so' marks a relationship between the way the drug made her feel and her actions. Eating a lot more is positioned as a logical consequence of the drug making her hungry. It also hints at unsuccessful news about her weight status. The patient then mentions weight in the conclusion to this narrative. She makes a strong assertion that she has gained weight: 'I've definitely put weight on' (line 45). With this assertion of weight gain the patient confirms the implication of lack of success first hinted at in line 5.

In this extract the patient produces a long response to the doctor's question, reporting a series of problems taking the drug Xenical and concluding with an assertion of weight gain. The patient hints at lack of success at the start of her answer, with 'tried' (line 5). She does not, however, make her assumed weight gain explicit until later. Delaying the explicit report of weight gain enables the patient to make reference to external problems and suggest that she is not personally responsible for weight gain. She displays it as something that happened to her despite her efforts to follow medical advice and lose weight. The patient's answer can be heard as an example of 'defensive detailing' (Drew 1998) in which a speaker builds up a case for something being reported as troublesome (*e.g.* weight gain) but includes various details to suggest she is not to be blamed for it. In doing so the speaker works to avoid possible moral censure. The way in which the patient shrouds her report of weight gain by first hinting at it before ultimately making it explicit also has some similarities to the delivery of 'bad news' in various conversational settings (Maynard 2003) and is found in several other cases in my data. Despite one hint at what might be a 'correct' mode of conduct, the doctor's utterances do not explicitly blame the patient for her 'bad news' about stopping the drug and gaining weight. In this way, the patient's work around responsibility and agency, which presents her problems as things she had no control over, can be seen as jointly accomplished.

Extracts 3 and 4 show typical ways in which patients produce answers that imply lack of success in weight-loss progress. In each case the patient reports mitigating factors that explain his/her reported weight gain. These are factors beyond the patient's personal choice/

control – in Extract 3 an operation and in Extract 4 a negative reaction to medication. In other examples in the data, these factors also relate to additional medical problems or the pressures of family life and work. By invoking these factors patients minimise their own agency in relation to weight gain. They therefore perform moral work by distancing themselves from issues that can be understood in the context as normatively negative: not exercising, eating too much, gaining weight etc. So whilst patients emphasise their agency in relation to behaviours associated with weight-loss progress, they minimise their agency when talking about behaviours associated with weight gain. A final point is that there appears to be a difference in the moral work performed by the patients in Extracts 3 and 4. In Extract 3 the patient produces a relatively straightforward report that announces weight gain immediately. In Extract 4 the patient produces a long, narrative response that delays reporting weight gain until after she has listed a series of mitigating factors. Attributing weight gain to a medically required operation (Extract 3) can be seen as normatively less problematic than attributing it to a personal decision to stop taking a prescribed drug (Extract 4). It is possible to see corresponding nuances in the moral work performed in these two extracts. The various issues of agency, effort and action observed throughout the analysis can also be seen as being connected to normative concerns surrounding obesity and patienthood, as is discussed next.

Discussion

This chapter discussed four typical examples of opening questions and responses in obesity-related medical consultations. Analysis revealed a distinct pattern in patients' responses and here I discuss how this pattern connects with moral concerns surrounding obesity and patienthood. I also highlight the contribution of this research to the sociology of obesity and discussions of healthcare practice.

The doctor's opening questions in these data can appear similar to general enquiry questions, such as 'How are you?', that we often ask at the start of social encounters. However, features of their delivery, such as timing and lexical choice, provide a hearing of these questions as relating specifically to the medical context and function to solicit information from the patient in order to begin the 'business' of the consultation. Patients treat them as such and produce answers relevant to the setting. In their answers patients report and/or assess their treatment status and behaviours between appointments. Their answers can be heard to imply either 'success' or 'lack of success' in making weight loss progress. The ways in which patients orient to the role of their own behaviours in achieving (or not) this progress forms a key pattern in the data. Patients implying success emphasise their agency in terms of efforts and actions which have led to continued exercise, improved health etc. By contrast, patients implying lack of success minimise their agency by invoking mitigating factors, such as not being able to exercise, or having a bad reaction to a drug, which caused weight gain. Through these different references to agency, patients perform moral work. They draw on normative understandings of successful and unsuccessful weight-loss behaviours to associate themselves with 'creditworthy' actions, and position responsibility for 'negative' ones away from themselves. In doing so they also implicitly construct weight loss as positive and the absence of weight loss as negative and potentially blameworthy.

By orienting to successful weight loss and weight-loss behaviours as positive and the absences of these features as negative, the patients in these data can be seen to invoke normative themes similar to those identified in existing sociological studies of obesity. As discussed earlier, these studies suggest that obesity symbolises moral failure through laziness, greed and lack of self-control. The obese individual is required to regain moral standing by making an effort to become thin and displaying self-control. The patients in these data orient to obesity as an undesirable status and consistently display that they are making an effort to lose weight. By indicating their willingness and commitment to listen to medical advice, take new medications, overcome obstacles etc, they display evidence of efforts to master their bodies. By enhancing their agency in relation to losing weight, they can be seen to credit themselves for moving away from a devalued, obese body. They can also be seen to avoid taking responsibility for blameworthy lack of success. With their responses, there-fore, patients invoke themes similar to some of the wider moral dynamics surrounding obesity. Furthermore, they work to reject censure that may be applied to them as obese individuals.

Patients can also be seen to portray themselves as normatively 'good' patients. Across all four extracts, they display that they have knowledge about their condition, follow medical advice and make efforts to become well. These displays are consistent with the behaviours and 'responsibilities' described by Parsons in the classic typology of the 'sick role' (Parsons 1956, 1975). The sick role describes a temporary state of legitimised 'devi-ance' in which individuals can be exempt from certain social obligations and not regarded as responsible for their condition (ill health). In return, those individuals are required to make efforts to exit the sick role and return to 'normal life' by seeking and co-operating with medical advice and demonstrating that they want to get 'better'. The patients in these data attend to these responsibilities in their talk. Patients implying successful weight-loss progress indicate efforts to exit the sick role via their own willingness to become well and to co-operate with medical advice. Patients implying lack of success suggest mitigating factors which justify their continued position within the sick role and may also (Extract 3) indicate their continued efforts to exit the role despite the existence of these obstacles. This may pre-empt any possible criticism that they have not been doing 'enough' to try to get better. By attending to the sick role requirements in this way, patients can also be seen to attend to the moral implications of failing to meet the responsibilities of patient-hood. It is possible to suggest that these moral implications have particular resonance in the medical obesity context since, as seen in the discussion of the policy literature at the start of the chapter, individuals with 'lifestyle' conditions may be seen to have caused their own ill health. This can threaten their privilege of not being held as responsible for their condition and may mean that any lack of medical progress may be seen as further evidence of 'undesirable' behaviour. Therefore, the moral work of displaying efforts to exit the sick role and of avoiding responsibility for weight gain may have particular relevance for obese patients.

A key point to be made is that the openings of consultations, and by extension the moral work performed in them, are jointly accomplished by the doctor and patient. Interaction is achieved through a process of collaboration; patient responses are con-tingent on the doctor's prior opening question (just as the question itself may be shaped by earlier talk, as in Extract 3). In all four extracts, the opening question solicits an answer from the patient without explicitly referring to weight. This enables patients to select a topic to refer to, and choose what information to report and in what order. Patients implying lack of success therefore have the opportunity to connect weight gain to mitigating factors, including reporting those factors first. All patients have the oppor-tunity to reference details that support the normative position they are taking in terms of efforts being made, mitigating factors and so on. This collaboration continues as the patient produces his/her answer. Many of the doctor's further utterances take the form of short tokens which acknowledge the patient's talk and encourage it to continue on the same topic. Furthermore the doctor neither explicitly accepts nor rejects the patients' self-assessments, and inferences to 'correct' behaviour (see Extract 4) are made implicitly.

By demonstrating how these questions and responses are achieved collaboratively, these findings indicate the benefits of taking an interactional, conversation analytic approach to medical consultations about obesity. Normative concerns about responsibility, effort and so on are not automatically 'there' in any given encounter; they are produced by the actions of those present. In obesity-related consultations moral issues are made visible through the talk between practitioner and patient. The visibility of these moral issues is bound up with practices of talk – for example, practices of information delivery, connections between questions and answers and the opening of medical encounters. This underlines the importance of recognising the role of interactions during medical consultations about obesity. Existing sociological studies treat obesity as a social and moral 'problem'; it is also possible to see that, in the medical context, interactional problems exist in connection with the condition. For example, patients encounter the 'problem' of how to frame their weight-loss progress when talking to the doctor and my data show that they respond to this by displaying that they are taking an active role in their treatment and, in line with current policy commitments, that they are committed to change and take some responsibility for their cure. These kinds of interactional findings can add to sociological understanding of obesity.

These findings also have relevance to healthcare practice. Exisiting CA studies (*e.g.* Garafanga and Britten 2003) note that practitioners can pay attention to the ways different opening questions shape the opportunities patients have to talk about their concerns. This study adds an awareness that opening questions may also shape opportunities for moral work occurring in these responses. Displays of moral worth are a constant feature in these data and appear to be part of the agenda that patients pursue when answering opening questions. It may be useful for practitioners to be aware that some questions enable this agenda to be pursued more easily than others. For example, the generally worded 'how are you?' type questions observed here can initiate the medical business of the consultation whilst enabling patients to respond on their own terms. My data show that when given this opportunity, patients tend to produce responses that attend to the moral implications of having lost or gained weight and construct their agency to enhance or reduce their personal responsibility for progress. They orient to these relatively open, non-constraining questions as opportunities to display or defend their moral status. By contrast, more specific questions such as 'how is your weight?' would request that patients report success or failure immediately without an opportunity to introduce mitigating factors first. Another relevant issue is the medical requirement that obese patients take some responsibility for their condition and cure. By attending obesity clinics, the patients in these data acknowledge their condition as a medical problem. However, the analysis shows that whilst they take responsibility for successes, they avoid responsibility for lack of success. It is worth conducting further analysis to investigate whether this avoidance may create tensions in the encounter, in particular in discussions over treatment interventions. More generally, policy initiatives that advocate 'good' communication in medical obesity settings (such as the NICE guidance discussed in the introduction) need to recognise the complexity of the interactions that occur between practitioners and patients. The simultaneous institutional and moral agendas existing in obesity-related consultations require further attention in interactional analysis and medical practice.

Acknowledgements

I would like to thank all the participants who agreed to take part in this study. I am also very grateful to the two anonymous referees, the editors, plus Robert Dingwall and Ruth Parry for their comments on various drafts of this chapter.

References

Aphramor, L. (2005) Is a weight-centred health framework salutogenic? Some thoughts on unhinging certain dietary ideologies, *Social Theory and Health*, 3, 315–40.

Atkinson, M.J. and Heritage, J. (eds) (1984) *Structures of Social Action: Studies in Conversation Analysis*. Cambridge: Cambridge University Press.

Ball, K. and Crawford, D. (2005) Socio-economic status and weight change in adults: a review, *Social Science and Medicine*, 60, 1987–2010.

Batnitzky, A. (2008) Obesity and household roles: gender and social class in Morocco, *Sociology of Health and Illness*, 30, 3, 445–62.

Boardman, J.D., Saint Onge, J.M., Rogers, R.D. and Denney, J.T. (2005) Race differentials in obesity: the impact of place, *Journal of Health and Social Behaviour*, 46, 229–43.

Bolden, G. (2006) Little words that matter: Discourse markers 'so' and 'oh' and the doing of other-attentiveness in social interaction. *Journal of Communication*, 56, 661–88.

Bordo, S. (1993) *Unbearable Weight: Feminism, Western Culture and the Body*. Berkeley: University of California Press.

Byrne, P. and Long, E. (1976) *Doctors Talking to Patients: a Study of the Verbal Behaviour of General Practitioners Consulting in their Surgeries*. London: Her Majesty's Stationery Office.

Chang, V. and Christakis, N. (2002) Medical modelling of obesity: a transition from action to experience in a 20th century American medical textbook. *Sociology of Health and Illness*, 24, 2, 151–77.

Crossley, N. (2004) Fat is a Sociological Issue: Obesity rates in late modern, 'body conscious' societies, *Social Theory and Health*, 2, 222–53.

Department of Health (2004) *Summary of Intelligence on Obesity*. London: The Stationery Office.

Drew, P. (1998) Complaints about transgressions and misconduct, *Research on Language and Social Interaction*, 31, 3 and 4, 295–325.

Garafanga, J. and Britten, N. (2003) 'Fire away': the opening sequence in general practice consultations, *Family Practice*, 20, 242–7.

Gard, M. and Wright, J. (2005) *The Obesity Epidemic: Science, Morality and Ideology*. London: Routledge.

Garfinkel, H. (1967) *Studies in Ethnomethodology*. Englewood Cliffs, N.J.: Prentice Hall.

Gill, V.T. (1998) Doing attributions in medical interaction: patients' explanations for illness and doctors' responses, *Social Psychology Quarterly*, 61, 342–60.

ten Have, P. (1989) The consultation as a genre. In Torode, B. (ed.) *Text and Talk as Social Practice*. Dordrecht/Providence, R.I.: Foris Publications.

Heath, C. (1986) *Body Movement and Speech in Medical Interaction*. Cambridge: Cambridge University Press.

Heritage, J. (1984) A change of state token and aspects of its sequential placement. In Atkinson, J.M. and Heritage, J. (eds), *Structures of Social Action*. Cambridge: Cambridge University Press.

Heritage, J. (1985) Analyzing news interviews: aspects of the production of talk for an 'overhearing' audience. In van Dijk, T. (ed.) *Handbook of Discourse Analysis, Volume 3, Discourse and Dialogue*. London: Academic Press.

Heritage, J. and Robinson, J. (2006) The structure of patients' presenting concerns: physicians' opening questions, *Health Communication*, 19, 2, 89–102.

Jefferson, G. (1980) On 'trouble-premonitory' response to enquiry, *Sociological Enquiry*, 50 153–85.

Jutel, A. (2005) Weighing health: the moral burden of obesity, *Social Semiotics*, 15, 2, 113–25.

Loureiro, M.L. and Nagya, R.M. Jr (2006) Obesity, weight loss, and physicians' advice, *Social Science and Medicine*, 62, 10, 2458–68.

Maynard, D. (2004) *Bad News, Good News: Conversational Order in Everyday Talk and Clinical Settings*. Chicago: University of Chicago Press.

Monaghan, L. (2005) Discussion piece: a critical take on the obesity debate, *Social Theory and Health*, 3, 302–14.

National Audit Office (2001) *Tackling Obesity in England*. London: The Stationery Office.

NICE, (2006) *Clinical Guideline 43, Obesity: Guidance on the Prevention, Identification, Assessment and Management of Overweight and Obesity in Adults and Children*. London: National Institute for Health and Clinical Excellence.

Parsons, T. (1951) *The Social System*. London: Routledge and Kegan Paul.

Parsons, T. (1975) The Sick Role and the Role of the Physician reconsidered. *Millbank Memorial Fund Quarterly*, 53, 257–70.

Pilnick, A. and Coleman, T. (2003) 'I'll give up smoking when you get me better': Patients' resistance to attempts to problematise smoking in general practice (GP) consultations, *Social Science and Medicine*, 57, 135–45.

Rich, E. and Evans, J. (2005) Fat ethics – the obesity discourse and body politics, *Social Theory and Health*, 3, 341–58.

Robinson, J. (2006) Soliciting patients' presenting concerns. In Heritage, J. and Maynard, D. (eds) *Communication in Medical Care: Interaction between Primary Care Physicians and Patients*. Cambridge: Cambridge University Press.

Sacks, H. (1992) *Lectures on Conversation Volumes 1 and 2*. Edited by Jefferson, G. Oxford: Basil Blackwell.

Saguy, A.C. and Riley, K.W. (2005) Weighing both sides: morality, mortality, and framing contests over obesity, *Journal of Health Politics, Policy and Law*, 30, 5, 869–923.

Sarlio-Lahteenkorva, S. (1998) Relapse stories in obesity, *European Journal of Public Health*, 8, 203–9.

Silverman, D. (1987) *Communication and Medical Practice: Social Relations in the Clinic*. London: Sage.

Sobal, J. (1995) The medicalisation and demedicalisation of obesity. In Maurer, D. and Sobal, J. (eds) *Eating Agendas: Food and Nutrition as Social Poblems*. New York: Aldine de Gruyter.

Sobal, J. (2003) The size acceptance movement. In Loseke, D. and Best, R. (eds) *Social Problems: Constructionist Readings*. New York: Aldine de Gruyter.

Strong, P.M. (1979) *The Ceremonial Order of the Clinic: Parents, Doctors and Medical Bureaucracies*. London: Routledge and Kegan Paul.

Throsby, K. (2007) 'How could you let yourself get like that?': stories of the origins of obesity in accounts of weight loss surgery, *Social Science and Medicine*, 65, 1561–71.

Warin, M., Turner, K., Moore, V. and Davies, M. (2008) Bodies, mothers and identities: rethinking obesity and the BMI, *Sociology of Health and Illness*, 30, 1, 97–111.

Webb, H. (2009) *Doctor-patient interactions during medical consultations about obesity*. University of Nottingham: unpublished PhD thesis.

World Health Organisation (2000) *Technical Report Series 894: Obesity: Preventing and Managing the Global Epidemic*. Geneva: World Health Organisation.

6

Progressivity and participation: children's management of parental assistance in paediatric chronic pain encounters
Ignasi Clemente

Introduction

This chapter analyses an overlooked aspect of children's ability to exert agency and control in paediatric encounters: how children answer clinicians' questions by inviting specific types of parental support and excluding others. Specifically, I examine how older paediatric patients initiate four types of actions, including the solicitation of parental assistance, as a means to overcome difficulties when answering questions during pain symptom accounts. Although at first glance children's solicitation of parental assistance may suggest that children are not competent respondents, I show that in fact they actively organise their symptom presentations by (1) deciding when to preclude or request assistance; (2) orienting to the preference for progressivity (*i.e.* the interactional pressure to complete the activity of answering, and moving along with the progress of the medical interview); and (3) using specific interactional strategies that simultaneously invite parental participation and limit it. Unlike previous research that has focused on how parents take over the role of respondent, I show that children can involve parents while maintaining their role as primary informant of their own symptoms, as well as managing the rights and responsibilities associated with this role.

Providing clinicians with symptom information, a fundamental aspect of the 'patient' category (Byrne and Long 1976, Heritage and Robinson 2006, Mishler 1984, Roter and Hall 1992, Stivers 2007b) is not easy: it involves accounting for the visit, assessing what information is medically relevant (Heritage and Maynard 2006), transforming one's experience into medically discrete symptoms (Kleinman 1988, Mishler 1984), and ultimately, managing one's self publicly (Goffman 1959). For children with recurrent non-malignant pain, this task is even more complex for two reasons: the difficulty of articulating an account out of long and complex medical histories of multiple (often misdiagnosed and mistreated) pain symptoms and the time pressure to produce this account before the clinician shifts to the parent or the parent takes over (Carter 2002, Clemente in press, Clemente *et al.* 2008, Nutkiewicz 2008). Thus, although the strategies identified in the present chapter are neither restricted to children nor to chronic pain patients, children's competence as symptom informants is even more noteworthy in the particular context of paediatric chronic pain treatment. More generally, my research suggests that clinicians can promote children's participation, and can access their symptom accounts directly in three specific ways: by building upon children's strategies for acting as symptom informants; by addressing the challenges associated with increased patient involvement in medical interactions; and by turning difficulties into opportunities for children to practise 'being a patient'.

Background

Paediatric communication is a dance of three partners (Gabe *et al.* 2004, Pantell and Lewis 1993, Tates *et al.* 2002a), even while one is momentarily silent. Yet researchers frequently adopt a dyadic approach, analysing separately communication between the doctor and parent and that between the doctor and child (Tates and Meeuwesen 2001). This dyadic framework leaves unexamined a fundamental aspect of paediatric encounters: the communication between the child and the parent, whether it is parental control of child talk (Aronsson and Rundström 1988, Tates and Meeuwesen 2001) or the negotiation for response to clinicians' questions (Stivers 2001). My analysis of children's management of parental assistance while answering clinicians' questions provides further evidence that no aspect of paediatric communication can be analysed as an isolated dyadic exchange, whether between child and clinician, parent and clinician, or even child and parent.

Children's limited participation has been described across numerous paediatric settings and conditions, including emergency care (Wissow *et al.* 1998), acute and routine outpatient care (Aronsson 1991, Stivers 2001, Tates *et al.* 2002b, van Dulmen 1998), family therapy (Cederborg 1997, Tannen 1983) and chronic illness (Beresford and Sloper 2003, Pyörälä 2004, Silverman 1987, Young *et al.* 2003). Some authors have reported that parents take the interactional floor and reduce children to the status of passive bystanders or 'non-persons' (Aronsson and Cederborg 1996, Cederborg 1997, Pyörälä 2004, Strong 1979), but other authors have observed higher levels of children's participation (Silverman 1987, Stivers 2001). Socio-historical and cultural changes in perceptions of children's competencies and expectations (James and Prout 1997, Meeuwesen and Kaptein 1996, Pufall and Unsworth 2004) help to explain different degrees of participation. Despite these differences, two findings recur across studies: children participate less than parents, and infants and young children participate less than older ones.

In this chapter, I situate children's participation, turn-by-turn, in the specific circumstances within which children's actions occur. The investigation of children's social actions 'from within', reveals 'the procedures by which participants themselves organise and make sense of their activities in a given social context', as well as how 'those empirical circumstances', or 'arenas of action', can be both enabling and constraining in terms of children's capacity to display social competencies' (Hutchby and Moran-Ellis 1998: 10).

The child-initiated actions examined here manage multiple risks that threaten children's role as primary informants of their symptoms. When a child does not answer in a timely fashion or displays difficulties in answering, a parent often answers (Stivers 2001). Parents face a dilemma: to wait to see if the child, the selected respondent, eventually answers, or to answer the question themselves and thereby move the interaction along (Stivers and Robinson 2006). Stivers and Robinson illustrate how participants often resolve this dilemma by prioritising the progressivity of the interaction: the non-selected speaker overrides the primary rights of the selected respondent in order to complete the activity at hand (*i.e.* answer the question). However, as I show here, parental override is not always the default outcome; the children themselves may initiate courses of action to retain, affirm, and take upon themselves both the rights and the responsibilities of answering.

My study makes a number of contributions to the study of childhood and 'patienthood', at the intersection between the interaction order (Goffman 1983) and other social systems, particularly the family and medicine. First, I advance research that approaches childhood as socially constructed and not biologically determined (James and Prout 1997) by providing a data-driven analysis of children's own ways to exert some agency and participate in their own healthcare. Instead of focusing on how adults encourage or discourage children's participation (Clemente in press, Clemente *et al.* 2008, Stivers 2007a, Tates *et al.* 2002a), I focus on what children do to overcome these limitations.

Secondly, I advance research on patients' contributions to the medical interview. With the growing interest in patient-centredness (Mead and Bower 2000, 2002, Stewart *et al.* 1995), this analytic 'spotlight on the patient (Drew 2001) complements research that has focused primarily on clinicians' patient-centred behaviours.

Thirdly, my spotlight on how the child patient incorporates and limits parental participation in the pain symptom account manifests the theoretical and clinical complexities of Seiffge-Krenke's 'one body for two' problem (1997): the permeable boundaries between the roles of parent-caregiver and child patient with different sets of knowledge over one ill body. I show that the category of patient (with its associated practices, rights, and responsibilities) cannot be unequivocally equated with one person. Furthermore, these findings underscore the importance of providing children with opportunities to learn through participation (Rogoff *et al.* 2003) and to practise 'being a patient' (Stivers 2007a), so as to promote proactive patient behaviours that will facilitate their transition to adulthood and to taking responsibility of their own healthcare.

Finally, the detailed analysis of the socially organised give-and-take between parents and children when answering clinicians' questions underscores the need to take into account the semi-autonomous character of the 'interaction order' (Goffman 1983). Analyses of paediatric medical encounters should include the fundamental interactional practices with which social life is organised. In the present case, this involves examining how participants orient their actions vis-à-vis the dilemma of sequence progressivity, that is, of the 'nextness' and contiguity of an answer after a question (Schegloff 2007). Under these interactional pressures, I illustrate how child patients not only manage to accomplish the task of answering, but also to reaffirm their primary rights as pain symptom informants.

Data and methods

The analysis presented here is based on 69 video-recorded outpatient intake visits at three tertiary care clinics in the US, specialising in paediatric pain, gastroenterology, and neurology. The data also included child and parent self-reported measures and semi-structured parent and child interviews that were collected at the time of recruitment and six months later. Parents completed IRB-approved written informed consent forms and children provided written assent. Findings from the other study components have been reported previously (Bursch *et al.* 2006).

Patients (64% White), 46 girls and 23 boys, 10–18 age range, mean of 14.3 years and median of 14 years) had complex medical histories of multiple pain symptoms over extended periods of time (an average of 48 months prior to their tertiary care visit, with 41% of patients presenting multiple pain diagnoses). Patients had been through numerous appointments: they averaged 19 medical visits within the last 12 months, and 51 per cent of all patients had been seen previously by at least six different doctors. In the majority of intakes (88%), patients were accompanied solely by the mother.

Eight clinicians (75% White), five women and three men, 34–64 age range) participated in the study. All the clinicians were physicians, except for a clinical psychologist who worked in tandem with a physician in the pain clinic and was present in 23 intakes (45% of pain intakes).

The qualitative findings reported here are based on an examination of the opening and history-taking phases of the medical interaction (Byrne and Long 1976, Heritage and Robinson 2006), and were analysed using conversation analysis (Goodwin and Heritage 1990, Heritage 1997). Conversation analysis looks for practices in social interaction that evidence systematic communication design. To be identified as a practice, particular elements of communication conduct must be recurrent, specifically situated, and attract responses that distinguish them from related or similar practices. A central feature of this analytical approach is grounding the analysis of the practices used to perform a social action (*e.g.* using the words 'ear infection' to suggest a diagnosis during problem presentation) through the examination of responses of other participants (Stivers 2002). Conversation analysis has been widely used to study communication in medical settings (Heath 1986, Heritage and Maynard 2006, Maynard 2003, Peräkylä 1995, Silverman 1987, Stivers 2007b, West 1984).

Results

When a clinician asks a question of a child patient, a default organisation of participation is set in motion: the clinician and the patient engage in mutual gaze, and the other participants often remain silent and look either at the clinician who has asked the question or at the child who is expected to answer. In selecting the child patient as the respondent for a question, the clinician displays to both child and parent a preference to hear from the child. Embedded in the action of asking a question of the child are the expectations that the child knows the answer, is capable of answering, has rights to answer, is motivated to answer, and will do so immediately after the clinician's question.

In this section, I analyse children's departures from this default organisation of participation as children deal with difficulties in providing answers. In particular, I identify four actions children initiate in the service of answering: answer searches, solicitations of corroboration, solicitations of an answer, and completions. In an answer search, children display having problems, but do not seek (yet) parental assistance with the production of an answer. Instead, children use this strategy to buy some time while they attempt to answer on their own. Children also solicit parental assistance either to corroborate or give an answer. Finally, in the context of a parent's answering, children carry out a number of different actions, such as accepting, rejecting, modifying, or simply outlasting the talk that a parent has produced to assist with the task of answering. In doing so, the child displays his/her right and responsibility to bring to completion the task of answering which s/he was originally asked to do. The following child-initiated actions are three among other departures from the 'default' sequence of clinician asking child a question and child answering it: children also ask parents to expand their answers or claim insufficient knowledge with an 'I don't know'; clinicians either pursue an answer with the child or shift to the parent; or parents self-select to provide unsolicited answers.

Answer search
The expectation that an interlocutor will answer, and will do so contiguously and without delay, is a cardinal presumption of asking a question (Heritage 2007, Sacks 1987, Schegloff 2007, Stivers and Robinson 2006). In my data set, the paediatric clinicians' strong commitment to having the child present his/her symptoms at the beginning of the medical encounter is expressed by giving long periods of time to children to produce an answer (Clemente in press, Clemente *et al.* 2008). Additionally, parents, as in other paediatric encounters, allow

children to try to respond first (Stivers 2001). However, the time that the child has to produce an answer is not unlimited: all participants display an orientation to time limitations. Clinicians may intervene with a second pursuit question or a repeat to deal with assumed problems of understanding; and parents, guided by clinician's child-centred waiting, may turn to look at the child to check for the cause of the delay.

More importantly, the children themselves display an orientation to the accountability of their non-response: children produce non-lexical speech perturbations following clinicians' questions, such as 'um', or a 'thinking face' gesture (Goodwin 1983, Goodwin and Goodwin 1986), or both, in order to display that they are trying to answer but do not have an answer yet. Non-lexical perturbations are typical of word searches and other forms of self-initiated repair (Schegloff 1979, 1984, Schegloff *et al.* 1977), in which the speaker signals to the other participants that although s/he has interrupted his/her production of talk, s/he is *not* (1) giving up his/her role as speaker, (2) abandoning the production of talk, and (3) inviting other participants to help with the word search. During a 'thinking face' gesture, participants interpret gaze aversion (*i.e.* the speaker looks at a middle distance indeterminate point or modifies the positioning of his/her head to avoid mutual eye contact) as signalling that there is a reason to wait. With these vocal and non-verbal displays, the current speaker initiates a new and distinct activity – involving recollection, estimation, or search for a word in the service of resuming his/her talk.

In Extract 1, an 11-year-old boy embodies the activity of searching for an answer non-verbally with a 'thinking face' gesture. In her symptom elicitation, the clinician tries to determine whether the child suffers from two different types of headache, as diagnosed by previous clinicians, or only one type, as the child claims. In lines 1–3, the clinician announces that she is abandoning her questioning about the two headaches and begins to elicit the headache symptoms. (The patient in each case is identified as PAT, the parents as MOM/DAD, and the clinicians as DOC, or DR1/DR2 if two are present.)[1]

Extract 1 Case 57

1	DOC:		Okay. Just going back to: (.) h <u>YO</u>u:r headache, and we won't
2			<u>c</u>all it <u>t</u>wo different kinds of headaches at this moment.
3			(.) cuz: if it's the <u>s</u>ame to <u>y</u>ou:, it's the <u>s</u>ame.
4			(1.6)
5	DOC:		Pounding?,
6			(1.0)
7	PAT:	→	((thinking face)) Mm: no:: it just (.) ((looks at doctor))
8			stays there.

After the clinician's request to confirm if pounding is one of his headache symptoms, the boy immediately engages in a 'thinking face' gesture (line 7). The boy withdraws his gaze from the clinician, avoids looking at his parents, and poses his gaze on no particular object in front of him. In the absence of non-lexical perturbations, his non-verbal 'thinking face' gesture makes it clear that he is actively engaged in answering. The patient indicates that there is no need for his parents or the clinician to initiate additional courses of action to deal with the delay, such as additional questions, prompts or unsolicited answers.

In Extract 2, we find a combination of multiple non-lexical perturbations and a complex choreography of gestures and body movements that include eye rubbing and covering, head lowering and raising, middle distance stares, playing with one's hair, and symmetrical hand movements. In line 1, after an extended period of social talk and a discussion of the patient's medical records, the clinician starts asking a 12-year-old boy questions about how his pain symptoms began. The boy answers the clinician's questions (lines 5 and 9), but does not launch an elaborated pain account.

Extract 2 Case 61

```
 1  DOC:          And what (.) .hh tell me a little bit about the pa:in. You had
 2                whooping cough.
 3                (0.3)
 4  DOC:          When you were Ni:ne?=
 5  PAT:          =Yeah.
 6                (0.5)
 7  DOC:          And that's when everything started?,
 8                (0.3)
 9  PAT:          Yeah.
10  MOM:          Yea:h.
11                (0.6)
12  DOC:          So what do you < remember >.
13                (0.3)
14  DOC:          Back when you were nine.
15                (0.5)
16  PAT:    →     ((places hands under chin)) Uh ug uhm (1.0) .hhhhh hhhhh (1.2)
17          →     ((rubs eyes)) u:::h (5.0) ((pulls hair back and places hands on
18          →     the top of head)) I remember (0.4) uhm (0.7) uh .h (1.1)
19          →     like I started to feel this pai:n in my back. (0.3) and (1.1) I
20          →     don't really remember it that well,
21  DOC:          Uh huh.
22  PAT:          Til I went to hospital,
23                (0.4) .hh[hhh
24  DOC:                   [And then what d'you < remember >,
25                (1.0)
26  PAT:    →     ((lowers head and places hands on the back of head)) Wuhh (0.5)
27                uh (2.5) ((raises head and covers eyes with hands)) when I was-
28                ((thinking face while pulling back hair)) (0.8) uh, (0.3) hhh
29                hhhhh (2.4) hhhh .hhh it jus- ((lowers head with hands on the
30                back of head)) (3.7)
31  DOC:          Should we let mom fill this out?
32  PAT:          ((still looking down with hands on the back of head)) Yeah.
33  DOC:          Oka:y.
34                (·)
35  PAT:          Sorry.
36  DOC:          O::h N↑o::.
```

When the clinician asks broader questions (lines 12 and 14), which are more burdensome and less likely to be answered (Clemente in press, Clemente *et al.* 2008, Stivers 2007a), the patient displays serious problems in framing a response. The child's delays, pauses, and non-lexical perturbations are punctuated by his constant movement of hands and head. With this complex non-verbal and verbal word searching behaviour, the child displays both that he is having difficulties and that he is actively engaged in trying to answer. Despite his numerous difficulties, he does not seek assistance from his mother. He only gives up his role of primary speaker at the clinician's explicit request for permission to talk to his mother (line 31). As Extract 2 also shows, the child's ability to engage in answer searches is contingent on the clinician's and parent's withholding of their own talk. In this sense, children's answer searches must be considered as collaborations, in which the child searches for an answer and clinicians and parents permit him/her to do so.

Solicitation of corroboration

Independently of whether the child engages in his/her answer search, children may initiate other actions in the service of answering clinicians' questions: soliciting parental assistance to corroborate a tentative answer that the child is producing, or to give an answer. We will first examine children's corroboration requests.

In a solicitation of corroboration, a child puts forward a candidate answer to be confirmed or disconfirmed by the parent. Children rely on gaze to initiate corroborations and occasionally use a final turn 'right?', a full-fledged question, or try-marked intonation (Sacks and Schegloff 1979). There are two types of corroborations: partial and full. In a partial corroboration, the child solicits corroboration of a single component of his/her answer, often inviting a parent to confirm a reference to a person (Enfield and Stivers 2007, Sacks and Schegloff 1979), place (*i.e.* location of a symptom or place of a medical appointment), time (*i.e.* date of a medical appointment, and onset or duration of a symptom), or medication. In Extract 3, a clinician asks a 16-year-old girl about recent changes in her leg pains (lines 1–3). The girl produces a first component of her extended answer and then runs into difficulties.

Extract 3 Case 42

```
 1  DOC:          So: during the past six mo:nths, have they stayed the sa:::me,
 2                > have they been getting < be:tter, or do they just kinda go up
 3                and do:wn.
 4                (.)
 5  PAT:          I:sto:pped having them for a whi:le,
 6  DOC:          Mm hm.
 7                (0.3)
 8  PAT:    →     .hh A::nd n::o:w like ((thinking face gesture lasting one
 9          →     second)) ((patient looks at mom)) two: mo:nths a:go:?
10  MOM:          Mm hm,
11  PAT:          ((patient turns head to clinician)) I: (.) began having them
12                again.
```

In lines 8–9, the patient first looks away from the clinician into a 'thinking face' gesture, and then looks at her mother to solicit corroboration that 'two: mo:nths a:go:?' is the appropriate description of when her leg pains returned. With the try-marked final upward intonation of her tentative reference, the patient solicits corroboration for that temporal reference and not for the other components of her answer. After mom corroborates it, the patient returns her gaze to the clinician and completes her extended answer (lines 11–12).

An example of a full corroboration can be found in Extract 4 below. A 13-year-old girl is answering questions regarding the periodicity and duration of her abdominal pain episodes. In line 1, the clinician asks the girl if her abdominal pain also occurs on weekends. After some initial non-lexical perturbations, the girl gives an extended answer, explaining to the clinician that pain occurrence depends on whether she is going somewhere or staying at home (lines 3–6).

Extract 4 Case 26

```
 1  DOC:           Do you have it on wee:kends?
 2                 (0.5)
 3  PAT:           U::h (1.1) it- depends. Not at ho:me. (let's say) I'm going out
 4                 or something, (0.8) to like (.) I dunno like a play or something
 5         →       ((patient starts turning her head)) I usually get ((patient
 6         →       makes eye contact with mother)) that.
 7  MOM:           Mmhmm.
 8                 (2.6)
 9  DOC:           U:h hu:h.
10                 (4.0)
11  DOC:           Tch so > when you go to < a pla:y or you're leaving the hou:[se:,
12  PAT:                                                                        [Mm
13                 hm,
14                 (1.0)
15  DOC:           °You'll get (.) belly pain,°
```

As she approaches the last part of her turn, the girl, who had been facing the clinician, begins to turn her head to her right, where mom is sitting (lines 5–6). As the girl says 'that' she makes eye contact with mom, who has been looking at her throughout the entire answer. As soon as mom produces her minimal form of agreement (line 7), both mother and girl disengage from each other, abandon the brief period of mutual gaze, and return to look at the clinician in front of them. The clinician unequivocally selects the girl as the respondent for his next question (lines 11 and 15), and the patient continues in her role of primary informant (lines 12–13).

Solicitation of an answer
In a solicitation of an answer, the child invites a parent to assist collaboratively with the production of an answer. In contrast to the corroboration requests discussed above, here the child contributes less (*i.e.* the child does not produce a candidate answer to be corroborated) and requests more (*i.e.* the child invites the parent to produce an answer, but retains the right to accept or reject it). Soliciting an answer can be done non-verbally, primarily relying on gaze, or in a combination of gaze and talk. Once again, we find two types of solicitations of answers depending on whether children solicit parental assistance with only a component of an answer or a full answer. For instance, a clinician asks a 14-year-old girl with cerebral palsy about the origin of her chronic back pain (data not reproduced here). The girl engages in a partial solicitation in the midst of her telling and asks for her mother's assistance only in naming the specialty of one of several doctors to whom she refers in her elaborated answer. Together with partial corroborations, partial answer solicitations are examples of solicitations within the boundaries of a turn of talk: the speaker grants another participant conditional entry into his/her own uncompleted turn (Goodwin 1986, Lerner 1996).

Full answer solicitations, on the other hand, take place at turn boundaries (*i.e.* before an answer is produced). In Extract 5, a full solicitation is done exclusively non-verbally, as in most solicitations in the present study. An 11-year-old girl with pain in multiple sites of her body comes with her grandparents to the clinic. In line 1, the clinician formulates a question about the approximate time for when her pain was worst. The clinician pursues an answer from the girl after her silences and incomplete answers (lines 2–5).

Extract 5 Case 38

```
 1  DOC:            .hh when was it (0.4) the worst.
 2                  (2.6)
 3  PAT:            Probably (in the middle).
 4                  (0.7)
 5  PAT:            Like, (0.4)
 6  DOC:            About when.
 7                  (0.3)
 8  PAT:            Uh like:, (0.3)
 9  DOC:            What month. < Do you [remember about?,
10  PAT:     →                          [((turns head from clinician to grandma))
11  GMA:            Befo:re Christmas I think. < Just before Christmas.
```

In line 10, as the clinician attaches a second, clarifying question to her initial question 'What month', the girl abandons mutual eye contact with the clinician, and turns to look at her grandmother (GMA). Without much delay, her grandmother answers the question looking at the girl and not at the clinician (line 11).

Answer completion
Children carry out different actions to limit parental participation during and after soliciting assistance, including accepting, rejecting, clarifying, modifying what a parent has said, and continuing with his/her own talk before the solicitation. With these actions, a child accomplishes answer completion and exercises his/her rights as primary respondent in charge of answering. Some of these children's actions are illustrated in the continuation of the 11-year-old girl's solicitation analysed in the previous extract. In Extract 6 below, we see that as soon as her grandmother provides the answer 'Befo:re Christmas I think', the girl abandons mutual eye contact with her grandmother, stares at a middle distance indeterminate point in a 'thinking face' gesture while she says 'A little-' (line 12).

Extract 6 Case 38

```
11  GMA:       Befo:re Christmas I think. < [Just before        Chris[tmas.
12  PAT:                                    [A little- (.)            [just before=
13  PAT:                                    [((thinking face))        [((looks at
14             [clinician))
15  PAT:       =[Christmas.
16  DOC:  Like- (.) after Thanksgiving.
```

The overlap between the girl's 'A little-' and her grandmother's talk occurs at turn completion (Jefferson 1984), when her grandmother adds a second and more precise temporal reference. Simultaneously, the girl's 'thinking face' gesture and initial 'A little-' indicate that she is not about to relay merely her grandmother's first answer, but that she is assessing its appropriateness. Indeed, 'A little-' evidences that the girl is attempting to modify her grandmother's first answer or produce a different one. In this context of competitive overlap characterised by hitches and perturbations (Schegloff 2000), the girl abandons her 'A little-' and moves to show the appropriateness of her grandmother's second answer with her full repeat (lines 12 and 15). With her full repeat, the girl manages to outlast her grandmother's talk, give her answer in the clear, and be the last person talking (Jefferson 2004). Despite the fact that the clinician has already overheard it, the girl's delivery of her answer to the clinician is a way to display her approval of her grandmother's second answer. Altogether, the girl's actions demonstrate that she is acting as primary respondent with full participant roles and not as animator or 'sounding box' of her grandmother's words (Goffman 1981, Goodwin and Goodwin 2004, Levinson 1987), as well as with rights to accept or reject answers of secondary informants, claim ownership of the sequence, and limit parental assistance.

A fundamental aspect of how children invite and limit parental assistance is found in the organisation of a solicitation. In most solicitations, the child abandons the default position of sitting facing and looking at the clinician, and adopts a transient position in which his/ her body continues to face the clinician, but the head is turned toward the parent. This 'torqued' body positioning (Schegloff 1998) frames the engagement between child and parent as temporary, since the child does not modify his/her sitting so as to face a parent in a more permanent positioning. This limited nature of solicitations is observable in Extracts 3, 4 and 6 above, in which the child brings her gaze back to the clinician as soon as the accompanying adult complies with the child's request.

In addition to the ecologically embodied organisation of solicitations, children can also resort to answer completions to ensure that parents do what they have been asked, no less and no more. A child may, after producing an initial answer solicitation (*e.g.* turning to look at a parent after the child is asked to give the date of a medical appointment), pursue it with a corroboration (*e.g.* proposing 'October?' as a candidate answer to be confirmed) after a parent fails to assist with the initial solicitation.

More often, children's answer completions are structured to ensure that a parent does not do more than s/he has been asked. Children's solicitations carry important risks for their participation as primary respondents. On the one hand, children initiate a solicitation because they are having difficulty providing an answer; the child risks being replaced as primary informant if s/he does not manage to produce an answer in a timely fashion. On the other hand, by inviting a parent to talk, the child's status as primary informant is also at risk: a parent may use the invitation to disagree with the child or to do more than the solicitation specifically requested.

The clinician's selection of the child as respondent to a subsequent question is crucial in deciding who will talk after answering is completed. A key function of children's completions is to influence the clinician's selection by reinforcing that the child is the original respondent to the question, and that the child is ready and willing to continue in the role of primary respondent. In Extract 7, a clinician asks a 12-year-old boy how much school he has missed because of his stomach aches (line 1). The child initiates first an answer search and then solicits the answer from his mother (line 4).

Extract 7 Case 25

```
 1  DR2:       So how much school are you missing,
 2             (0.7)
 3  PAT:       U:m,
 4  PAT:       ((patient looks at mom))
 5             (4.0)
 6  MOM:       He's missed some half days. <he's missed u-like one whole day
 7             since he'd been on the medication.
 8  DR2:       Mm hm.
 9  MOM:       But I'm pushing him to go to school.
10             (0.5)
```

11	DR2:	Mn hm,
12	MOM:	Cuz we took- We were off <u>two</u>: months (0.7) for the do:ctors.
13	DR2:	Mm [h:m.
14	MOM:	[Wh::en uh we saw doctor Bayer the first time. She pulled'im
15		out and the doctors before they had him off a week at a time.
16	DR2:	Mm h::m,
17	MOM:	.hhh hhh So we were <u>ou</u>:t for over two months. hh
18		(3.1)
19	DR2:	°Okay°=
20	PAT:	→ =Now I'm back on the- back at school and stuff.
21	DR2:	Good.
22		(0.5)
23	DR 1:	Tch so u:m (.) I was <u>n</u>oticing here that you- (.) wer- have been
24		having problems vomiti:ng, did <u>t</u>hat start befo:re the ab<u>do</u>minal
25		pain or about the same time.

Mom takes this opportunity to give an extended answer, which she delivers looking at the clinicians and not at her son. After some back and forth, mom concludes her answer with a summary statement prefaced with 'So' (line 17), which is acknowledged as moving to closure by the clinician's sequence shift-implicative 'Okay' (Beach 1993). After this exchange, the child produces a second move to close, returning to his present situation vis-à-vis school (line 20), and the sequence is closed by the clinician's assessment (line 21). By returning to his current situation the child displays that the task of answering is now complete and that the clinician is to make the next move (Robinson and Heritage 2005). The child not only indicates his willingness to relinquish the interactional floor; more importantly, the child indicates that he is the one with the rights to relinquish the floor. He succeeds in reminding the clinicians that he is ready to continue as the primary informant, and one of the clinicians selects him as respondent in the next question (line 23).

Discussion

I have identified four strategies with which older children (10–18 years) overcome difficulties in answering clinicians' questions and reaffirm their rights as clinician-selected respondents. In an answer search, a child displays that s/he is having problems answering but forestalls parental assistance at this point. In a solicitation of corroboration, the child invites a parent to confirm or reject the answer that the child is producing. In a solicitation of an answer, the child invites the parent to assist with the collaborative production of an answer. In an answer completion, the child re-positions him/herself vis-à-vis what the parent has contributed to the task of answering, and vis-à-vis his/her role of initial respondent selected to answer. Although these actions often co-occur, they are nevertheless independent phenomena.

These practices are evidence of children's ability to manage the expectations and responsibilities associated with the role of a primary symptom informant. These actions, distinct from answering but done in the service of answering, illustrate how children locally organise the symptom presentation in two ways. First, children initiate new courses of action, whether on their own or by enlisting others' support, to accomplish responses to questions. Secondly, they use these actions to manage risks to their primary respondent status. If a child does not answer in a timely fashion or displays difficulties in answering, the clinician may switch to a parent or the parent may start talking to help the child. On the other hand, if the child invites the parent to talk, the parent may go on to disagree or to contribute more than s/he has been asked. By initiating these four strategies, children minimise the risks of losing their role as respondent while actively contributing to the progressivity of the clinical information gathering.

To a large degree, these child-initiated strategies are successful because they invite specific types of parental support and exclude other forms of parental participation. When a child initiates an answer search, s/he is prospectively limiting parental participation by withholding and discouraging it. Answer solicitations limit parental participation by framing parental assistance as temporally limited: the child and parent adopt unstable positions of body torque to look at each other while continuing to orient their lower bodies towards the clinician. This transient position is abandoned as soon as the parent assists the child.

Finally, answer completions limit parental participation both retrospectively and prospectively: they frame what the parent has said as responsive to an action embedded within the child's answer, act as a reminder that the child is the original primary informant, and display the child's resumption of his/her role as primary informant (and thus, selectable to answer a clinician's next question). In doing so, children establish themselves in the position of primary informants with full rights to talk and organise talk locally, and establish parents in the position of secondary informants with *limited* rights to talk, as long as the clinician retains the child as primary respondent. A child exercises his/her primary respondent rights to ask for help if deemed necessary; to frame parental talk not as an alternative answer, but as ancillary talk provided to assist him/her; and to sanction the appropriateness of such assistance, by accepting, rejecting, or modifying it.

Conclusion

Relying on a triadic child-parent-doctor communication perspective (Stivers 2001, Tates and Meeuwesen 2001), I have identified four practices, including children's solicitation of parental assistance, with which children locally organise the presentation of pain symptoms and manage the expectations and responsibilities associated with this fundamental aspect of 'patient role'. My description of these previously unexamined child-initiated actions sheds light on children's competence as symptom informants, within the empirical circumstances that both enable and constrain children's ability to display their social competences (Hutchby and Moran-Ellis 1998). Indeed, my analysis of children's efforts to overcome these constraints reveals that children with long and complex histories of pain symptoms not only accomplish the task of answering, but also manage risks that threaten their roles as primary informants: they discourage adults from jumping in to help them and ensure that parents do not do more than what they have been asked to do. I argue that children succeed in affirming their rights as clinician-selected primary informants because these child-initiated strategies invite specific types of parental support and exclude other forms of parental participation. At the same time, this dynamic give-and-take between parents and children shows how the 'patient' role cannot always be equated with one person: although the child is the patient, parents carry out role-associated activities (Tates *et al.* 2002a).

Children, like their parents, experience difficulties in answering (Stivers 2007a) and organise their actions with an orientation to the 'interaction order' (Goffman 1983) that prioritises completing the activity at hand and moving along with the progress of the medical interview (Stivers 2001, Stivers and Robinson 2006). However, instead of being occasions for parents to become primary informants, children's difficulties can open up opportunities for informal learning through participation (Rogoff *et al.* 2003), so children can practise 'being a patient' (Stivers 2007a) with clinicians and parents as collaborators. Since patients' proactive roles in their medical visits are fundamental to effective healthcare (Frosch and Kaplan 1999, Greenfield *et al.* 1988, Kaplan *et al.* 1989), future studies should continue to identify strategies that promote children's participation in clinical encounters across different types of care and conditions: including patients' own strategies, as well as adults' patient-centred and child-centred behaviours. Once identified, specific strategies to promote children's participation can be tested for effectiveness at the clinical level and disseminated via professional and patient education (*e.g.* brochures for chronically ill children describing methods of effective communication with clinicians). Furthermore, given that children's ability to accomplish the task of answering is contingent on clinicians' and parents' collaboration, future studies should also examine the relationship between clinicians' degree of child-centredness, parents' degree of support, children's deployment of proactive behaviours, and children's developmental trajectories. Studies should investigate, for instance, whether younger children solicit parental assistance more often than older ones, or whether children's solicitations are more related to clinicians' and parents' behaviours than to child age. At a health policy level, future studies should continue to examine the practical and ethical dilemmas of involving chronically ill children in the management of their own health (Bluebond-Langner *et al.* 2005), balancing the emphasis on promoting children's participation with an understanding of the responsibilities that increased participation places on these children as patients.

Acknowledgements

Research for this chapter was supported by the National Institute of Mental Health: Grant No. NIMH/R01 MH63 779, P.I.: M. Jacob. I would like to express my gratitude to all the members of the UCLA Center for the Study and Treatment of Pain. I am particularly indebted to John Heritage for his generous contributions, both intellectual and practical, at every stage of this chapter. I also wish to thank Marcia Meldrum and Marian Katz for their helpful editing advice, and Lonnie Zeltzer for her mentorship and unremitting support. I am also grateful to Andrea Maestrejuan for her careful reading and Iris Halldorsdottir for her exquisite transcription. In the final stages of the writing of this chapter, my thinking about children's participation in healthcare encounters has been influenced by my work, generously supported by the Division of Occupational Science and Occupational Therapy at the University of Southern California, in the project *Boundary Crossings: Re-Situating Cultural Competence* (NCMRR, NICHD); 2-R01HD38878-06; P.I.: M. Lawlor).

Note

1   For transcription conventions see Jefferson 1974.

References

Aronsson, K. (1991) Facework and control in multi-party talk: a paediatric case study. In Marková, I. and Foppa, K. (eds) *Asymmetries in Dialogue*. Hemel Hempstead, UK and Savage, MD, USA: Harvester Wheatsheaf Barnes and Noble Books.

Aronsson, K. and Cederborg, A.C. (1996) Coming of age in family therapy talk: perspective setting in multiparty problem formulations, *Discourse Processes*, 21, 2, 191–212.

Aronsson, K. and Rundström, B. (1988) Child discourse and parental control in pediatric consultations, *Text*, 3, 159–89.

Beach, W.A. (1993) Transitional regularities for casual 'okay' usages, *Journal of Pragmatics*, 19, 325–52.

Beresford, B.A. and Sloper, P. (2003) Chronically ill adolescents' experiences of communicating with doctors: a qualitative study, *Journal of Adolescent Health*, 33, 3, 172.

Bluebond-Langner, M., DeCicco, A. and Belasco, J. (2005) Involving children with life-shortening illnesses in decisions about participation in clinical research: a proposal for shuttle diplomacy and negotiation. In Kodish, E. (ed.) *Ethics and Research with Children. A Case-Based Approach*. Oxford and New York: Oxford University Press.

Bursch, B., Tsao, J.C.I., Meldrum, M. and Zeltzer, L.K. (2006) Preliminary validation of a self-efficacy scale for child functioning despite chronic pain (child and parent versions), *Pain*, 125, 1–2, 35–42.

Byrne, P. and Long, B. (1976) *Doctors Talking to Patients. A Study of the Verbal Behaviours of Doctors in the Consultation*. Exeter: Royal College of General Practitioners.

Carter, B. (2002) Chronic pain in childhood and the medical encounter: professional ventriloquism and hidden voices, *Qualitative Health Research*, 12, 1, 28–41.

Cederborg, A.C. (1997) Young children's participation in family therapy talk, *American Journal of Family Therapy*, 25, 1, 28–38.

Clemente, I. (in press) Preserving the child as a respondent: dilemmas of patient-centered questioning in a pediatric pain tertiary care clinic, *Communication and Medicine*.

Clemente, I., Lee, S.H. and Heritage, J. (2008) Children in chronic pain: promoting pediatric patients' symptom accounts in tertiary care, *Social Science and Medicine*, 66, 6, 1418–28.

Drew, P. (2001) Spotlight on the patient, *Text*, 21, 1/2, 261–68.

Enfield, N.J. and Stivers, T. (2007) *Person Reference in Interaction*. Cambridge: Cambridge University Press.

Frosch, D.L. and Kaplan, R.M. (1999) Shared decision making in clinical medicine: past research and future directions, *American Journal of Preventive Medicine*, 27, 11, 1139–45.

Gabe, J., Olumide, G. and Bury, M. (2004) 'It takes three to tango': a framework for understanding patient partnership in paediatric clinics, *Social Science and Medicine*, 59, 5, 1071.

Goffman, E. (1959) *The Presentation of Self in Everyday Life*. New York: Doubleday.

Goffman, E. (1981) *Forms of Talk*. Philadelphia: University of Philadelphia Press.

Goffman, E. (1983) The interaction order: American Sociological Association, 1982 Presidential Address, *American Sociological Review*, 48, 1, 1–17.

Goodwin, C. (1986) Gestures as a resource for the organization of mutual orientation, *Semiotica*, 62, 1/2, 29–50.

Goodwin, C. and Goodwin, M.H. (2004) Participation. In Duranti, A. (ed.) *A Companion to Linguistic Anthropology*. Oxford: Basil Blackwell.

Goodwin, C. and Heritage, J. (1990) Conversation analysis, *Annual Review of Anthropology*, 19, 283–307.

Goodwin, M.H. (1983) Searching for a word as an interactive activity. In Deely, J.N. and Lenhard, M.D. (eds) *Semiotics*. New York and London: Plenum Press.

Goodwin, M.H. and Goodwin, C. (1986) Gesture and coparticipation in the activity of searching for a word, *Semiotica*, 62, 1/2, 51–75.

Greenfield, S., Kaplan, S.H., Ware, J.E., Yano, E.M. and Frank, H.J.L. (1988) Patients' participation in medical care: effects on blood sugar control and quality of life in diabetes, *Journal of General Internal Medicine*, 3, 448–57.

Heath, C. (1986) *Body Movement and Speech in Medical Interaction*. Cambridge: Cambridge University Press.

Heritage, J. (1997) Conversation analysis and institutional talk: analyzing data. In Silverman, D. (ed.) *Qualitative Analysis: Issues of Theory and Method*. London: Sage.

Heritage, J. (2007) *Constructing and navigating epistemic landscapes*, Paper presented at the 102nd Annual Meeting of the American Sociological Association, New York City.

Heritage, J. and Maynard, D.W. (eds) (2006) *Communication in Medical Care. Interaction between Primary Care Physicians and Patients.* Cambridge University Press: Cambridge.

Heritage, J. and Robinson, J.D. (2006) The structure of patients' presenting concerns: physicians' opening questions, *Health Communication,* 19, 2, 89–102.

Hutchby, I. and Moran-Ellis, J. (1998) Situating children's social competence. In Hutchby, I. and Moran-Ellis, J. (eds) *Children and Social Competence: Arenas of Action.* London and Washington, D.C.: Falmer Press.

James, A. and Prout, A. (eds) (1997) *Constructing and Reconstructing Childhood: Contemporary Issues in the Sociological Study of Childhood.* Falmer Press: London; Washington, D.C.

Jefferson, G. (1974) Error correction as an interactional resource, *Language in Society,* 2, 181–99.

Jefferson, G. (1984) Notes on Some Orderliness of Overlap Onset. In D'Urso, V. and Leonardi, P. (eds) *Discourse Analysis and Natural Rhetorics.* Padova, Italy: CLEUP Editore.

Jefferson, G. (2004) A sketch of some orderly aspects of overlap in natural conversation. In Lerner, G.H. (ed.) *Conversation Analysis: Studies from the First Generation.* Amsterdam and Philadelphia: John Benjamins.

Kaplan, S.H., Greenfield, S. and Ware, J.E. (1989) Assessing the effects of physician-patient interactions on the outcomes of chronic disease, *Medical Care,* 27, S110–27.

Kleinman, A. (1988) *The Illness Narratives: Suffering, Healing, and the Human Condition.* New York: Basic Books.

Lerner, G.H. (1996) On the 'semi-permeable' character of grammatical units in conversation: conditional entry into the turns pace of another speaker. In Ochs, E., Schegloff, E.A. and Thompson, S.A. (eds) *Interaction and Grammar.* Cambridge: Cambridge University Press.

Levinson, S.C. (1987) Putting linguistics on a proper footing: explorations in Goffman's concept of participation. In Drew, P. and Wootton, A. (eds) *Erving Goffman: Explorations in the Interaction Order.* Cambridge: Polity Press.

Maynard, D.W. (2003) Bad *News, Good News: Conversational Order in Everyday Talk and Clinical Settings.* Chicago and London: The University of Chicago Press.

Mead, N. and Bower, P. (2000) Patient-centredness: a conceptual framework and review of the empirical literature, *Social Science and Medicine,* 51, 7, 1087–110.

Mead, N. and Bower, P. (2002) Patient-centred consultations and outcomes in primary care: a review of the literature, *Patient Education and Counseling,* 48, 1, 51–61.

Meeuwesen, L. and Kaptein, M. (1996) Changing interactions in doctor-parent-child communication, *Psychology and Health,* 11, 6, 787–95.

Mishler, E. (1984) *The Discourse of Medicine: Dialectics of Medical Interviews.* Norwood, N.J.: Ablex Pub. Corp.

Nutkiewicz, M. (2008) Diagnosis versus dialogue: oral testimony and the study of pediatric pain, *Oral History Review,* 35, 1, 11–21.

Pantell, R.H. and Lewis, C.C. (1993) Talking with children: how to improve the process and outcome of medical care, *Medical Encounter,* 10, 3–7.

Peräkylä, A. (1995) *AIDS Counselling: Institutional Interaction and Clinical Practice.* Cambridge: Cambridge University Press.

Pufall, P.B. and Unsworth, R.P. (2004) Introduction. In Pufall, P.B. and Unsworth, R.P. (eds) *Rethinking Childhood.* New Brunswick, NJ: Rutgers University Press.

Pyörälä, E. (2004) The participation roles of children and adolescents in the dietary counseling of diabetics, *Patient Education and Counseling,* 55, 3, 385–95.

Robinson, J.D. and Heritage, J. (2005) The structure of patients' presenting concerns: the completion relevance of current symptoms, *Social Science and Medicine,* 61, 2, 481–93.

Rogoff, B., Paradise, R., Arauz, R.M., Correa-Chávez, M. and Angelillo, C. (2003) Firsthand learning through intent participation, *Annual Review of Psychology,* 54, 175–203.

Roter, D.L. and Hall, J.A. (1992) *Doctors Talking with Patients/Patients Talking with Doctors: Improving Communication in Medical Visits.* Westport, CT, US: Auburn House/Greenwood Publishing Group, Inc.

Sacks, H. (1987) On the preference for agreement and contiguity in sequences in conversation. In Button, G. and Lee, J.R.E. (eds) *Talk and Social Organization.* Clevedon: Multilingual Matters.

Sacks, H. and Schegloff, E.A. (1979) Two preferences in the organization of reference to persons and their interaction. In Psathas, G. (ed.) *Everyday Language: Studies in Ethnomethodology*. New York: Irvington Publishers.

Schegloff, E.A. (1979) The relevance of repair to syntax-for-conversation. In Givón, T. (ed.) *Syntax and Semantics*. New York: Academic Press.

Schegloff, E.A. (1984) On some gestures' relation to talk. In Atkinson, J.M. and Heritage, J. (eds) *Structures of Social Action*. Cambridge: Cambridge University Press.

Schegloff, E.A. (1998) Body torque, *Social Research*, 65, 3, 535–96.

Schegloff, E.A. (2000) Overlapping talk and the organization of turn-taking for conversation, *Language in Society*, 29, 1, 1–63.

Schegloff, E.A. (2007) *Sequence Organization in Interaction: a Primer in Conversation Analysis I*. Cambridge: Cambridge University Press.

Schegloff, E.A., Jefferson, G. and Sacks, H. (1977) The preference for self-correction in the organization of repair in conversation, *Language*, 55, 2, 361–382.

Seiffge-Krenke, I. (1997) 'One body for two': the problem of boundaries between chronically ill adolescents and their mothers, *Psychoanalytic Study of the Child*, 52, 340–55.

Silverman, D. (1987) *Communication and Medical Practice: Social Relations in the Clinic*. London: Sage.

Stewart, M., Brown, J., Weston, W., Donner, A., McWhinney, I., McWilliam, C. and Freeman, T. (1995) *Patient-centred Medicine: Transforming the Clinical Method*. London: Sage.

Stivers, T. (2001) Negotiating who presents the problem: next speaker selection in pediatric encounters, *Journal of Communication*, 51, 2, 1–31.

Stivers, T. (2002) Presenting the problem in pediatric encounters: 'symptoms only' versus 'candidate diagnosis' presentations, *Health Communication*, 14, 3, 299–338.

Stivers, T. (2007a) Practicing Patienthood: when doctors turn to children in primary care encounters, Unpublished Mimeograph. Max Planck Institute for Psycholinguistics: Nijmegen, the Netherlands.

Stivers, T. (2007b) *Prescribing Under Pressure: Parent-Physician Conversations and Antibiotics*. Oxford and New York: Oxford University Press.

Stivers, T. and Robinson, J.D. (2006) A preference for progressivity in interaction, *Language in Society*, 35, 3, 367–92.

Strong, P.M. (1979) *The Ceremonial Order of the Clinic: Parents, Doctors, and Medical Bureaucracies*. London and Boston: Routledge and Kegan Paul.

Tannen, D. (1983) Doctor/mother/child communication: linguistic analysis of pediatric interaction. In Fisher, S. and Todd, A.D. (eds) *The Social Organization of Doctor-patient Communication*. Washington, D.C.: The Center for Applied Linguistics.

Tates, K., Elbers, E., Meeuwesen, L. and Bensing, J. (2002a) Doctor-parent-child relationships: a 'pas de trois', *Patient Education and Counseling*, 48, 1, 5–14.

Tates, K. and Meeuwesen, L. (2001) Doctor-parent-child communication: A (re)view of the literature, *Social Science and Medicine*, 52, 6, 839–51.

Tates, K., Meeuwesen, L., Elbers, E. and Bensing, J. (2002b) 'I've come for his throat': roles and identities in doctor-parent-child communication, *Child Care Health and Development*, 28, 1, 109–16.

van Dulmen, A.M. (1998) Children's contributions to pediatric outpatient encounters, *Pediatrics*, 102, 3, 563–68.

West, C. (1984) *Routine Complications: Troubles with Talk between Doctors and Patients*. Bloomington, IN: Indiana University Press.

Wissow, L.S., Roter, D., Bauman, L.J., Crain, E., Kercsmar, C., Weiss, K., Mitchell, H. and Mohr, B. (1998) Patient-provider communication during the emergency department care of children with asthma, *Medical Care*, 36, 10, 1439–50.

Young, B., Dixon-Woods, M., Windridge, K.C. and Heney, D. (2003) Managing communication with young people who have a potentially life threatening chronic illness: qualitative study of patients and parents, *British Medical Journal*, 326, 7384, 305–10.

7

Embedding instruction in practice: contingency and collaboration during surgical training

Marcus Sanchez Svensson, Paul Luff and Christian Heath

Introduction

There has been a longstanding interest in the sociology of health and illness concerning medical education and training. Some of the most influential ethnographic studies in the field, including for example Becker *et al.* (1961), Freidson (1970) and Bosk (1979), were concerned with the ways in which expertise, practice and a clinical mentality were established both through formal training and working with others. It is recognised that social interaction, interaction with patients, peers, other colleagues and staff, is fundamental to learning how to accomplish particular activities in the highly contingent circumstances of healthcare delivery. These concerns resonate with a more recent body of research, broadly characterised as the 'practice turn', found in particular within cognitive science and social anthropology, exemplified by the influential contribution of Lave and Wenger (1991), within fields associated with learning and education (*e.g.* Ball and Lampert 1999, Cobb *et al.* 2001) and in quite a different way within studies of healthcare (*e.g.* Timmermans and Angell 2001, Goodwin *et al.* 2005, Prentice 2007). Once again these contributions stress the importance of interpersonal communication and social interaction as the principal vehicle in and through which people are encompassed within, and sustain, 'communities of practice'; that is, the ways of accomplishing highly specialised activities in concert with others in ordinary everyday situations. Despite the substantial contribution of these and related studies to our understanding of 'situated learning', less attention has been paid to the forms of interaction that occasion instruction and learning and enable students, trainees and fellow clinicians to observe, attempt, and become familiar with technical procedures and practices. In this chapter we seek to explore these issues with regard to the surgical operation. The complexity of many surgical procedures, the contingencies of particular cases, the potential risk to patients, and the necessity to perform the task in close collaboration with others, poses particular challenges to both teaching and learning.

A number of recent studies have begun to explore how specialised and professional ways of seeing are interactionally configured and disseminated within working environments, including the operating theatre and other medical settings (see for example Goodwin 1994, Hindmarsh and Pilnick 2002, Pomerantz 2003, Mondada 2006, Koschmann *et al.* 2007, Hindmarsh *et al.* forthcoming). We draw on these and related studies to consider the collaborative accomplishment of instruction and the ways in which momentary insights enable trainee surgeons to witness, follow and comprehend the deployment of technical procedures with regard to the contingencies of specific cases. In particular whilst recent studies have primarily focused on how the body features in practices of displaying, assessing and understanding, certain phenomena (*cf.* Koschmann *et al.* 2007, Hindmarsh *et al.* forthcoming), we explore how momentary revelations of the 'surgical field' provide the resources to enable students and trainees to follow, comprehend and, on occasions, contribute to, the concerted production of a complex medical procedure. In this regard, we also briefly consider how instruction and training during surgery rely upon the ability of other professionals, including nursing staff and anaesthetists, to anticipate, prepare for, and remain sensitive to these moments or episodes of teaching and to enable the surgeon to interweave the demands of education with the practicalities of the task on hand.

Methods and data collection

Our data consist of video recordings of two 'naturally occurring' surgical operations gathered in a leading ear, nose and throat hospital in central London. These recordings are part of a larger study of work, interaction and collaboration in operating theatres (Sanchez Svensson 2005) – a study that involved about 30 days of fieldwork including field observations, informal interviews and a corpus of 40 hours of video recordings.

These materials were collected following ethical clearance from the Health Trust and the hospital involved in the study, and adhered to guidelines provided by the UK's Economic and Social Research Council (ESRC). We also discussed the study and data collection with the clinical staff and patients involved. The agreement was that the materials could be used as long as patients could not be identified from any images or texts that were published by the researchers.

The video recordings, augmented by conventional fieldwork, have enabled us to consider how tasks and activities in such complex work settings are accomplished through the interplay of embodied conduct, talk and the use of various tools and technologies, to analyse the interactional and collaborative production of surgical operations and training. One particular advantage of video was that it also enabled us to hold a series of joint 'data analysis sessions' with clinicians, where we discussed extracts from the recordings. These joint sessions proved invaluable to help us to become familiar with the more technical aspects of particular procedures and their performance as well as the background to certain activities and interventions.

We draw on ethnomethodology and conversation analysis and the burgeoning corpus of research concerned with the interplay of talk, visual conduct and the use of tools and technologies that has come to be known as 'workplace studies' (see for example Engestrom and Middleton 1998, Luff *et al.* 2000, Heath and Luff 2000). Our interest is in the ways in which 'occasioned viewings' are critical to enable trainees to see and inspect certain phenomena at a particular moment, but also for their ability to follow and make sense of the progressive accomplishment of the operation and the deployment of a procedure. This poses certain challenges to an analytic commitment primarily concerned with the interactional production of short, circumscribed sequences of action. In this regard, whilst we focus in this chapter on the collaborative accomplishment of moments of insight and instruction, we also briefly consider subsequent episodes of talk and interaction, and the ways in which the occasioned interventions provide the resources for the trainees to comprehend the progressive aspects of the operation.

The operating theatre as an ecology for instruction

The operating theatre is a work setting that has developed both as a platform for a technical activity and as an arena for learning and development. The contemporary versions of apprenticeship in the operating theatre involve a structured training programme during which the trainees work hard to obtain sufficient experience from practice and pass the necessary examinations. In the United Kingdom, for those who follow the surgical path, basic surgical training involves initially learning those aspects of medicine and generic skills common to all varieties of medical practice. After two years of basic surgical training the trainee then takes a post in one of the surgical specialities. This phase of training, called 'higher surgical training', is undertaken in the specialist registrar grade where trainees expand their clinical experience, assume increasing responsibilities and develop a specialist interest. Higher training takes five or six years and once complete and all examinations passed, the trainee can become a specialist registrar and apply for a post as a consultant.

There is a longstanding recognition within medical education of the importance of clinical experience and practical case knowledge. One of the more significant aspects of the training is the opportunity to join the senior surgeons in the actual environment of the operating theatre (see Figure 1). The more formal knowledge gained from reading textbooks and handbooks or attending lectures provides the student or trainee with relatively abstract knowledge concerning the ways in which cases are managed and the ways task specific skills and competencies are applied. It is widely recognised that surgery requires a fine mix of intellectual, technical and manual skills and that these skills can only be acquired through the opportunity to observe and discuss actual procedures and how they are applied, in collaboration with others, in actual cases. Indeed, it is recognised that each and every case is in a sense unique and poses particular challenges to the performance of the task and its application.

In teaching hospitals senior members of the surgical team have the responsibility to enable trainees to learn from the case. This may involve the surgeon in showing trainees how to perform particular procedures during minor and routine cases, and in some cases providing more experienced trainees with an opportunity to perform an incision or other minor or less critical parts of the operation under the supervision of the surgeon. Either way, it is important that trainees are able, within the constraints of the emerging task and the environment of the operating theatre, to witness and follow the operation, both as the surgeon prepares the surgical site and applies (a) specific technique(s) to the particular case on hand. In other words, the student or trainee is required to participate as an observer.

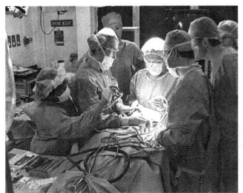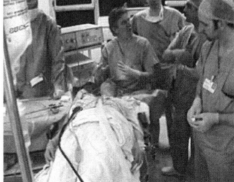

Figure 1 *In each of the cases the surgeon is central, surgical trainees stand next to the bed and medical students stand behind. In the left image a scrub nurse (on the left) holds an instrument ready for use; in the right image, an anaesthetist (on the right) monitors the condition of the patient*

'Intelligent' or 'informed' observation relies upon the ability of the surgical team to selectively render visible the performance of the surgical procedure and specific aspects of the case on hand. In this way, the trainee not only develops a familiarity with particular practices and procedures but becomes sensitive to, and aware of, the contingent deployment of those procedures with regard to particular cases.

Recognising the problem and its transformation

The surgical site is a relatively circumscribed domain, consisting in many cases of less than a couple of square centimetres. In order to maximise its availability and visibility to the surgeon, trainees and colleagues in the operating theatre frequently find themselves in positions where the surgical site is inaccessible, even though it may lie in close proximity. In many forms of surgery there is no other way to access the surgical field, unlike the cameras and accompanying monitors used in micro-surgery that enable the site to be displayed to all who happen to be present. Moreover, in most cases trainees will not have hitherto witnessed the performance of the particular procedure, and even if they have observed the general procedure in question on a previous occasion, they may well be unfamiliar with the ways in which a surgeon deals with the contingencies or idiosyncrasies of a particular case. As Pope (2002) suggests, surgeons bring preferences, past experiences, sensory responses and abilities to deal with the contingencies of surgical work. If the presence of trainees in the operating theatre is to have any educational value, it is critical that that they can not only witness aspects of the operation but are able to make sense of the contingent application of the procedure within the developing course of the operation. The surgeon, therefore, in co-operation with other members of the surgical team, has to selectively reveal aspects of the surgical site and the procedure so as to enable the trainees to make sense of, and 'intelligently' follow, the activities on hand despite their limited access to the operation. Moreover, this has to be accomplished so as to preserve the integrity of the task(s) on hand and the proper, professional practice upon which it relies. This resonates to some extent with the ways in which Bosk (1979) describes how surgeons allow room for the learning experiences of the trainees, without putting the patient at risk.

Let us consider an example. The surgical team is involved in clearing and widening the interior areas of the patient's throat. Some time before, the patient underwent an operation involving the removal of the larynx where the surgeon performed a tracheotomy. This involves making an artificial opening called a stoma in the front of the neck, and bringing the upper portion of the trachea up to the stoma and securing it, providing a permanent and alternative way for air to get to the lungs. Since the operation, the inner area of the throat has become tight, making it difficult for the patient to breathe and causing a number of infections. One of the problems that can emerge in such cases is when connective tissue – granulation tissue – replaces a clot in the healing wound. In order to improve the patient's breathing by clearing the airway and widening the windpipe, the surgeon uses particular instruments: a suction tube to remove tissues and secretion (mucus) and a dilator to widen the narrow parts of the throat. As part of this procedure the surgeon also uses a bronchoscope to see the interior of the throat and examine the progress of the intervention. The bronchoscope is a long telescopic lens that is inserted through the aperture in the throat to enable visual examination.

On this occasion two surgical trainees, Mark and Nick, have joined the surgeon. Nick is still in basic surgical training and has less experience of actual cases in the operating theatre; he knows about the procedure from the textbooks and seminars but has not witnessed it being performed. For him, as it is for all surgical trainees, this is not only an opportunity to learn about the procedure but to experience its performance with regard to the circumstances and contingencies of this particular case.

We join the action in the operating theatre as the surgeon begins the procedure. The surgeon (Sean) takes the bronchoscope, leans over the patient and inserts the bronchoscope through the airway opening. The surgeon begins to examine the interior of the throat with the trainee patiently waiting behind his hack. The surgeon then explains what he can see (Case 1 – Transcript 1).

Referring to a discussion that occurred just prior to the procedure commencing, the surgeon informs the trainee that he is now looking at 'the little she::lf:' (la). It is this little

Case 1 – Transcript 1

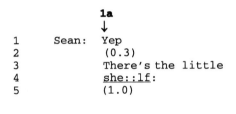

```
                            1a
                            ↓
1       Sean:   Yep
2               (0.3)
3               There's the little
4               she::lf:
5               (1.0)
```

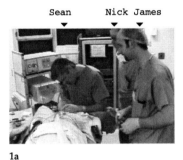

1a

```
                        1b
                        ↓
6       Sean:   You can  see  where it  s:o
7               na:rrows
8               (3.0)
9               (you  see  the)  shelf  and
10              mucus there
11              (1.0)
```

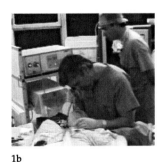

1b

```
                1c
                ↓
12      Nick:   m:mm
```

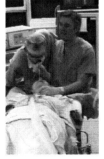

1c

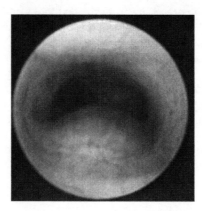

Figure 2 *An example image of the trachea and the narrowing pathway through a bronchoscope*

shelf, caused by an outgrowth that is where the airway tube meets the trachea (see Figure 2), that is causing the patient's breathing problems, and the surgeon provides further resources to enable Nick to discover and see the problem for himself.

In response to Sean's invitation 'You can see where it s:o na:rrows', Nick moves nearer to the surgical field (1b), and bends down over the instrument and examines the throat (1c). As he looks into the bronchoscope, Sean encourages him to see the shelf and the surrounding mucus ('(you see the) shelf and mucus there'). Nick's glance down the bronchoscope, coupled with his considered response 'm:mm', and immediate withdrawal, serves to display to the surgeon that he has seen the problem and recognised it. In this way, in producing a minimal, yet apparently adequate, recognition of the particulars of this problem, Nick enables Sean to immediately begin the procedure, the principal task on hand.

The surgical procedure consists of the surgeon clearing and broadening the throat by successively inserting a series of rods (dilators) of different sizes. By providing the trainee with an opportunity to view the throat prior to the intervention, the surgeon enables Nick to understand and follow the procedure with regard to specific qualities of this case: for example, the degree of narrowing and scale of the outgrowth and surrounding secretion that form this particular blockage and the particular qualities of this growth that have caused difficulties for the patient and her ability to lead a normal life. Moreover, the surgeon can draw upon the earlier viewing and identification of the problem to discuss different approaches to the problem, the results from previous operations, the improvements that they can later observe, and what may be expected and anticipated in the longer term.

Having seen and inspected the growth, secretion and the narrow path of the airway, the trainee is able to make sense of a procedure that involves inserting successive dilators of an increasingly large size into the airway to make it progressively larger. The scale of the dilators, and the way in which they are inserted, can be seen with regard to characteristics of this particular case. During the procedure, the surgeon intermittently uses the bronchoscope to inspect the progress of the operation and assess whether the throat has been cleared and broadened. The surgical field, and its transformation, remains largely invisible to the student, but on the occasions where he is invited to view the progress, it is only intelligible by what is known about the specifics of this case and by virtue of the contrast with the original state of the throat.

Case 1 – Transcript 2

```
 1      Sean: How (doe)s it look no::w
 2            (0.2)
 3            eh
 4            (.)
 5            Nick you see with the (ge)
 6            with the mucus
 7            di::stu::rbed
 8            (0.5)
```

2a
↓

```
 9      Nick: Yeah=
10      Sean: =It's looking half
11            reasonable now
12            (0.5)
13      Nick: Yeah yeah
```

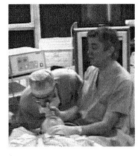

2a

2b
↓

```
14      Sean: at one time there was a
15            sort of window across
16            there
17            (0.4)
```

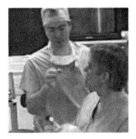

2b

2c
↓

```
18      Sean: and it was (down to a
19            minimum)
20            (0.4)
21            Much better than it was
```

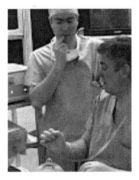

2c

Five minutes into the operation, the surgeon invites the trainee to view the improvement that successive dilations have made (see Case 1 – Transcript 2 above).

Having encouraged the trainee to glance through the bronchoscope the surgeon attempts to get him to look at how the mucus has been disturbed and how now it is 'looking half reasonable'. He then provides a contrast with the way in which it had appeared on a previous occasion and the extent of narrowing. Until this point, the trainee has had the opportunity to inspect the difficulty prior to the deployment of the procedure. He is only now able to look and see the ways in which the dilators have transformed the area surrounding the little shelf. In this way, not only can the trainee compare and contrast the effect of the procedure on the airway, but is able to see for himself what constitutes for the surgeon 'looking half reasonable'. In other words, the initial insight and the surgeon's accompanying description provide the resources for the trainee to follow and make sense of the procedure and assess how it has transformed the problem with regard to the particulars of this case.

Interestingly, as our transcript reveals (see Transcript 2 above), not only does the trainee affirm his understanding of the current state of the throat (2a) but as the surgeon continues to talk he seeks to demonstrate his understanding. The trainee stands up and makes a gesture with his right hand to show the width of the passageway (2b). In the light of this gesture and whilst he talks about the previous state of the throat, the surgeon produces a similar hand gesture of his own (2c) confirming the characterisation provided by the trainee. The trainee shakes his head as if to show his appreciation of the seriousness of the earlier condition. Before continuing with the case the surgeon concludes that it is now 'much better than it was'.

The ways in which the trainee responds to the assessment and his inspection of the throat and its transformation, provides the surgeon with a sense of the ways in which the trainee has seen and understood the effect of the procedure and the qualitative changes that have been accomplished in this case. The shaping of his fingers illustrates a broader and wider area down the throat, contrasting with the much narrower passage seen earlier. In contrast, the surgeon then uses the gestural characterisation of the trainee to elucidate how this transformation, on this occasion, stands in relation to the severity of the patient's problem on a previous occasion. In other words, whilst enabling the trainee to witness and to follow this procedure and inspect its effects, the surgeon goes to some trouble to delineate this operation within the career of the patient's difficulties and their surgical interventions.

The timely revelation of a problem's characteristics

To enable junior staff and trainees to follow complex procedures and their specific application in particular cases, it is necessary for the 'problem' in question to be seen at certain stages of the activity's accomplishment. Once seen, it is then possible to understand the contingencies that may emerge when performing a particular procedure, and to become familiar with, or be sensitive to, the ways in which a procedure has to be deployed with regard to a particular case and the difficulties it may afford. It is not unusual, however, for particular 'problems' to be almost invisible, certainly to the untrained eye, and significant time and effort are often directed towards exposing the problem prior to undertaking surgery. It is critical that junior doctors and trainees are able to view the specifics of the exposed problem before the procedure takes place; they are able to understand why the procedure is performed, on this occasion, in this particular way. In a sense therefore, the indexical or occasioned properties of the 'problem' are part and parcel of understanding the procedure and its routine, yet contingent, accomplishment.

Consider the following fragment. We join the action as the surgeon clears mucus around a tumour (an oesteoma) in one of the frontal sinuses (a cavity in the frontal bone just above the eyebrows). The surgeon (Maria) has exposed the anterior of the sinus, elevated the bone overlaying the sinus and is using a drill and various other instruments to remove the mucus and to gain access to the tumour. It has taken some time to expose the tumour and render it accessible for surgery. However, in this case, even though the tumour has been exposed, it has grown in such a way that it has become integrated with the bone structure

Case 2 – Transcript 1

Jane   Maria   Peter

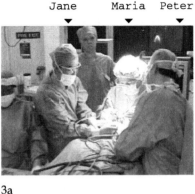

```
              3a                    3b
              ↓                     ↓
 1    Maria:  Can you see the line there
 2            (1.2)
 3            the    little    line    there
 4            (lying) around it
 5    Jane:   Yes
 6    Maria:  Do   you   see   it   at   the
 7            bottom there
 8            (1.0)
 9            that little V:::
10    Jane:   mm
11            (1.0)
```

3a

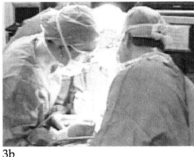

3b

```
12    Maria:  Okay
13            (0.2)
                        3c
                        ↓
14    Maria:  thats where the oesteoma
15            (is) against the back wall
16            (1.0)
17            It's very ⌈ very tight
18    Jane:            ⌊ yeahs
```

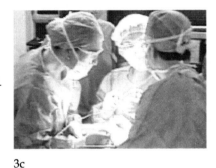

3c

deep inside the cavity of the frontal sinus and this will prove challenging for its removal. Two surgical trainees (Jane and Peter) are attending the operation and providing assistance where necessary (3a). The surgeon stops drilling and places the suction tip in the particular area of interest and produces the utterance: 'Can you see the line there'. The question occasions a reorientation by Jane and Peter; they move forward and turn towards the surgical field (3b).

The trainees' reorientation to and inspection of the surgical field, whilst occasioned by the question, does not provide sufficient resources to enable the surgeon to recognise that they have seen the line and location of the oesteoma. A second or so later, she specifies the location of the line in relation to the oesteoma, 'the little line there (lying) around it' (lines 3–4), and Jane responds with 'yes' (line 5), but Peter, aside from looking more closely, produces no response. The surgeon makes a further attempt to enable Peter, and perhaps Jane, to discover the line in relation to the location of the oesteoma in the cavity of the frontal sinus – 'do you see it at the bottom there?', No vocal response is forthcoming, and both trainees look more closely towards the area of the oesteoma. Once again, the surgeon provides a further specification of the line that lies around the oesteoma in the bottom of the cavity – 'that little V:::' – and what the two trainees should be looking for; a specification that provides a guide as to how it might be found and seen. Again, it receives an acknowledgement from Jane, but no verbal response from Peter. A moment later, when the surgeon delivers the actual statement 'that's where the oesteoma (is) against the back wall', she turns directly towards Peter (3c). Her description is accompanied by a gesture in which she shapes her hand into a representation of the tumour and its location in the cavity of the frontal sinus (3c). The gesture and its accompanying description illustrate what should be seen, and provide Peter, if not also Jane, with the resources to enable them to retrospectively make sense of the tumour and its position within the cavity.

The trainees' sense and recognition of the oesteoma is accomplished through the surgeon's progressive attempts to align their orientation to enable them to see what is almost hidden, a series of actions that is shaped with regard to the emerging participation of Jane and Peter. The very ways in which the location and character of the oesteoma is revealed is fashioned with regard to the visible and vocal conduct of the trainees. Her successive attempts to reveal the line and oesteoma are built though a series of actions that specify a particular alignment and secure an appropriate display that the objects have indeed been found and seen. They progressively emerge with regard to the seeming absence of a sequentially appropriate response from the trainees, in particular Peter, who both fails to claim or show that he has seen the little line and recognised its significance. The surgeon's attempts to secure particular forms of participation and particular ways of orienting to the surgical field, are sensitive to the different alignments of the two trainees in the developing course of producing the activity.

Interestingly, however, this progressive alignment of the participants towards the visual scene of the surgical field appears not to be primarily concerned with revealing the oesteoma. Whilst they have earlier been able to see parts of the oesteoma, the surgeon now encourages the two trainees to see not only where it is, but to locate the object within the particular structure of the cavity and its contents. The identification of 'the little line' and 'at the bottom there', and as characterised as 'that little V:::', progressively reveals the oesteoma's position at the rear of the sinus, tucked against the back wall. The revelation of the oesteoma in this way orients the two trainees to the specifics of this case and thereby to its implications for the application of the procedure that the surgeon will perform. It attempts to provide the resources to enable the trainees to recognise the ways in which the procedure is (and will be) shaped with regard to the contingencies at hand, in particular the difficulties of removing a tumour from a relatively inaccessible location. Her last assessment 'It's very very tight' underscores the difficulties that she is now facing and how the procedure should be understood with regard to the particular contingencies of this case, specifically the location of the tumour.

Given the absence of any explicit response from Peter, it is interesting to notice how he, a few minutes later (see Case 2 – Transcript 2) just as the surgeon has finished a round of drilling near the location of the tumour, appears to comment on the location of the oesteoma and the problem it entails, barely audibly noting that it is 'very thick'. The remark appears to display an understanding of the difficulties associated with the size of the bone

Case 2 – Transcript 2

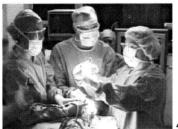

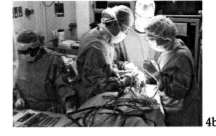

4a

4b

```
1     Peter:   (very thick)
2              (0.1)
3     Maria:   Yeah what she's got: ah on the scan::
4              (0.2)
5              you can see she's got a very big ah sort of (0.5)
6              anterior (0.3) ah frontal septum¹
7              (0.5)
8              °if you look on the scan° (She's got) a thick frontal
9              bone with a sort of (0.4) ah quite thick ah septum into
10             the anterior cranial fossa²              4a
11             (0.4)                                     ↓
12    Maria:   and then you got a relatively small frontal sinus and
13             that little bit of (0.2) s: septation³ becomes part of
14             the intersinus septum which is integrated into the
15             osteoma
16             (0.1)
17             that's the problem and that's what we are on here.
18             (0.5)
19             What I am doing is drilling around it      4b
20             (0.3)                                      ↓
21             and you can just see:: (1.0) the:: (1.0) freer please
22             (0.2)
23              you can just see there::: (1.0) the:: (1.5) juncture
24             (1.0)
25             (just there)
26             (0.5)
27             between the osteoma
```

Note:

[1] A septum is a thin partition or membrane that divides two cavities or soft masses of tissue.

[2] A fossa is a depression or hollow in a bone.

[3] A septation is the division or partitioning of a cavity into parts by a septum

structure and the location of the tumour being deep inside the sinus. The remark occasions a lengthy description from the surgeon, as she explains the surrounding anatomy and the pathology of the problem, and the difficulties the location of the tumour poses for access and removal. During this description, a highly technical description that is critical to the trainees' ability to follow the procedure and understand the particular difficulties in this case, the surgeon temporarily suspends the principal surgical task.

Revealing the location of the oesteoma and drawing attention to its 'tightness' serves retrospectively to illuminate, and perhaps account for, the difficulties that the surgeon has faced in accessing the tumour and preparing the surgical field. It also provides the trainees with a sense of the specific characteristics and contingencies that will inform the application of the surgical procedure and the difficulties that it may entail. It enables the trainees to embed the procedure within the practicalities and constraints of this case, and retrospectively and prospectively to make sense of the particular actions undertaken by the surgeon. The perception and determination of the oesteoma's location, and the trainee's ability to comprehend how the procedure is being deployed on this occasion and the difficulties faced by the surgeon, are accomplished in and through the interaction, interaction that provides the trainees with access to, and a way of seeing, the oesteoma at this stage or moment of the proceedings. These revelations, through which trainees are provided with momentary access to aspects of the surgical field, are positioned to provide resources to enable deployment of the particular procedure to be intelligible and accessible, even though it may partially be hidden from view.

Supporting instruction: preserving the integrity of the procedure

In the previous case, Peter's comment is immediately followed by a lengthy description from the surgeon concerning the complexities of the case. In this account she relates details of the case to a scan displayed in front of the team, and encourages the trainees to re-examine and inspect the surgical site, comparing the actual problem with the scan of the tumour that has informed the intervention. Maria describes particular characteristics of this case and gestures using both hands to capture the large size of the frontal septum, the small size of the frontal sinus and the relationship between the two. Maria then points to the region of the patient's head saying 'and that's what we are on here', picking up the suction tool. The shift from the characterisation of the case, drawing on the scan, to the actual osteoma encourages both Jane and Peter to turn towards the surgical site and inspect the features described by Maria. As they turn towards the surgical site, Maria then describes the specific part of the procedure she is undertaking 'What I am doing is drilling around it'. Maria starts to use the suction tool as she says 'and you can just see:: (1.0) the:: (1.0) freer please (0.2) you can just see there:::'. Maria then shows the trainees the region around the osteoma. To enable the trainees to more closely inspect the oesteoma and its location, the surgeon requires a freer – an instrument for elevating or lifting bone structures. The utterance 'freer please' (line 21 in Case 2 – Transcript 2, see arrow 4b), embedded within this lengthy description, is for the scrub nurse (Susan) standing to Jane's right. The nurse passes the freer in the pause following 'you can just see there:::'.

During Maria's long description of the problem, Susan, having placed the drill ready for the next part of the operation, begins cleaning another instrument, occasionally glancing at the scanned image on the display. As Maria competes the description of the problem and says 'and you can just see::', Susan then turns to scan the trolley where the instruments are laid out. When the surgeon asks for the freer, she immediately picks it up from the table and passes it to Maria. The timely and unproblematic passing of the instrument, its deployment just at the moment it is relevant to the illustration, demonstrates the way in which the scrub nurse is both following, and orienting to, the surgeon's characterisation of the problem in the course of its production. The instrument is ready on hand, and ready not simply for the next stage of the procedure but ready to render that the problem is visible, accessible, to the trainees.

At major teaching hospitals surgical operations can include a significant number of participants. As well as the surgeon, one or two surgical trainees and two or three students, there will be at least one scrub nurse, and one or maybe two anaesthetists. Providing instruction or insight into a surgical procedure or practice may require actions from one of the other participants, particularly from those involved in the performance of the operation such as the scrub nurse or an anaesthetist. Those participants, other than the surgeon and the trainees, may have to remain sensitive not only to the progress of the procedure, but to the instruction and informing that arises, so as to enable moments of insight and demonstration to be unproblematically accomplished.

It is worthwhile to return to the throat operation discussed in the first case. When we enter the action (see Case 1 – Transcript 3 below), the surgeon (Sean) is undertaking the procedure but has temporarily stalled the activity to discuss further details of the case with the two trainees (Nick and Mark). The procedure, successively inserting the dilators into the patient's throat, requires the patient to be manually ventilated by the anaesthetist. Here, a small tube is placed in the hole in the patient's throat, the same hole used for inserting the dilators and bronchoscope during the surgical procedure. This tube is connected to a small bag that enables the anaesthetist to manually pump oxygen to the patient's chest. To insert the dilators or bronchoscope the tube is removed. During this period, the

Case 1 – Transcript 3

Sean Mark   Nick

```
 1   Sean:   That is all gone now
 2           (0.4)
 3   Mark:   Is it?
 4           (0.2)
 5   Sean:   Yeah
 6           (0.2)
 7           seriously (0.2) there is no
 8           granulation
 9           (0.4)
10           little bit mucus around

             5a
              ↓
11   Sean:   but (2.0) no actual
12           °granulation°
13           (2.0)
```

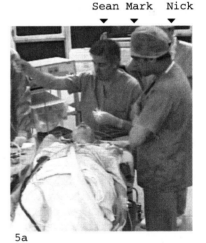

5a

```
14   Sean:   O::kay
15           (0.3)
16           you can hold that end for me
17           that would be gre::a:t
18           (0.2)
19           and we'll just pop in again
20           (1.0)

             5b
              ↓
21   Sean:   gently
```

James

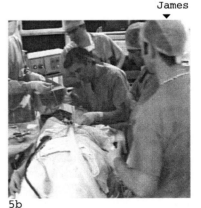

5b

patient is receiving no oxygen and it is critical therefore that the tube is replaced at regular intervals. If the patient receives no oxygen for more than 60 seconds then brain damage can occur.

When Sean in our extract (see Case 1 – Transcript 3) says 'Yeah (0.2) seriously (0.2) there is no granulation' (lines 5–8, image 5a) he turns towards the instrument trolley to his right, picks up the bronchoscope and the suction tube and asks the scrub nurse to hold the tube (lines 16–17). He then introduces the ventilation tube ('and we'll just pop in again' – line 19) for the anaesthetist (James) to manually ventilate the patient, so they are ready to proceed with the next stage of the operation.

By manually ventilating the patient, by squeezing the bag, the anaesthetist displays that he is sensitive to this juncture in the operation. It is interesting to note how initially his orientation, away from the surgical scene, seems to be designed not to draw any attention. He occasionally turns towards the surgical scene to monitor the discussion and to watch for the opportunity to ventilate the patient. By ventilating the patient at a suitable and witnessable opportunity he not only produces the actions that are critical to the safety of the patient but avoids disrupting the instructional activity.

The same kind of sensitivity is shown by the trainees. As the surgeon says 'little bit mucus around' (line 10) and starts picking up the instruments, Mark moves to his right and slightly away from the surgical scene. Nick then follows, moving to stand behind Sean and Mark (5b). The trainees, in particular Mark, seem to recognise the upcoming transition from the talk and visual conduct of the surgeon. They position themselves to facilitate the upcoming procedure, providing the surgeon with the space, 'the elbow room' to coin the phrase used by Hughes (1958), to perform the procedure. The conduct of the trainees defers to, and serves to preserve, the integrity of the surgical activity.

Just after Sean puts the tube back in, James (the anaesthetist), who has been standing a little back from the bed, moves in and gives the ventilation bag a squeeze to supply the patient with oxygen. The surgeon produces a long summary of the current progress of the procedure, at one moment making it possible for one of the students to see this in the light of what he has previously seen. Sean then goes on to the next round of dilation. Whilst continuing to engage with the trainees, and preparing for the next stage of the operation, the surgeon is also sensitive to the prospective needs of the anaesthetist, inserting the ventilation tube in such a way to give him time to prepare and implement one round of ventilation before the next stage of the procedure. The surgeon himself is also not only concerned with the progress of his own activity, but is sensitive to the ability of others to undertake their tasks and responsibilities and thereby preserve the integrity of the ongoing surgical procedure.

In surgical operations moments of explicit surgical training are interwoven within the ongoing surgical procedures. The transitions into and out of these moments are delicately managed by the participants in the operation – not only by the surgeon and trainees, but also by other members of the clinical team. In various ways anaesthetists and nurses help configure their own activities to enable moments, sometimes episodes, of demonstration and instruction to be unproblematically interleaved within the concerted accomplishment of the operation, preserving the professional integrity of the procedure and its accountability, whilst enabling trainees to observe and in some cases participate in the principal task on hand. In various ways, moments and episodes of instruction and demonstration place contingent demands upon the production of the specialised activities of other members of the surgical team, and as we have begun to see, place demands upon the ways in which they orientate to and understand the particular surgical procedures and the opportunities and occasions they afford for learning. It is unfortunate perhaps that, as far as we are aware, so little analytic attention has been paid to the ways in which the different participants within surgical teams enable instruction and demonstration and the sorts of competencies and resources on which the smooth accomplishment of these episodes rely.

Discussion: formal procedures and their occasioned application

It has long been recognised that the ability to learn highly complex medical tasks relies upon both formal instruction and the opportunity to 'participate' in the accomplishment of everyday healthcare practice. It is argued, for example, that through engagement with more senior practitioners within ongoing practice, students and trainees acquire the skills and competencies, in communities of practice, that are required to perform these complex tasks in organisationally relevant and appropriate ways (Lave and Wenger 1991).

In her insightful study, Pope (2002) draws upon interviews and observations of surgical work to identify three ways in which surgical work can be considered contingent: with regard to the case, to the particular surgeon and to other external factors. For example, Pope points to the different ways in which surgeons' decisions both before and during surgery are shaped by such matters as the particulars of the patients' circumstances, the skills of their assistants and even the size of their own hands. Pope raises concerns with relying too much on surgeons' own reports of the contingencies they face as it may unduly prioritise their accounts of their skills and tacit practices. Nevertheless, she suggests, following others (Berg 1997, Wood *et al.* 1998), that by taking contingency seriously the conventional boundaries between practical and technical knowledge may need to be rethought.

By considering the ways in which surgical work is accomplished in practice we can see how surgeons manage these contingencies from moment-to-moment through interaction with their colleagues. Examining those occasions when instructions and insights are provided throws light not only on how their knowledge and skills are deployed but also on how practitioners learn from, and about, the contingent application of formal procedures in particular cases – how 'situated learning' is accomplished in practice.

Save for a few insightful studies, such as those concerned with how surgeons provide 'tacit guidance' when providing training in manual tasks (Prentice 2007), how practitioners manage the internal boundaries of a community of practice (Goodwin *et al.* 2005), and how 'professional visions' are configured within medical environments (Mondada 2006, Koschmann *et al.* 2007, Hindmarsh *et al.* forthcoming), we have little understanding of the significance of, or practice that underpins, 'situated learning'. In the case at hand, we can begin to see how trainees are not simply provided with an opportunity to observe or discuss the operation, or to handle the instruments and engage in a specific part of a procedure, but with the resources to enable the deployment of procedures to be seen and considered with regard to the particulars and the particular demands of the case. Trainees need to be provided with the resources to be able to witness and follow a surgical procedure, but also to have a sense of why it is done in this way on this occasion; in other words they need a sense of how the procedure is performed with regard to the specific case and practicalities. These viewings are not simply accomplished so that an object or feature can be seen at this moment, but seeing the 'phenomena' provides the means to understand the contingent and occasioned deployment of the procedure. In other words, the surgeon, in concert and collaboration with colleagues, provides trainees with ways of embedding a formal procedure with the reasoned and relevant contingencies of the case on hand; in such ways, a new member comes to know and skilfully apply rules of an organisation (see for example Weider

1974). It is the ability to recognise these reasoned and relevant contingencies, and thereby deploy a procedure, that is critical to the appropriate and accountable performance of medical practice.

The ways in which trainees are provided with the opportunities to discuss cases and with the resources to see, and make sense of, particular phenomena and practices, might appear to rely on the differential status of the participants in a formal training situation: the surgeon, a more senior consultant with teaching responsibilities, and trainees, less experienced members who participate only to receive insight and knowledge about the particular case. It might also be thought that the activities of the trainees are principally concerned with listening to and observing the surgeon or providing relevant support. However, there are a number of aspects of teaching and learning situations in the operating theatre that raise some interesting issues with regard to, our understanding of apprenticeship and situated forms of learning, at least in this particularly complex setting.

First, we can see how moments of instruction have to be positioned not only with regard to the proper performance of the task at hand, as a formally organised activity, but with consideration to what trainees may need to know at certain moments to retrospectively and prospectively make sense of, and (intelligibly) follow, the action and the procedures of occasioned deployment. The timing and place of the insight and instruction provides the resources for rendering the procedures visible and intelligible with regard to the particular case at hand, whilst simultaneously preserving the integrity of the operation and its emerging and contingent demands. Secondly, trainees rely on ways of seeing the surgical phenomenon and the occasioned application of the procedure that 'progressively' emerges, so that for example, seeing this now recasts what has happened and in turn provides a scheme of interpretation with which to see and make sense of subsequent problems, actions and the like. These moments of insight and instruction form a critical element of gestalt that enables an emergent retrospective–prospective sense of the activity in the course of its accomplishment. They are not simply moments of looking, but by virtue of seeing here and now they enable an informed and cumulative sense of the action and the case to emerge. Thirdly, the occasioned production of these insights and instructions by the surgeon necessitates timely and relevant contributions from a range of participants. Scrub nurses and anaesthetists, for example, orient to the requirements of providing instruction and in various ways serve to support these occasioned interventions or breaks from the activity at hand. Being a good trainee involves deference to the emerging demands of the principal activity: the operation. Nevertheless, differing contributions from a number of participants with a range of expertise are co-ordinated to accomplish the task at hand whilst also reflexively rendering visible the ways in which the task is produced.

To disregard the 'situation' of 'situated learning' renders epiphenomenal the social and the interactional organisation through which demonstration and instruction is accomplished within the demanding circumstances of a complex medical procedure. It also undermines our ability to understand what is taught and learnt in these circumstances, in particular the ways in which formal procedures and practices are applied, performed and configured with regard to the contingencies of the case at hand, and the relevant scheme of contingencies that might properly inform the procedure's deployment.

Acknowledgements

We would like thank everyone in the Royal National Ear, Nose and Throat Hospital in London for granting us access to their workplace and for their willingness to talk about their work. We are particularly grateful to Dr. David Enderby and Dr. Maxim Nicholls. We are very grateful for the comments and suggestions from Dirk vom Lehn, Katie Best and other members of the WIT Research Centre and Hillevi Sundblom for their support with the issues and materials discussed here. We would also like to thank the editors of the book and the anonymous referees for their insightful and very helpful comments on the chapter. Research on this chapter was undertaken as part of the various projects including two EU projects COSI and PALCOM.

References

Ball, D.L. and Lampert, M. (1999) Multiples of evidence, time, and perspective: revising the study of teaching and learning. In Lagemann, E.C. and Shulman, L.S. (eds) *Issues in Education Research: Problems and Possibilities*. San Francisco: Jossey-Bass Publishers.

Becker, H., Geer, B., Hughes, E. and Strauss, A. (1961) *Boys in White: Student Culture in Medical School*. Chicago: University of Chicago Press.

Berg, M. (1997) *Rethinking Medical Work*. Cambridge MA: MIT Press.

Bosk, C. (1979) *Forgive and Remember: Managing Medical Failure*. Chicago: University of Chicago Press.

Byrne, P. and Long, B. (1976) *Doctors Talking to Patients: a Study of the Verbal Behaviours of Doctors in the Consultation*. London: HMSO.

Cobb, P., Stephan, M., McClain, K. and Gravemeijer, K. (2001) Participating in classroom mathematical practices, *Journal of the Learning Sciences*, 10, 1 and 2, 113–64.

Freidson, E. (1970) *Profession of Medicine: a Study of the Sociology of Applied Knowledge*. New York: Dodd-Mead.

Goodwin, C. (1994) Professional vision, *American Anthropologist*, 96, 3, 606–33.

Goodwin, D., Pope, C., Mort, M. and Smith, A. (2005) Access, boundaries and their effects: legitimate participation in anaesthesia, *Sociology of Health and Illness*, 27, 6, 855–71.

Hall, R. and Stevens, R. (1995) Making space: a comparison of mathematical work in school and professional design practices, in Star, S.L. (ed.) *The cultures of computing*. London: Basil Blackwell.

Heath, C.C. and Luff, P. (2000) *Technology in Action*. Cambridge: Cambridge University Press.

Hindmarsh, J., Reynolds, P. and Dunne, S. (forthcoming) Exhibiting Understanding: the body in apprenticeship. *Journal of Pragmatics*.

Hindmarsh, J. and Pilnick, A. (2002) The tacit order of teamwork: collaboration and embodied conduct in anaesthesia, *The Sociological Quarterly*, 43, 2, 139–64.

Hughes, E.C. (1958) *Men and Their Work*. Glencoe: Free Press.

Koschmann, T., LeBaron, C., Goodwin, C., Zemel, A. and Dunnington, G. (2007) Formulating the 'Triangle of Doom', *Gesture*, 7, 1, 97–118.

Lave, J. and Wenger, E. (1991) *Situated Learning: Legitimate Peripheral Participation*. Cambridge, MA: Cambridge University Press.

Luff, P.K., Hindmarsh, J.J. and Heath, C.C. (eds) (2000) *Workplace Studies: Recovering Work Practice and Informing System Design*. New York and Cambridge: Cambridge University Press.

Middleton, D. and Engestrom, Y. (1996) *Cognition and Communication at Work: Distributed Cognition in the Workplace*. Cambridge: Cambridge University Press.

Mondada, L. (2006) Bilingualism and the analysis of talk at work: code-switching as a resource for the organization of action and interaction, in Heller, M. (ed.) *Bilingualism. A Social Approach*. Basingstoke: Macmillan.

Pomerantz, A. (2003) Modelling as a Teaching Strategy in Clinical Training: When Does It Work? in: Glenn, P., LeBaron, C. and Mandelbaum, J. (eds) *Studies in Language and Social Interaction: In Honor of Robert Hopper*. Mahwah, NJ: Lawrence Erlbaum Associates.

Pope, C. (2002) Contingency in everyday surgical work, *Sociology of Health and Illness*, 24, 4, 369–84.

Prentice, R. (2007) Drilling surgeons: the social lessons of embodied surgical learning, *Science, Technology and Human Values*, 32, 5, 534–53.

Richardson, D. (2006) Training of general surgical residents: what model is appropriate? *American Journal of Surgery*, 191, 296–300.

Sanchez Svensson, M. (2005) *Configuring awareness: work, interaction and collaboration in operating theatres*. Unpublished PhD thesis. University of London.

Silverman, D. (1987) *Communication and Medical Practice: Social Relations in the Clinic*. London: Sage.

Strong, P.M. (1979) *The Ceremonial Order of the Clinic*. London: Routledge and Kegan Paul.

Timmermans, S. and Angell, A. (2001) Evidence-based medicine, clinical uncertainty, and learning to doctor, *Journal of Health and Social Behavior*, 42, 4, 342–59.

Weider, D.L. (1974) *Language and Social Reality: The Case of Telling the Convict Code*. The Hague: Mouton.

Wood, M., Ferlie, E. and Fitzgerald, L. (1998) Achieving clinical behaviour change: a case of becoming indeterminate, *Social Science and Medicine*, 47, 1729–38.

8

Creating history: documents and patient participation in nurse-patient interviews

Aled Jones

Introduction

Over 13 million patients were admitted to hospital for in-patient care within the National Health Service (NHS) in England and Wales during 2006–07 (HES 2007) and each patient had their care needs assessed by a registered nurse (RN) or student nurse. These 'nursing admission assessments' therefore form a significant part of nurses' routine daily work pattern in hospitals. Nursing assessments usually take place at the patient's bedside forming one part of a hectic admission process which sees patients also undergo a medical assessment and various interventions such as blood pressure measuring, height and weight recording and blood taking.

In this chapter I explore the work of nurses when initially assessing the health and social care needs of adults undergoing admission into hospital. The simultaneity of the patient's entry into hospital with the need for nurses to gather assessment information regarding the individual, has led to the synonymous use of multiple terms to describe these activities. During this study, for example, nurses stated that they were 'admitting a patient', 'assessing a patient', 'taking the history', 'interviewing a patient' – with each term relating to the same activity.

Nursing literature is unequivocal regarding the significance of the admission process for the nurse-patient relationship being forwarded as *the* important area of nursing work to be performed when a patient enters hospital (Latimer 2000). Furthermore, the assessment interview has long been identified by nurses as an opportunity to encourage patients to participate in their care (Crawford and Brown 2004, King 1971). For example, Sully and Dallas (2005: 74) refer to the admission interaction as a phase of nursing work which offers opportunities 'to develop a partnership' with patients (2005: 74). Similarly, Tutton's (2005) interview study reported that nurses viewed history taking as fundamental 'to the process of participation' (2005: 149) creating an opportunity 'for knowing what was important to them' (2005: 148).

The above descriptions of the admission interview are typical of those found in the nursing literature which largely focuses on verbal communication during the admission interaction. However, nursing in general, and the admission process in particular, sees nurses routinely writing in and reading a variety of patient records and other kinds of documents. Systematic reviews of nurses' record keeping and recording systems (Currell and Urquhart 2004, Moloney and Maggs 1999) report there to be a lack of credible research which examines the interactional practices of nurses and patients when records are being consulted or filled. Similarly, Heath *et al.* (2003) and Timmermans and Berg (2003) draw attention to the disregard in sociological research for the ways in which people, in ordinary, everyday circumstances, use tools and technologies, objects and artefacts, to accomplish social action and interaction.

Recently, authors such as Ventres *et al.* (2006), Kaner *et al.* (2007) and McGrath *et al.* (2007) have explored the effects of medical records on the interaction of physicians and patients. However, few studies examine the use of seemingly mundane technologies such as paper-based or electronic patient records (EPR) and their detailed effects on healthcare talk and interaction. In addition, studies rarely attempt the fine-grained analysis of talk in non-primary care contexts or contexts involving nurses.

Study aims

The data presented here provide a rare glimpse into the interactions of nurses and patients during episodes of acute hospital care. The aim of this chapter is to explore nurses' use of mundane technology (paper-based nursing record) during the admission process of patients into hospital and whether the use of such technology affects the extent of patient participation during the admission process. What emerges from the analysis is a better understanding of the interactive and interdependent relationship within nursing assessment interviews between the spoken words of nurses, the written word of the assessment document and the spoken words of the patients' contributions. The analysis will subsequently inform a discussion regarding nursing practice during admission interviews, as well as contribute to the debate regarding record keeping at a time of great change where hospital records, such as those used during the admission process, are soon to be completed in electronic format.

Background – patient participation

The image of the consumer stands at the heart of attempts by policy makers to reform health systems to meet the demands of a 'modern' world in which citizens are assumed to have greater involvement and confidence in challenging clinician authority (Newman and Vidler 2006). In the UK and beyond, such a conception has been a central feature of the increasing value placed on patient participation (and patient involvement and partnership) at all levels of healthcare delivery. For example, patient participation has been prioritised in a plethora of supra-national (WHO 2005), national (NHS Executive 1996) and sub-national (Welsh Assembly Government 2003) government policy documents.

Professional bodies and regulators of nursing practice in the UK have also identified patient participation and involvement as central to good nursing practice. For example, Royal College of Nursing (2003: 3) identifies a 'commitment to partnership' with patients as one of its six defining characteristics of nursing. The Nursing and Midwifery Code of Professional Conduct (NMC 2008: 2) recommends that nurses should uphold 'people's rights to be fully involved in decisions about their care'. However, despite the many writers and policy documents advocating patient participation within the context of nursing care, there is little consensus about what participation means.

Fieldwork for my study was undertaken at hospitals using Dougherty and Lister's (2004: 36) manual of clinical nursing procedures as a 'best-practice' guide. The manual offers guidelines on various aspects of nursing practice including 'communication and assessment'. For example, the assessment interview 'should progress logically, ensuring meaning for the participants' whilst also providing nurses with an opportunity to 'gain an understanding of the patient's priorities for care' (2004: 30). Overall, the procedure manual characterises the initial interview as an interaction which enables the gathering of patient information whilst also facilitating the establishment of a therapeutic nurse-patient relationship. Whilst patient participation during initial assessment is not explicitly mentioned, the manual does state that effective assessment 'should be a process in which the patient ideally plays an active role' (2004: 25).

The procedure manual therefore avoids presenting guidelines to nurses about participation during patients' admission (or any other phase of care). In so doing, the manual reflects a wider trend in nursing literature and policy documents which encourages patient involvement during the admission phase but avoids offering specific guidance. The lack of specific guidelines is probably indicative of the potentially complex nature of participation and care giving in practice settings. For example, hospital wards, such as those recruited into this study, admit adult patients suffering from a wide variety and severity of illness which result in varying opportunities for patient participation. Such potential complexity would quickly make redundant specific guidelines for use on acute medical wards, for example.

What remain, therefore, are literature and policy documents that exhort nurses to involve patients. Sahlsten *et al.*'s (2008: 9) in depth analysis of the patient participation literature describes the defining attributes of patient participation as including interaction where 'The nurse displays genuine interest and empathy' and 'where the patient volunteers information without being asked, or is invited to do so by means of open questions'. Sahlsten and colleagues' defining attributes neatly capture how nursing literature has traditionally portrayed patient participation as being dependent on a command of relevant communication skills (interest and empathy, the use of open questions, etc.). As such, they provide a useful conceptual 'baseline' for further exploration in this study.

Peräkylä and Vehviläinen (2003) have called on conversation analysts to explore the relationship between professional-client interaction and organised knowledge (referred to as 'stocks of interactional knowledge' or SIKs) that are found in textbooks and policy documents. In particular, they propose that conversation analysis (CA) findings can provide a more detailed picture of practice than that described in SIKs. In doing so, CA can add a new dimension to the understanding of practices described within abstract or general documents. The intention in this chapter therefore is to create a dialogue between nursing SIKs which describe patient participation and the actual practices of nurses, in the hope of adding a new dimension to the understanding of practices described by an SIK.

Methods

Sample and recruitment

This study focused on three acute hospital sites in the UK with data being collected from five hospital wards in total (two medical wards and one ward from general surgery, neurology, cardiology). All patients recruited were classified as 'unscheduled admissions', having been admitted to the wards via a referral that day from a primary care practitioner or the accident and emergency unit. The initial admission interviews were carried out by registered nurses within two hours of the patient arriving on the ward. It is inevitable that nurses also assessed patients during subsequent interactions but the study's attention was maintained purely on the initial admission interview which, as discussed earlier, has been presented in the literature as a prominent and important event within which information is gathered and rapport with the patient established.

The method used is conversation analysis (CA) as applied to the study of institutional interaction (see Drew and Heritage 1992). Twenty-seven admission interviews were observed, audio-taped (621 minutes of talk) and transcribed, whilst 25 nursing documents produced as a result of these interviews were photocopied and analysed; no nurse or patient was recorded/observed more than once. There were no explicit inclusion/exclusion criteria adopted for recruitment to this study, and a purposive sampling approach was undertaken, with the researcher choosing cases that illustrated the process under scrutiny (Silverman 2005). Relevant ethical approval for the study was granted and data anonymised before publication.

Prior to audio recording a total of 45 admission interviews were observed during 175 hours of participant observation on the wards. The need for a period of field-work became clear during preliminary visits to clinical areas. Particularly apparent during these visits was the complexity of activities undertaken during the assessment interview and the range of distributed activities which feature, sometimes only momentarily, in the accomplishment of the work in question. Therefore, various forms of data were collected using 'field methods' (ten Have 2004: 127). Observations, note taking, documents which were perused and copied, all helped to sketch the overall features of the setting, while the audio record-ings were collected to identify the spoken strategies used to actually 'do' the assessment interview.

Notes were taken during the admission process (*e.g.* 'nurse writing in notes', 'patient points to left side of head') and a summary report of each admission was written up imme-diately at its completion. The report was a particularly useful record of the interaction between nurse and patient, allowing more detail to be added to the notes taken during the admission and leading to a fuller consideration of nurses' and patients' conduct.

My observations built upon previous studies that had utilised observational data to understand doctor-patient work in primary care settings (Heath 1986, Ruusuvuori 2001). These studies reveal how participants co-ordinate tasks with the actions of others, how they monitor each other's conduct and its relevance, and how attending to the medical record shapes and constrains interpersonal communication. During the course of this study it became apparent that nurse-patient interaction was similarly influenced on occasion through nurses attending to or reading the admission record during the admission interview. In particular, the close working of nurses with the assessment document, appears at times, to limit the patient's voice and restrict opportunities for patient participation.

Analysis

Analysis involved repeatedly listening to the tapes and reading through the transcriptions, based on Jefferson's (1984) orthography, which were produced as soon as possible fol-lowing recording. The analysis of talk was augmented by the field-data detailed above. For example, photocopies of the nursing notes gave an insight into what nurses wrote during the admission. Timing the admission interview with a digital stopwatch enabled handwritten fieldnotes regarding gestures, laughter or nurses reading the notes to be co-ordinated with the transcripts at a later stage. For example, a fieldnote entry such as 'NW 3.12' was subsequently translated into 'nurse writing in the notes at 3 minutes and 12 seconds' of the admission interview. The overview of the admission, which I wrote at its completion, also enabled me to access useful supplementary information during analysis. Such additional data proved invaluable in the absence of video-recording, the use of which proved impractical for a variety of reasons associated with the acute-care nature of the settings.

Topical organisation of talk: One feature of the admission interaction was the extent to which the topics discussed during admission followed the sequence of topics as they appeared on the admission document being completed by the nurse at the time of the interview.

Extract 1: SB 1 – 3 minutes into assessment of surgical patient admitted for 'observation re. abdominal pain/distension'

25	n	any problems with your bowe[ls or w]aterworks
26	p	[no-no]
27		(6.0) ((nurse writing in notes))
28	n	and you manage to wash and dress yourself
29	p	yeh yeh
30		(8.0) ((nurse writing in notes, patient looking through window))
31	n	and you're walking about ok [you] don't get short of breath [walki]ng
32	p	[yeh] [no-no]
33	n	walking around or anything
34		(7.0) ((nurse writing in notes))
35	n	sleeping what you're like with your =
36	p	= well you know it's off and on you know not good not bad ((short
38		laugh)) you know we both sleep for about three to four hours and then
39		we're awake you know so:::
40		(4.0) ((nurse writing in notes 'sleeps 3–4 hours'))
41	n	(do you do anything?) with religion or anything
42	p	uh:: > > no < <

When reading Extract 1 with Figure 1 (below), we can see how the nurse asks the patient questions concerning bowels/waterworks and hygiene 'and you manage to wash and dress

Topic sequence during assessment.	Layout of the assessment form.		
The sequence of topic areas discussed - numbers correspond to boxes that are filled in on the form (right).	**Roper's model of nursing** *For assessment of patient on admission*		
1 Language spoken	**Maintaining safe environment**	**Communicating**	**Breathing**
2 Any problems with diet?			
2 Drinking fluids well?	*Not discussed*	*1*	*5*
2 Weight loss?			
3 Any problems with bowels or waterworks?	**Eating & drinking**	**Eliminating**	**Personal cleansing and dressing**
4 Manage to wash and dress yourself			
5 Walking about ok, no short of breath walking?	*2*	*3*	*4*
7 What are you like sleeping?			
8 Do you do anything with religion?	**Controlling body temperature**	**Mobilising**	**Working and playing**
9 Any hobbies?	*Not discussed but 'no problems' entered*	*5*	*9*
10 You've come in with abdominal pain?			
11 Do you smoke at all?	**Expressing sexuality**	**Sleeping**	**Dying**
11 Alcohol?	*Not discussed*	*7*	*8*
'There we are' – interview completed.			
	Pain	**Health promotion**	**Named nurse**
	10	*11*	*Not discussed*

Figure 1 *Sequence of nurse-patient talk (SB1) compared to layout of the admission document*

yourself' (line 28 relating to 'Personal cleansing and dressing' on the document) before moving on to the unconnected topics 'and you're walking about ok' (line 31 – 'Mobilising' on the document), sleeping (line 35) and religion (line 41).

As was noticeable across the dataset, the nurse's action of reading and writing in the admission document (Extract 1 lines 27, 30, 34, 40) seemed to influence topic-ordering during the assessment interview. However, this is not to suggest that the document 'controlled' the interaction, as Figure 1 also shows that the nurse chooses to skip certain topics (*e.g.* 'controlling body temperature' is not discussed before 'mobilising') and covers some topics out of the order presented on the assessment form. It is therefore worth noting that the choice of how to specifically question patients regarding these topics is at the discretion of individual nurses. The assessment form merely reminds the nurse of the details that might be noted during admission and lists them in a prefixed order, but does not dictate the practical shape the gathering of the patient information might take. Indeed, the topic headings merely mapped out the topic areas for discussion as nurses rarely followed the exact order of the topics as written on the assessment sheet.

Concerns have previously been noted about how nurses' and physicians' use of paper or computerised templates tends to 'crowd out' the patient's voice (Berg and Bowker 1997, Harris *et al.* 1998, Rhodes *et al.* 2006). These concerns have led to guidelines recommending that nurses should not follow assessment frameworks too rigidly as they may prevent nurses from critically thinking about the significance and type of information they are gathering from patients (Dougherty and Lister 2008). It is evident from the data presented in this section that, on the whole, topic selection during the admission interview is guided by the admission framework, rather than being rigidly followed by nurses. However, in the next section data are explored which suggest that nurses, on occasion, follow the admission framework more rigidly. It will be shown that a more rigid adherence to the admission template has implications both for the type of information that is gathered from patients and for the patient's voice within the interaction.

Delaying patient descriptions of their illness history to fit with corresponding areas of the nursing record: The previous section discusses how the assessment document functions as an informal prompt sheet for the topics to be covered during the patient's admission and that the patients' 'activities of daily living' were assessed as a series of single, unconnected topic areas (bowels, hygiene, walking). However, patients rarely experience symptoms of illnesses or problems with daily living activities as single events or as clearly defined topic areas. Regardless of this, nurses repeatedly directed the interaction according to the particular area of the paperwork (and the one topic) that was being completed at that time. The focus on one topic at a time was problematic for patients as seen in the following extract, where a nurse is admitting a patient onto the neurology ward for investigations into recurring headaches.

Extract 2: Mb2 – Delayed discussion of headaches, 11 minutes into the admission.

176	n	YOU DO a lot round the house then to help is it-
177	p	well (.) mu::muck in- with the daughters come in =
178	n	= do they oh ok
179	p	wu since April I can't (.) bloody do much cos I (.) =
180	n	= alrigh
181	p	because these headaches come straight away-
182	n	...°right ...

183		(0.8)
184	n	what type of accommodation do you live in↑
185	p	we've gorra council house

2 minutes later, following discussion/recording of patient's occupational status (retired) and confirmation of his General Practitioner's details.

208	n	right (.) reason for admission
209		(1.6)
210	p	hu:headac[hes]
211	n	[hu] (.) headaches right how long have you been having these
212		headaches
213	p	uhm since last April

In Extract 2, the nurse whilst completing the 'Social factors' part of the form asks the patient a question regarding his house cleaning arrangements. In the course of answering, the patient discusses needing assistance with the house work ('I can't bloody do much' – line 179) in relation to his reasons for being admitted ('these headaches' – line 181). Therefore, the patient clearly introduces 'headaches' at this point as a relevant consideration which limits his ability to 'do much'. However, in this case it paves the way for a further question on 'social factors' concerning 'accommodation'. Previous CA studies reveal that acknowledgement tokens, such as the nurse's 'right' (line 182) and subsequent pause (line 183) are 'closure implicative' (Jefferson 1972: 317) and pave the way for the introduction of another topic. In this case, however, a topic is re-introduced, namely the discussion of 'social factors' such as 'accommodation' (line 184).

The subject of headaches, however, is re-introduced later in the admission as the nurse asks 'reason for admission' (line 208 – corresponding to the box 'Reason for admission/referral'). Interestingly, the question is met with a considerable silence (1.6 seconds) suggesting that the patient experiences some difficulty with the preceding talk (Pomerantz 1984). Furthermore, fieldnotes written immediately afterwards noted how 'exasperated' the patient appeared during this stage of the admission.

One possible reason for the difficulty is that the patient had already clarified that 'headaches' were a major concern and constituted the reason for admission. The pause may also display the patient's expectation that the nurse takes into account what had been said beforehand, an expectation related to the notion of 'recipient design'. Boyd and Heritage (2006) note that the principle of recipient design is critical to the achievement of rapport in healthcare interaction, as questioning patients in a way that is orientated to their responses to previous questions 'will generally tend to be heard as sensitive, concerned, and caring' (2006: 164).

Extract 3 demonstrates a similar occurrence, featuring a different interview and nurse on the neurology ward, where a patient is being admitted for 'investigations into ?prolapse disc'.

Extract 3: VG432 – 9 minutes into admission – delayed discussion of sleep

211	n	are you able to sleep with the pain
212	p	oh:: I'm no good sleeping like (.) I'm up at 3
213	n	have you been taking tablets to help with the sleep
214	p	the GP wouldn't give me sleeping tablets and when I go to bed =
215	n	= right you've come in for tests into pain in your back

216		(9.0) ((nurse writing in notes))
217	n	right have you had any falls at all

6 minutes later following discussion of mobility, hygiene, diet and elimination

499	n	how are you with sleeping
500		(2.0)
501	p	I::: uh I'll go to sleep (.) wake up (.) for a bit like =
502	n	= mmhuh↑

Whilst discussing 'reason for admission' (back pain) the nurse asks the patient 'are you able to sleep with the pain' (line 211). The patient proceeds to explain that sleeping is difficult (line 212), adding that the GP refused to prescribe sleeping tablets (line 214). However, the discussion of sleep/bed time is terminated by the nurse stating the reason for admission (line 215) and withdrawing eye contact via the act of writing 'admitted for investigation re. back pain' in the notes. Six minutes later the nurse re-introduces the topic of sleep (line 499), resulting in a delay component of two seconds before the patient hesitantly begins to answer.

Patients therefore display difficulties when previously disclosed information is revisited during the assessment interview. As they never see a copy of the assessment form, patients have no way of knowing that earlier discussion of 'headaches' or 'sleep' are re-introduced by nurses in an attempt to co-ordinate talk with the sequence of topics appearing on the paperwork. Fieldnotes suggest that this feature of the assessment interview proved irritating to the patients, and it may well be that patients expect nurses to be sensitive to earlier answers. Interestingly, critics of standardised research interviews have similarly found that a lack of recipient design during interviews produces awkward interactions (Maynard and Schaeffer 2006, Woofitt and Widdicombe 2006).

The influence of reading and writing in the notes on patient interaction: As already noted, the assessment was frequently punctuated by nurses writing in the patient's admission documents. For example, Extract 4 (below) sees the nurse and patient discussing the patient's previous medical history before the nurse's gaze moves towards the notes placed on the table in front of her where she writes in the 'previous admissions' box 'Hysterectomy 24 years ago'.

Extract 4: VR206 – 4 minutes in, patient admitted to medical ward for shortness of breath

51	p	I had a hysterectomy
52	n	when was that
53	p	hu::: twenny four years ago now twenny five
54	n	°oh alright° ok
55	n	(10) ((writing in notes))
56	n	any other medical problems
57	p	uhm (.) yeh my ( ) (on-going?) problems (swelling?)
58	n	your ankles still swell do they
59	p	yeh and my blood pressure is quite high my blood pressure
60	n	(4.0) ((writing in notes))

Following the 10 seconds it takes for the nurse to write in the notes (line 55), supplementary questions on the related theme of 'other medical problems' are introduced, followed by the patient's answers which are immediately written in the notes. Although none of the nurses explained to patients that periods of interaction would sometimes be followed by periods of writing, the patients' conduct was sensitive to nurses' interactions with the notes as they rarely interrupted or questioned nurses whilst they wrote. Therefore, nurses' re-direction of gaze (away from the patient) when writing in the notes had significant consequences for the production of patient talk. However, rather than assuming that the use of nursing notes remain stable throughout interactions, Heath and Hindmarsh (2002: 118) recommend that the use of objects such as nursing records be examined to understand how they 'come to gain their particular significance at specific moments within courses of action'. With this in mind, the following extracts demonstrate specific moments where the nursing records achieve particular significance during the admission interview.

Extract 5: TDJ034 – opening turns of admission to medical ward, the patient being interviewed by the nurse following assessment by the doctor.

1	p	what's this for now↑
2	n	we're just going to admit you
3		((nurse shuffles the forms and bangs them on the desk))
4		(1.5) ((nurse reading the notes))
5	p	[you shouldn't have to]
6	n	[you remem-member] =
7	n	mmh
8	p	= shouldnt have to readmit me ther-the Dr came to clerk me this morning
9	n	°ahh°
10		(10) ((nurse reading through notes and organising the paperwork))
11	n	°right° (.) can I have your telephone number
12	p	zero two three

The patient mistakenly reports there to be no need for the nurse to repeat the admission process as she has already been admitted by the ward doctor (see line 8). Whilst joint medical-nursing admissions do occur in some hospitals, it was not the case here. The nurse's hushed utterance (ahh – line 9) is followed by his engagement with the notes in such a way that is influential within the interaction. For example, the patient's behaviour is sensitive to the re-direction of the nurse's gaze (line 10) as no further discussion of the need to 'readmit' occurs whilst the notes are consulted. The silence which accompanies the nurse's reading is only broken when the nurse asks for the patient's telephone number (line 11), an utterance that simultaneously starts the disputed admission interview and silences the patient's queries about the need for 're-admission'. Overlooking the opportunity to explain the separate nursing and medical admission processes, the nurse then proceeds with a full assessment of the patient from this point onwards.

Extract 6 also demonstrates how reading the notes alters the course of the interaction, this time when a patient attempts a discussion of his cancer and treatment options.

Extract 6: DWA95 – 6 minutes into admission to a surgical ward for ongoing cancer treatment

47	n	did he get you to sign a consent form
48	p	no =
49	n	= sorry about that
50	p	not yet (.) so I think this is uh::m (.)°I can't° this is ( ) cancer in
51		the uh colon I had removed a tumour [remo]ved
52	n	[mhuh]
53	p	about uh > > twelve months ago < < by Mr Y and he's passed me on
54		now to Mr X so I don't know whether its all related with the cancer
55		in the uhm (.) oesopha::g
56	n	oesophagus
57	p	oesophagus yeh (.) so they're trying to burn it away now
58	n	righty ho
59		(10) ((nurse reading/looking at notes))
60	p	I don't know whether I've got much to worry about at my age (laughs
61		a bit) I think they're anxious for me to get a telegram from the Queen
62		((patient laughs for 1.2 seconds))
64		((nurse laughs for 1.5 seconds)
65		(4.0) ((nurse looking at notes))
66	n	so you've had a right hemicolectomy in the past didn you
67	p	yes

Towards the end of an explanation of recent hospital treatment which begins on line 53, the patient appears to 'probe' for more information towards the end of this turn, stating 'I don't know whether it's all related with the cancer ...' (lines 54–55). The nurse does not 'hear' this as a probe, for example by responding to or exploring the patient's concerns; instead, she helps with the pronouncement of terminology (line 56). The patient continues describing his treatment 'they're trying to burn it away now' (line 57) followed by the nurse's response 'righty ho' (line 58), an idiom associated with attempts to close interaction (Beach and Dixson 2001), and disengagement of eye contact to read the notes (2001: 59).

A deviation from the norm, however, occurs, as the patient breaks the silence accompanying the nurse's reading by repeating an earlier theme of uncertainty, stating 'I don't know if I've got much to worry about at my age' (line 60). The patient continues by speculating that his imminent treatment is motivated by others': ('they') wish him to 'get a telegram from the Queen'. Both laugh at this point, with the nurse's laugh marginally outlasting the patient's before trailing off into another four seconds of silence as the nurse reads the notes. This short period of reading leads to the re-starting of the interview with an unrelated point 'so you've had a right hemicolectomy. ...' (line 65). The word 'so' can be heard as a direct effect of the nurse reading the notes, and has the immediate effect of orientating the interaction to what was just read (Beach and Dixson 2001) in contrast to what was just discussed and laughed about (cancer and prognosis). Further talk about cancer treatment and prognosis remained unvoiced during the remainder of the interview.

Extract 6 sees the patient offer an account of his previous hospital experience which is unrelated to a question. Such 'off-topic' departures can be used by patients to accomplish a range of ancillary tasks, for example they can be used to introduce features of the patient's life-world which are matters of significance or preoccupation. Heritage and Stivers (1999) propose that departures exist in defiance of the restrictive agenda of physicians' questioning, providing insights into what was 'on the patient's mind' (1999: 165). The off-topic departure in Extract 6 can be heard in the same way, with the talk, temporarily at least, being focused on the patient's own preoccupations and topics rather than the nurse's.

Patient-initiated departures have the potential to offer nurses different interactional possibilities where patients lead the discussion. Yet what is emerging is that the initial assessment constitutes an environment in which patient-led talk is most often curtailed. As a result, what was 'on the patient's mind' is not responded to during the admission, which according to nursing literature and policy at least, appears to be the ideal forum for such discussion. One possible reason for this could be related to a question of relevance. Off-topic expansions neither respond to a prior question nor offer clarification of an earlier response. As the nurses' actions suggest, they therefore have little relevance to the form-filling task at hand.

Documentation reduces patient participation: In this section I compare the entries written into the nursing record with the 'raw material' (Hak 1992: 145) of the actual spoken interaction used to produce the record. In particular, the comparison will show how patients' utterances are transformed into a written 'nursing history'. Guidelines produced by the UK nursing regulatory body specify that the nursing record should demonstrate a full account of the patient's assessment in addition to being factual, accurate and 'recorded in terms that the patient/client can understand' (Nursing and Midwifery Council 2007: 2).

With this in mind, Extract 7 provides a typical stretch of interaction where the nurse and patient are discussing the topic of sleep.

Extract 7: EGH 239 – 14 minutes into admission to a cardiology ward for investigations into chest pain

247	n:	How-how long do you sleep (.) for ↑
248		(3.2)
249	p:	°Uh:: I wake quite early uhm:: °
250	n:	How many hours do you sleep at night?
251	p:	Well I try and get 8 hours but its not- its not always 11 o'clock umh
252		(0.6)
253	n:	Broken sleep is it↑
254	p:	I sleep til seven probably yeh yeh
255		(0.5)
256	n:	How many hours a night rough::ly↑
257	p:	(0.5) Say seven um I think
258		(7.8) ((n writes in notes))
259	n:	Righty ho (.) so you're a retired gentleman

Of interest here is that the above interaction about the patient's sleep is written onto the assessment sheet by the nurse as 'Sleeps 7hrs a night'. Looking at the transcript and listening to the tape, it is clear that the written version of the patient's sleep (entered into the 'Sleeping' section of the form) does not capture the nuance of the verbal description of the patient's sleep pattern. The transcript shows a series of qualifiers ('probably' line 254, 'I think' line 257) which together with the pauses between questions (lines 248, 252) and equivocation (line 249) suggest that the patient may regard the nurse's questions as problematic. Indeed the patient appears to reject the original premise of the question (How long. ...) by attempting an answer that initially avoids any quantification of the length of sleep.

However, the question of how long the patient sleeps is repeated a further two times (lines 250 and 256). Each repeat of the question follows a response by the patient which draws upon personal experience to describe a night's sleep (lines 249 and 251), answers which are declined until a more objective quantification of time is produced (7 hours line 257). What becomes apparent is that the repeating of the question is due to the nurse pursuing a category of answer (number of hours) which is different from the category of answer (quality of sleep pattern) actually given by the patient. The initial question regarding how duration of sleep is repeated until this category of answer is provided.

A review of the 'Sleeping' section of the assessment documents collected during this study showed that all documents contained a quantification of sleep rather than a description of sleep pattern. However, it is important to note that the discussion of quantity rather than the quality of patients' sleep in Extract 7 is not 'caused' by the assessment tool; it is instead the result of the way nurses choose to implement the record at this particular time. Whilst other nursing records specifically determine the type of content allowable (certain sections of a fluid chart can only be filled using metric numerical data e.g. 20 mls), the assessment sheet only pre-structures broad topic areas rather than the exact type of information to be collected. In this way the assessment sheet can be seen as a mediating rather than a determining presence during the interaction.

As already touched upon, the information about 'sleeping' that is finally recorded in the patient's notes is not a direct reflection of the patient's utterance but the outcome of the nurse's interpretation of the nature of a permissible response and her pursuit of such a response. While the statement 'sleeps 7 hours a night' may be technically correct the patient's actual experience, which he tried to volunteer, was lost. A comparable restriction of patient histories is noted in Berg's (1996) study of doctor-patient consultation. Berg noted that writing down one line summaries of complex medical and social issues produced a particular rendering of patients' histories that appeared more manageable on paper than when communicated verbally by the patient.

Discussion

Assessing the impact of paper-based technology on nurse-patient interaction is timely, as the UK health service moves towards the use of EPRs. Policy makers have favourably contrasted EPRs to current paper-based records which they describe as antiquated, inefficient and a threat to patient safety (WAG 2003). However, nurses have consistently adopted a negative stance towards EPR, with a particularly enduring concern being that electronic systems restrict the patient's voice and individuality (Darbyshire 2004, Kirshbaum 2004, Lee 2006, Rhodes et al. 2006, Rodrigues 2001). For example, Rhodes et al. (2006: 374) state that moves towards the use of computerised templates in nursing 'risk emphasising diagnostics over therapeutics and diminish the patient to a minor supporting role'. Somewhat ironically, therefore, this study shows that nursing practice using 'old' paper-based technology limits patient participation and the patient's voice in similar ways to those attributed to 'new' electronic technologies.

Therefore, an alternative consideration of the use of technology in nursing and in other areas of healthcare practice is required, one which follows on from Timmermans and Berg's (2003) plea neither to over- nor under-estimate the role of technology in healthcare and which focuses not only on templates (computerised or paper), but on the practitioners who use them. Ventres *et al.* (2006) provide a fine example of one such study that considers the practitioner more fully than most. Their recent ethnographic findings discuss how 'physician style' was a major determinant of how EPR technology was used in encounters with patients. For example, those doctors with an 'interpersonal style' were led more by patient narratives than those with an 'informationally focused' style who positioned themselves at the computer monitor and asked computer-guided questions.

Borrowing Ventres' terminology, the nurses in this study utilised an 'information focused' style of interaction asking 'template-guided' questions. It is impossible in this study to categorically state why the nurses utilised a 'template-guided' style of interaction with patients which appears at odds with best-practice guidelines for the assessment. In these busy and time-scarce clinical environments nurses' use of the admission template certainly aided in managing the recurring task of taking a patient's history.

An easy answer would be to cite the admission document template itself, a position that would reverse the historical tendency that sees nurses view such technologies as neutral objects which have little tangible effect on actual care-giving (Barnard 2002). For example, one could point to the way in which the interaction follows the overall shape of the template, and the way in which detailed answers given by patients were sometimes reduced to a few words and figures that fitted into, for example, the 'Sleeping' box. In other words, one could claim the document controlled the interaction. Yet, at other times nurses could be seen to skip or change the sequence of topics appearing on the document (as shown in Figure 1) and the template makes no practical recommendations about how nurses should interact with patients during its completion. Overall, the admission document could not function without the nurses working with it, the implication of which is that no one element is in control, nurses, patients or the assessment template.

Viewing the assessment documents as only one of many factors that influence interaction between nurses and patients is an alternative to the somewhat naive notion that technologies such as paper documents act with 'super technological powers' to control the actions of all others (Timmermans and Berg 2003: 100). Yet, such technological determinism is still evident in literatures and policy documents concerning management and information technologies. For example, the case for introduction of the Electronic Patient Record in Wales is partially made by policy makers who describe how 'antiquated paper-based systems' frustrate 'effective record keeping and potentially threaten the quality of care and patient safety' (Welsh Assembly Government 2003: 59). Explanations rarely consider exactly how the use of paper-based systems (could) exert these effects.

What the data do show is that the initial assessment interview, which has been forwarded as an important area of nurse-patient interaction within which patients are supposed to be active participants, sees patients largely take the role of passive responders. There is, however, little consensus about what patient participation is (Collins *et al.* 2007); at the same time there is mounting evidence that whilst some patients expect greater involvement during healthcare, others want little (Barratt 2005).

The kinds of guidance that nurses are given regarding communication with patients during initial admission interviews and how to provide opportunities for their participation should therefore be more informed by a better understanding of the interactional dynamics of, and the contextual influences on, nurse-patient encounters. For example, evidence suggests that many health professionals lack the requisite skills and that the contexts of care delivery (including socio-economic influences and work pressures) bring their own constraints (Collins *et al.* 2007), all of which are important factors which textbooks and policy documents do not currently address. Therefore, in any nurse-patient encounter, the particular constraints that govern how patients are involved and the extent of their influence on interaction are likely to shift from one moment to the next. Making this point clear in 'best-practice' guidelines would better highlight the potential for patient participation regardless of the presence of electronic or paper-based templates, the constraints of time, and so on.

Conclusion

Most hospital nurses in the UK still operate with paper rather than electronic technology, thus the data provide a timely insight into current nursing practices. The imminent introduction of EPRs into hospitals provides a challenge to all health professionals, and nurses have raised concerns regarding the introduction of EPRs on the grounds that electronic records will 'crowd out' the patient's agenda, resulting in the 'de-individualisation of care' (Lee 2005: 345). However, on the evidence of this study, nurses' decisions to shape the assessment interview around the structure and layout of the assessment document serve to suppress the expression of patient concerns whilst minimising patient participation.

Berg and Bowker's (1997) work on medical interaction suggested over a decade ago that instead of focusing on either the tool or the work practice it is their interrelation that is central. The analysis here similarly suggests that other factors need further consideration rather than merely focusing on the technology which accompanies the interaction. Nurses' use of paper-based or electronic records needs to be seen by nurse managers, researchers and policy makers as a social action embedded within a larger system of activity. This socio-technical view of nursing work, therefore, undermines the previously rationalist, technology-centred writing so pervasive within the nursing literature. A more balanced approach towards technology and its effects on nursing work suggests further research is needed into how nurses learn to use and then apply their understanding of paper-based (and electronic) technology to their daily practice. Such work would provide an invaluable adjunct to the current plethora of studies which focus on nurses' attitudes and perceptions regarding the introduction of specific information management technology.

Acknowledgements

My thanks to the reviewers and the editors for their valuable comments on earlier versions of this chapter. Thanks also to the patients and nurses who agreed to take part in this study, and to the RCBC (Wales)/The Health Foundation Fellowship scheme which allowed time to be dedicated to the writing of this chapter.

References

Barnard, A. (2002) Philosophy of technology and nursing, *Nursing Philosophy*, 3, 1, 15–26.
Barratt, J. (2005) A case study of styles of patient self-presentation in the nurse practitioner primary health care consultation, *Primary Health Care Research and Development*, 6, 327–38.
Beach, W. and Dixson, C. (2001) Revealing moments: formulating understandings of adverse experiences in a health appraisal interview, *Social Science and Medicine*, 52, 25–44.

Berg, M. (1996) Practices of reading and writing: the constitutive role of the patient record in medical work, *Sociology of Health and Illness*, 18, 4, 499–524.

Berg, M. and Bowker, G. (1997) The multiple bodies of the medical record: toward a sociology of an artifact, *Sociology Quarterly*, 38, 511–35.

Boyd, E. and Heritage, J. (2006) Taking the history: questioning during comprehensive history-taking. in Heritage, J. and Maynard, D. (eds) *Communication in Medical Care. Studies in interactional Sociolinguistics 20*. Cambridge: Cambridge University Press.

Collins, S., Britten, N., Thompson, A. and Ruusuvuori, J. (eds) (2007) *Patient Participation in Health-care Consultations*. Buckingham: Open University Press.

Crawford, P. and Brown, B. (2004) Communication. In Mallick, M., Hall, C. and Howard, D. (eds) *Nursing Knowledge and Practice Foundations for Decision Making*. 2nd Edition. London: Balliere Tindall.

Currell, R. and Urquhart, M. (2004) *Nursing Record Systems: Effects on Nursing Practice and Health Care Outcomes*. The Cochrane Library. Issue 4.

Darbyshire, P. (2004) 'Rage against the machine?': Nurses' and midwives' experiences of using computerized patient information systems for clinical information, *Journal of Clinical Nursing*, 13, 1, 17–25.

Dougherty, L. and Lister, S. (2004) *The Royal Marsden Manual of Clinical Nursing Procedures*. Oxford: Blackwell Science.

Dougherty, L. and Lister, S. (2008) *The Royal Marsden Manual of Clinical Nursing Procedures. Student Edition* Oxford: Blackwell Science.

Drew, P. and Heritage, J. (eds) (1992) *Talk at Work. Interaction in Institutional Settings*. Cambridge: Cambridge University Press.

Hak, T. (1992) Psychiatric records as transformation of other texts. In Watson, G. and Seiler, R. (eds) *Text in Context. Contributions in Ethnomethodology*. Newbury Park: Sage.

Harris, R., Wilson-Barnett, J., Griffiths, P. and Evans, A. (1998) Patient assessment: validation of a nuring instrument, *International Journal of Nursing Studies*, 35, 303–13.

ten Have, P. (2004) *Understanding Qualitative Research and Ethnomethodology*. London: Sage.

Heath, C. (1986) *Body Movement and Speech in Medical Interaction*. Cambridge: Cambridge University Press.

Heath, C. and Hindmarsh, J. (2002) Analyzing interaction: video, ethnography and situated conduct. In May, Y. (ed.) *Qualitative Research in Action*. London: Sage.

Heath, C., Luff, P. and Sanchez Svenson, M. (2003) Technology and medical practice, *Sociology of Health and Illness*, 25, 3, 75–96.

Heritage, J. and Stivers, T. (1999) Online commentary in acute medical visits: a method of shaping patient expectations, *Social Science and Medicine*, 49, 1501–17.

HES (2007) Headline Figures 2006–07. Accessed 18th July 2008 from http://www.hesonline.nhs.uk/Ease/servlet/ContentServer?siteID=1937&categoryID=193.

Jefferson, G. (1972) Side sequences. In Sudnow, D.N. (ed.) *Studies in Social Interaction*. New York, NY: Free Press.

Jefferson, G. (1984) On the organization of laughter in talk about troubles. in Atkinson, J.M. and Heritage, J. (eds) *Studies in Conversation Analysis*. Cambridge: Cambridge University Press.

Kaner, E., Heaven, B., Rapley, T., *et al.* (2007) Medical technology and communication: a video based process study of the use of decision aids in primary care consultations, *BMC Medical Informatics and Decision Making*, 7, 2, 1–11.

King, I. (1971) *Toward a Theory of Nursing: General Concepts of Human Behaviour*. New York: Wiley.

Kirshbaum, M. (2004) Are we ready for the electronic patient record? Attitude and perceptions from staff from two NHS trust hospitals, *Health Informatics Journal*, 10, 4, 265–276.

Latimer, J. (2000) *The Conduct of Care*. Oxford: Blackwell Science.

Lee, T. (2005) Nurses' concerns about using information systems: analysis of comments on a computerized nursing care plan system in Taiwan, *Journal of Clinical Nursing*, 14, 344–53.

Lee, T. (2006) Nurses' perceptions of their documentation experiences in a computerized nursing care planning system, *Journal of Clinical Nursing*, 15, 11, 1376–82.

Lipsky, M. (1980) *Street-level Bureaucracy: Dilemmas of the Individual in Public Services*. New York: Russell Sage Foundation.

Maynard, D. and Schaeffer, N.C. (2006) Standardisation-in-interaction. The survey interview. In Drew, P., Raymond, G. and Weinberg, D. (eds) *Talk and Interaction in Social Research Methods*. London: Sage.

McGrath, J., Arar, N. and Pugh, J. (2007) The influence of electronic medical record usage on non verbal communication in the medical interview, *Health Informatics Journal*, 1, 32, 115–18.

Moloney, R. and Maggs, C. (1999) A systematic review of the relationships between written manual nursing care planning, record keeping and patient outcomes, *Journal of Advanced Nursing*, 30, 51–7.

Newman, J. and Vidler, E. (2006) Discriminating customers, responsible patients, empowered users: consumerism and the modernisation of health care, *Journal of Social Policy*, 35, 2, 193–209.

NHS Executive (1996) *Patient Partnership: Building a Collaborative Strategy*. Leeds: NHS Executive.

Nursing and Midwifery Council (2007) Record Keeping. Accessed 21/04/09 from http://www.nmcuk. org/aDisplayDocument.aspx?documentID=4008.

Nursing and Midwifery Council (2008) *The Code: Standards of Conduct, Performance and Ethics for Nurses and Midwives*. London: NMC.

Peräkylä, A. and Vehviläinen, S. (2003) Conversational analysis and the professional stocks of inter-actional knowledge, *Discourse and Society*, 14, 6, 727–50.

Pomerantz, A. (1984). Agreeing and disagreeing with assessments: some features of preferred/dispre-ferred turn shapes. in Atkinson, J.M. and Heritage, J. (eds) *Structures of Social Action*. Cambridge: Cambridge University Press.

Rhodes, P., Langdon, M., Rowley, E., *et al.* (2006) What does the use of a computerised checklist mean for patient-centred care? The example of a routine diabetes review, *Qualitative Health Research*, 16, 353–78.

Rodrigues, J. (2001) The complexity of developing a nursing information system: a Brazilian experi-ence, *Computers in Nursing*, 19, 98–104.

Royal College of Nursing (2003) *Defining Nursing*. London: Royal College of Nursing.

Ruusuvuori, J. (2001) Looking means listening: coordinating displays of engagement in doctor-patient interaction, *Social Science and Medicine*, 52, 1093–198.

Sahlsten, M., Larsson, I., Sjöström, B. and Kaety, P. (2008) An analysis of the concept of patient participation, *Nursing Forum*, 43, 1, 2–11.

Silverman, D. (2005) *Doing Qualitative Research. A Practical Handbook*. 2nd Edition. London: Sage.

Sully, P. and Dallas, J. (2005) *Essential Communication Skills for Nursing*. Edinburgh: Elsevier Mosby.

Timmermans, S. and Berg, M. (2003) The practice of medical technology, *Sociology of Health and Illness*, 25, 3, 97–114.

Tutton, E. (2005) Patient participation on a ward for frail older people, *Journal of Advanced Nursing*, 50, 2, 143–52.

Ventres, W., Kooienga, S., Vuckovic, N., *et al.* (2006) Physicians, patients and the electronic health record: an ethnographic analysis, *Annals of Family Medicine*, 4, 2, 124–31.

Welsh Assembly Government (2003) *Putting Patient and Public Involvement into Practice*. Signposts 2. London: OPM.

WHO (2005) *Health promotion in Hospitals: Evidence and quality management*. Copenhagen: World Health Organisation.

Woofitt, R. and Widdicombe, S. (2006) Interaction in interviews. In Drew, P., Raymond, G. and Weinberg, D. (eds) *Talk and Interaction in Social Research Methods*. London: Sage.

9

Listening to what is said – transcribing what is heard: the impact of speech recognition technology (SRT) on the practice of medical transcription (MT)

Gary C. David, Angela Cora Garcia, Anne Warfield Rawls and Donald Chand

Introduction

Automation and information technologies are increasingly being applied to all aspects of healthcare with the aim of lowering costs and improving the quality of treatment. Part of this effort is the projected $10 billion that will be spent over the next five years toward creating a US-based national health information network, with the expectation that the investment in 'electronic health records and new technology will reduce errors, bring down costs, ensure privacy, and save lives' (speech by President Barack Obama, February 24th, 2009). At the same time, as Mark Chassin, President of The Joint Commission (a non-profit healthcare accreditation organisation), notes 'Patient safety can be jeopardised when technology is not carefully planned, integrated, fixed, or updated' (Roop 2009: 11). Thus, while technology has the promise of improving healthcare, that its application will automatically result in doing so is not a foregone conclusion.

With this growing interest in using automation and information technology in healthcare has come emergent research on its actual use, focusing on tools such as speech recognition (Shneiderman 2000, Borowitz 2001, Mohr *et al.* 2003) and electronic medical records/electronic health records (Berg 1998, Clarke *et al.* 2001, Greatbatch *et al.* 1995, Heath and Luff 2000, Hing *et al.* 2007). This research has documented essential work practices and social competencies that need to be supported by new technologies in order for technical implementations to succeed (*e.g.* Greatbatch *et al.* 2005, Heath and Luff 2000). To date, however, these studies have focused primarily on doctors (particularly radiologists) and nurses, and not on the work practices and skilled knowledge of the MTs who have been, and in conjunction with SRTs still are, primarily responsible for the creation of medical records.

In this chapter we explore how MTs do the work of editing 'back-end' (BESR – edited after they are dictated) speech recognition-generated documents. In doing so, we will illustrate how the work of MTs is far more complex than just typing what is spoken in voice files. Their work requires complex professionally-informed interpretive acts that in turn require sustained attention to the social order properties and content of the doctor's dictation, knowledge of medical terms and procedures, and an understanding of interactional processes, conventions of dictating, and of producing monologic speech acts. The MTs attention to these social order properties of the doctor's (dictator's) speech has direct implications for understanding the impact not only of the implementation of back-end systems, but also of front-end systems (FESR – edited as they are written) in which there is no transcriptionist involved.

While such technologies are marketed as a cost-effective and timely way to produce medical records, they may actually slow down the work and involve the potential risk of removing third-party quality assurance from the process. We conclude that, while new technologies have a role to play in the creation of healthcare documentation, such production technologies (and their implementation) should in most instances focus on facilitating and supporting, rather than replacing, the work of medical transcription done by skilled human workers.

Medical transcription, speech recognition, and record production

In medicine, the patient medical record has become a critical component of nearly all aspects of healthcare. Medical records emerged to support specialisation and co-ordination in medicine, making information about patients available to the increasing number of personnel involved in treatment and payment (see Timmermans and Berg 2003). This was not always the case – as the country general practitioner had little use for such extensive documentation. As healthcare becomes more complex, the importance of medical records continues to increase. In facilitating co-ordination between groups, medical records operate as important 'boundary objects' (Star 1999, Star and Griesemer 1989) that cross organisational boundaries and can be accessed by a variety users, including doctors, reimbursement agents, insurance companies, legal professionals, medical researchers, billing coders, audit contractors, and the patient. Given this diverse and distributed community of use, the comprehensive detail and integrity of the record has become very important.

Records are not simply reports of 'what happened', but accounts created for social purposes and uses, situated in various institutional contexts and without which neither co-ordinated action, or even compensation for services, may be possible. Garfinkel (1967: 186–207) noted in his study of record-keeping practices in a psychiatric clinic that, while records are created by individuals, they must be recognisably valid as competent accounts in organisational terms. He called this 'institutional accountability'. Similarly, medical records are not just for the originating doctor, but must also be recognisable and meaningful to other healthcare professionals. Formatting such documents according to widely recognisable standards – in institutionally accountable terms – is essential to their usability and validity. While a limited number of people may be present for a given medical encounter, the number of potential 'witnesses' to the event increases when the encounter becomes an accessible record.

Despite the centrality and importance of medical records, and the growing interest in them, relatively little research has been done on the process of their creation. Most attention has been given to the new technologies, while the skilled practices and social competencies of MTs have received relatively little attention. To the extent that the work practices of MTs add significant value to the medical record, systems that replace them could have a negative impact – unless they take the competencies of MTs into account. That the vast majority of MTs are women, at a time when the pay and status of women are still unequal, may have contributed to their current invisibility. However, their actual visibility has also changed. In the past MTs worked directly in the hospital or clinic setting, sometimes sitting in operating theatres taking dictation during surgeries. This is however no longer the case for most MTs. New technologies (improved information networks, computers, digital voice files) have resulted in most MTs telecommuting (with approximately 72 per cent of MTs worldwide working from home (David *et al.* 2008)).

Thus, their figurative invisibility has now become literal in their absence from the health-care setting.

Arguably the most significant change to the work of creating medical records has been the introduction of SRTs to create a written transcript of a doctor's dictated notes on a medical encounter. There are two ways that SRTs perform their role: synchronous recognition ('front-end' speech recognition – FESR) or asynchronous recognition ('back-end' speech recognition – BESR). Dictation typically occurs when doctors orally record (through a telephone, cell phone, microphone, or into a handheld tape recorder) a version of what occurred in the medical encounter, including any supplemental 'relevant' information from past encounters, lab reports, etc., which they decide is important for patient care (and billing). With synchronous recognition (FESR), speech is immediately transformed into text, which can be viewed by the dictator as s/he speaks. With asynchronous recognition (BESR), the digitised voice file is processed after the dictation is completed, and then transformed into a written version.

Both methods require editing. The difference is that with FESR editing is possible at the same time of the dictation, while with BESR editing is only possible after the entire record has been dictated. Another important difference lies in who does the editing. With FESR, the original dictator (often a doctor) is typically the one to edit and check the document for accuracy; in BESR it is typically the MT who performs the editing function by listening to the original dictation voice file and comparing it to what was produced by the SRT system (while also checking for dictator accuracy). Thus, in BESR, the MT performs two checking functions: (1) checking the accuracy of the SRT, and (2) checking the accuracy of the dictator.

Technology vendors have advocated both synchronous and asynchronous uses of SRTs for the production of cheaper, faster, and more accurate medical records. The extent of these claims varies by vendor, and their comparability is complicated by the different methodologies used by each company to justify their product (*Speech Recognition Adoption* 2008). While companies differ in whether the technology is offered as a replacement of medical transcription or as a tool for assisting the process, a consistent claim across the speech recognition industry is that SRTs can reduce costs due to faster turn-around times of medical documentation, higher efficiency, and increased accuracy. One hospital is reported (Wright *et al.* 2007) to speak of eliminating all transcription costs. An article entitled 'Less paper, less fuss, better patient care' reported greater efficiency and better patient care as a result of implementing health information technology (Schock 2007). SRT vendors (*e.g.* M*Modal, eScription, and Nuance) provide case studies that support the claim that their products will deliver on their promises, presenting SRT either as an important transcription aid, or as a complete replacement of those who do transcription.

Despite these promises, the literature reveals that results of SRT implementation have been mixed. Conn (2005: 38) reports that while 'technology is supposed to make medical transcription obsolete ... the demise of the medical transcription industry is greatly exaggerated'. This is due to the lack of accuracy found in SRT systems. Because of problems with accuracy and ease of use, 'experts confirm that outside of radiology and pathology, relatively few physicians have adopted the technology' (Goedert 2006: 44). While SRT has its place, van Terheyden (2005: 45), the Chief Medical Officer of a SRT company, notes that 'it is neither a panacea nor the Holy Grail'.

Part of the problem stems from the way in which SRTs are able to perform their work. SRTs generally treat transcription as a process independent of social and professional competencies. In order to produce a clean transcript SRTs treat hesitations, repeats and many other social order properties of speech as 'disfluencies' (see Extract 1). In cases of ambiguity SRTs do not leave out or flag terms as problematic. Instead, they 'choose' a word, often based on 'mathematic probabilities of when and how often words will appear in a particular context' (AHIMA 2003: 1). SRTs cannot create order in a file if the dictator has failed to record explicit and clear directions for this. Similarly, they cannot correct dictator errors, correct punctuation – or treat a repeat as a correction – without direction.

The work of doing medical transcription involves a complex set of tasks (see David, Chand and Garcia 2008, Garcia *et al.* 2008). MTs not only type what is dictated. They verify the spelling of medical terms and orient complex social order properties in the dictation, as well as recognise repeats, hesitations, and corrections in the monologue. They also flag critical medical errors and organise the transcript to meet the requirements of an organisational and legal record. In addition they can discern voice inflections for punctuation, convert spoken language into grammatical written language, filter background noise and distractions in the voice file, and check specific elements in the dictation against the larger context of the record. In cases of ambiguity they are trained either to omit or flag the questionable item. MTs are able to accomplish these tasks not only because of their training[1] in anatomy and physiology, pharmacology, legal issues, laboratory testing, and a range of medical specialisations, but because of their knowledge of mundane procedures and routine practices of interaction and spoken language. Through the application of this combination of professional and mundane social knowledge, the transcriptionist generates a record that complies with medical and legal standards – rather than just reproducing a sound file in written form. Transcription involves essential knowledge work based on social practices and is not just manual labour (*i.e.* typing).

The extent to which work is perceived as largely 'manual' or 'knowledge' work often is important when determinations are made whether technology can or should replace and/ or restructure work. Work that is considered more manual than knowledge based is typically at greater risk of being impacted by technology implemented as 'labour saving'. In fact, the most seemingly menial jobs can require extensive professional sense-making practices. As Rose (2004: xxvi) notes, 'In the rhetoric of the "new economy", communication skills, general problem-solving skills, or the ability to work in teams are privileged, and more likely to be treated as knowledge work, while more specific mechanical skills – associated with conventional blue-collar work – tend to be perceived as less valuable'. Research examining workplace practices has demonstrated that much knowledge and professional sense making goes into work that is deemed 'routine' and 'mundane'. For instance, Suchman (2000) in her study of legal secretaries found that informed judgment had to be exercised in examining and coding documentation related to a legal case. As Whalen, Whalen and Henderson (2002: 239) note, 'the traditional topics of "work routines" and "routinisation" need to be respecified in order to take into account how any "routine" is a contingently produced result.' In the end, attempts to 'save labour' through technological standardisation can have the impact of actually impeding work due to an interference with essential work skills, practices and routines.

The implementation of labour-saving technology, and more general standardisation of work, has also been linked to a deskilling of workers. Braverman's classic studies (1955, 1974) of automation questioned the extent to which technology contained the promise for a better society or sowed the seeds for social problems. Leo Marx (1987) questioned whether technology brings progress, or whether people are becoming increasingly disenchanted with the unfulfilled promise, and sometimes unethical application, of technology. Many studies address the impact of technology on work and deskilling (Garson

1988, Zuboff 1988, Orlikowski 1992, Harper *et al.* 2000). As Castells (1996: 263) notes, 'The effects of these technological changes on office work are not yet fully identified, because empirical studies, and their interpretation, are running behind the fast process of technological change'.

The impact of labour-saving technology on healthcare specifically has become an important topic for examination. Ritzer and Walczak (1988: 13) observe 'Not only are advanced technologies coming to control physicians, they are also helping to reduce the physician's authority over patients'. Greatbatch *et al.* (2005) found the implementation of a telephone triage system, while providing a certain structure to the performance of work, did not explicitly dictate (or standardise) how that work was actually delivered. Rather, nurses continued to try and exercise their professional beliefs and practices, which could pose significant challenges to technological implementation.

While there are some industry studies, however problematic, on the accuracy of the SRT, little research exists on the impact of SRT technologies on the actual work of creating medical records. To understand the impact of SRT on how MTs do their work, this chapter examines the use of an asynchronous SRT system (back-end BESR) by MTs in an acute healthcare setting. We examine how the technology integrates into the existing workplace practices of MTs (part of a larger study on medical transcription and the production of healthcare documentation). While SRTs can be an effective tool, the data also reveal potential limitations and dangers of over-reliance on SRTs. The technology not only impacts on how the work gets done, but has potential effects on the quality and the integrity of the resulting medical record.

Data and methods

The research reported here is part of a larger ongoing ethnographic project investigating the production of healthcare documentation. Fieldwork has involved observations and participation with both MTs and their professional associations, and with professionals and taskforces in the SRT industry. The project is rooted in an ethnomethodological (EM) approach that focuses on 'the ordinary "methods" through which persons conduct their practical affairs' (Lynch 1993: 5). Founded on the work of Harold Garfinkel (1967), the central argument is that all meaningful social objects and practices, including work, are constituted by social order properties and 'depend for their coherence on constant attention to, and competent display of, shared member's methods (ethno-methods) rather than on formal structures, or individual motivation' (Rawls 2008: 701). In the case of MTs the voice file and its socially ordered properties – as oriented and recognised by MTs – are the focus of analysis. EM is concerned with what Garfinkel (1996: 6) calls the 'What More' can be understood about the production of any local order phenomena beyond that which can be rendered through formal analytic approaches. Our research seeks to uncover the details of 'transcription-at-work'.

Along with attention to the detailed production of work, project data also included an online survey of MTs (n = 3807), 33 interviews with persons in the MT industry, eight MT focus groups, and fieldwork and observations of MTs and dictators using speech recognition technology, doctors using front-end SRTs, and audio and video of the process. In addition, the first author has been involved as an observer and participant on numerous SRT industry committees related to quality assurance, performance metrics, and the adoption of SRT. All subjects were made aware of the project's goals, and interviews and focus group participants signed participant confidentiality statements.

To demonstrate the challenges associated with SRT transcription and the MT work of editing that transcript, we conducted a single case analysis of an MT, working at a regional New England hospital, who was using a back-end speech recognition engine to edit a physician dictation. The dictation was made by a neurologist recording an encounter with a patient hospitalised for head pain.[2] As in studies of conversation using a single episode of interaction (Schegloff 1987), we examine a single case to understand in detail the features of the human machine interaction that occurs between the dictator, the technology, and the MT. To do so, we transcribed a version of the dictated voice file (VF) that attempted to capture as many details of the sound file as possible – with a focus on preserving elements of its character as a sound file – without reducing it all to words, punctuation and other social conventions of speech. The entire 19 minute 32 second dictation was transcribed using conversation analytic[3] (CA) notations (see Jefferson's transcription system in Atkinson and Heritage 1984). As in CA generally, punctuation in our VF transcript records punctuation marks where they can be clearly heard – rather than where they belong grammatically. The VF transcription was then analysed alongside the SRT-generated draft report (before MT editing), and the final edited medical record (the creation of which by the MT was observed in the worksite).

The creation of medical records is a social act (see Heath 1982), and therefore can be analysed as such. By observing in close detail the way the SRT 'hears' and transforms spoken words to text, and performs the formatting instructions included in the dictation, we can examine how the SRT performs. Similarly, as we analyse the MT's correction of the SRT's transcript in light of the doctor's dictation, the skills, knowledge, and practices used by MTs become visible.

Examining a single case of making a medical record

Natural features of dictation and speech recognition
The ability to recognise and treat speech disfluencies (such as hesitation markers (*e.g.* 'uh'), pauses, drawing out of speech, 'tisking' sounds, changes in pitch, emphasis, and repeats/stutters) as meaningful social order properties of speech (*i.e.* indicating correction, punctuation, reordering) is a social skill necessary for communication. The sequential positioning of these features can impact on how turns of talk are understood and how words are heard.

While the capabilities of SRT systems vary, one common feature is filtering out speech disfluencies – eliminating them from the transcript altogether. While some speech disfluencies are indeed unnecessary, others make a significant contribution to the sense of talk. For instance, the SRT can inadvertently omit the indefinite article 'a' when it is pronounced as 'uh' rather than 'ā'. The SRT sometimes misses the significance of error repair (when the dictator repeats a word to correct an error in dictation). SRT technology is not always successful in differentiating between consequential and inconsequential disfluencies, tending to filter too much. SRT are marketed as having the ability to 'learn' from past mistakes. But as Shriberg (2001: 153) points out 'speech recognition models are often trained on read or highly constrained speech'. Subsequent corrections by the MT only successfully 'train' the SRT when the corrections are consistent. If the same mistake is corrected in the same way a number of times, then the SRT will 'learn' to produce the corrected term whenever it identifies the original term in a sound file. Both this ability and the need for the MT to attend to it introduce problems of their own.

Extract 1 demonstrates some of these issues.

Extract 1: Lines 20–21 of Dictation (all line #s refer to VF master transcription)
(VF is our transcription, followed by the SRT and MT versions)

VF   (0.2) no history of uh seeing zig zag lines, white or dark spots in front of her
       eyes in front of his eyes, (0.4) .h h no uh photophobia (0.3)
SRT   .... no history of seeing Z.
       5. Dark spots in front of her eyes in from his eyes. No photophobia.
MT   ... no history of seeing zig/zag lines, bright or dark spots in front of his eyes.
       There was no photophobia ...

There are a number of points to note here. The SRT drops the 'uh' before 'seeing', as it is supposed to. But, then it also removes part of the description of symptoms, rendering 'zig zag lines, white or' as 'Z. ((new line))'. The SRT then treats some part of the disfluent speech as punctuation and begins a new sentence and a new line – with an additional space – with the terms '5. Dark'. This creates format problems in the document. The SRT also misses a common dictator error; the doctor confusing and then subsequently correcting the gender of the patient. The doctor first says 'her eyes' then corrects this mistake to 'his eyes'. The SRT changes the repeated words 'in front' before 'her eyes' and 'his eyes' to 'in from' when they occur the second time. Not picking up on the error repair format, the SRT adds confusion and error to the transcript. Lastly, in recognising 'No photophobia' the SRT begins a new sentence as indicated by the dictator, but does not correct it to a complete sentence. In so doing it performed appropriately, but the resulting record does not look as competent as it might.

The MT, by contrast, is able to recognise the error correction format, and clean the draft: treating 'zig zag' as a meaningful term, not as a repeat that should be eliminated; retaining the words 'white or' instead of eliminating them; and turning the words 'no photophobia' into a grammatical statement. The MT, orienting the social order properties of language and making use of both professional training and ordinary human speech competencies, is able to produce a more accurate, grammatical and organisationally presentable document.

Extract 2 displays similar problems with disfluency resulting in format issues.

Extract 2: Lines 33–35 of Dictation

VF   .h next line uh (2.0) h uh next line um (1.5) past medical history (5.0) .hh
       unremarkable (0.2) except number one. number two, .hh he describes that
       accidentally he shot his uh (0.2) .h left hand
SRT   Knee and past medical history.
       Unremarkable except
       1.
       2. He describes that he does extend he short his left hand ...
MT   **Past Medical History**
       1. Unremarkable.
       2. He describes that accidentally he shot his left hand ...

First, the doctor provides the instruction 'next line', which the SRT follows. But, when the doctor repeats the instruction, the SRT renders the second instance of 'next line' as 'Knee', thus not only missing the repeat – but rendering the repeat as a section header – but without proper section header format (bold) and content. These headers are important as they often guide the reading of the record when readers are searching for information.

The doctor then dictates the patient's medical history out of order. After the direction for a major header 'past medical history' he begins the medical history without a number sequence and then makes the correction. The utterance '.hh unremarkable (0.2) except' is followed by the words 'number one. number two'. The SRT does its job of recognising what was said, but does not correct it. The SRT hears a command for 'number one' followed immediately by a command for 'number two' – and types the transcript as such. Finally, while the SRT is able to filter out various hesitation markers and in-breaths that are not relevant to the record, it misses the essential information about the gun accident, rendering it as 'he does extend he short his left hand'.

The MT formats the header to conform with expectations regarding document form, and then orients the number sequence to the requirements of a medical history. The MT also removes the word 'except' from the record and corrects the description of the gun accident. Generally, the MT applies professional knowledge of the information that needs to be contained in the record, knowledge of the preferred format, and mundane reasoning skills regarding social order properties of the dictation, to make the final version of the record.

Doctors rely on MTs to 'fill in the blanks' and understand how the record should look. SRTs do not possess the same ability. While they can often recognise words, they are not able to orient to social ordered properties of those words (the properties of a list, the properties of a correction), nor can they orient to expectations regarding document format without direction. MTs, employing social competencies, are able to treat the dictation as an 'intendedly unified object'; a social *gestalt*, and thus to compose the information into a complete, unified and organisationally accountable social object.

Punctuation, instructions, and dictation

While some dictators provide directions for punctuation, doctors typically rely on MTs to provide punctuation as needed to make the record a readable and socially and organisationally competent document. To accomplish this, MTs rely on their hearing of the dictator's intonation, their understanding of the content and the social order properties of speech, and their knowledge of how the finished document should look. SRTs sometimes add punctuation at appropriate points, but problematic placements and elisions of punctuation often occur. SRTs work from a rule-based application of grammar, whereas MTs have a social and situated understanding of sense-making practices.

In Extract 3 the SRT's use of punctuation creates errors in the transcript.

Extract 3: Lines 23–24 of Dictation

VF   (0.7) at thuh ee ar he had head cee tee scan which was reported as unremarkable .hh followed by a spinal tap which revea:led uh .h u:h unremarkable u:h cee ef es (0.4) s: studies. (0.8) .h next line since his admission ...

SRT   Sensory ER he had a head CT scan which was reported as unremarkable followed by a spinal tap which revealed unremarkable CSF. Studies since his admission ...

MT   In the Emergency Room he had a head CT scan which was reported as unremarkable followed by a spinal tap which revealed unremarkable CSF studies.
Since his admission. ...

The SRT adds the word 'sensory' at the beginning of the first line. Then at the end of the second line puts a full stop after CSF and begins a new sentence with 'Studies.' This breaks up a test result 'CSF studies'. In the dictation, 'studies' has audible 'period intonation', making it hearable as the last word in the utterance. The SRT's failure to insert a 'period' (full stop) after 'Studies' is odd given that it 'hears' and implements the 'next line' command which follows this word. A line break in the middle of a sentence is unlikely. The MT hears 'CSF' as belonging with 'studies', and then hears 'next line' not only as an instruction to begin a new line, but also to insert a space creating a new paragraph. In addition to correcting the beginning of the utterance and changing it into a competent sentence, the MT performs two analytical functions that the SRT does not: hearing the punctuation intonation in the doctor's voice, and applying formatting commands with an orientation toward overall document formatting requirements.

The issue of misplaced punctuation may seem minor. However, any error in a record can raise suspicion regarding the accuracy of its content. As errors increase, the readability of the record can go down. In a narrative example reported by MTs at the same facility the authors were told that a physician dictated 'Since she was transfused she notes she definitely feels stronger'. However, the SRT system rendered, 'Since she was transfused she notes that she ***does not*** feel stronger' (emphasis added). Such an error is particularly worrisome because there is nothing noticeably wrong with the sentence itself to indicate there might be a problem, yet it inaccurately portrays patient condition.

Furthermore, patient care is just one use of medical records, and errors that may not have consequences for patient care can have significant repercussions in a legal setting, or in billing. Consequently, the organisational goal is to have a record with few, if any, errors.

Not marking eroneous recognition: numbers and lab values
When an MT cannot decipher an utterance, she is trained to leave it blank or otherwise 'flag' it as unclear. There are two ways the SRT approaches sounds it treats as speech (not disfluencies) but that are difficult to decipher. The first is not transcribing them and marking them nontranscribable with the word '<skip>'. The second is to transcribe the speech incorrectly. The SRT does not currently seem to have the capability to mark a term it does transcribe as tentative.

SRTs sometimes have problems with numbers, whereas identifying relations between numbers in combination constitutes an ordinary human competency for the MT. Extracts 4 and 5 demonstrate this:

Extract 4: Lines 50–51 of Dictation

VF	... pulse is fifty <u>eight</u>:. .h temperature ninety seven point four
SRT	... pulse is 50, 8, temperature 97.4
MT	... pulse is 58. His temperature is 97.4.

Extract 5: Lines 73–74 of Dictation

VF	( ) is one point zero two (and calcium) is ten point two and uh (5.0)
SRT	... creatinine is 1.0 and calcium is 9.2 ...
MT	... creatinine is 1.02 and calcium is 10.2.

In Extract 4, the doctor's emphasis on the word eight (indicated by underlining in the VF transcript) may have caused the SRT to hear it as separate from the number begun as 'fifty'. However, in Extract 5, the SRT transcribes a creatinine level of 1.02 as '1.0' and a calcium level of 10.2 as '9.2'. Elsewhere in the record, the SRT transcribed a hematocrit level of 41.3 as '41.37' and lymphocyte 7% as 'lymphocytes seven was sent'. These are potentially significant errors for test results that the MT was able to notice and correct.

Incorrect lab values can cause major complications for patient care. It is common for dictators to speak rapidly through lab values, and MTs who have access to labs or a patient's medical history can use that information to clarify unintelligible dictation. A SRT does not have that ability, and therefore relies solely on what the dictator says.

Furthermore, MTs are trained to know the normal range of lab values. If lab values do not match the rest of the record (as when abnormal values are given for an otherwise normal patient), MTs can double check this information (when they have access), or at least flag the potential source of error.

Correcting the dictation

A number of factors work against the goal of creating an intelligible and presentable medical record. The chief challenge can be the dictator. A 2004 study by AHDI found that 27 per cent of errors in medical records were linked to dictator mistakes: including reversing left and right, changing genders, dictating the wrong lab values, and confusing patients and patient numbers. The MTs interviewed describe dictation marred by doctors eating and drinking while dictating, talking on cell phones, driving cars, exercising on treadmills, or transcribing in noise-rich environments.

Correcting the doctor's dictation is one of the most important functions of the MT – and one in which both professional training and social competence play a large but often unacknowledged role. Working with SRT systems can interfere with this function if the MT becomes focused on correcting the SRTs mistakes, and also 'training the system,' and not on the dictator's mistakes. Training the SRT basically means that the system can become 'smarter' when a word is corrected and the system 'learns' to recognise the dictated word in relation to the correction. However, this only works if the correction is consistently applied in the same manner. For an MT, accuracy can become a matching process between the SRT transcription and the dictation. The question of whether the original dictation was in fact correct can get lost. MTs have told a number of stories about how the SRT typed the name of a drug correctly, but the doctor had dictated the wrong drug. The MT noticed because the condition being described would not be treated by the drug named in the dictation. When the MT is distracted from the task of checking the doctor's dictation for mistakes in order to verify and check what the SRT has transcribed and correct it consistently, medically important dictator errors can be missed.

In addition to these difficulties, our survey and ethnographic data reveal that problems can result because the technology changes how the work is done. In interviews, MTs have talked about the brain working differently when transcribing dictation from when editing SRT generated documents. One MT explained it as 'funnelling the voice file through your fingers (when transcribing from a voice file) versus through your eyes (when editing a SRT document)'. Others speak of 'following what the technology produces versus following their own knowledge'. As a result, when working from an SRT-generated transcript, MTs can end up paying more attention to whether the draft matches the dictation than focusing on whether what the dictator said makes sense. This divided attention can result in missing important errors in the dictation.

The response to the new technologies by MTs is mixed. Some MT instructors worry that new MTs will be intimidated by the technology and consequently less likely to correct what the 'machine tells them'. Some MTs report that they like using SRT and that it increases their productivity. However, editing does not always 'save labour' and MTs also report increased exhaustion because of the intense focus necessary to read text while listening to voice files. One report indicated that the focus required was similar to driving in a blizzard, in which constant attention is needed. Our survey revealed mixed enthusiasm for SRTs, with about equal percentages of those who responded to a question regarding experience with SRTs indicating that they could 'take it or leave it' (30%) or saw it as 'helpful in making me more productive' (27.9%).

It is clear that SRTs have a place in creating healthcare documentation; the task now is to determine what that place is.

Conclusion: automating versus supporting medical transcription

Whalen and Vinkhuyzen (2000:93), in their study of the use of expert systems in technological diagnostic work, argue that the 'expert system design should be founded upon the demonstrably indispensable aptitude and competence of users, and more responsive to the socially organised features of their activities'. While expert systems are often claimed to make experts out of non-experts through the extraction of knowledge from actual experts, such systems do not in fact accomplish this goal (see Whalen 1995). It is not that expert systems have no use, or do not work. But, their relevance is situated and involves essential social competencies. It is important to identify the conditions under which they do work.

Because of their limitations, technological implementations aimed at the production of medical records will need to take into account the abilities, work practices and particularly the social competencies regarding language use and interaction of those who are involved in their creation. In writing about the problematic nature of SRT-generated transcripts, van Terheyden (2005: 42) comments that '[w]ritten language may need punctuation – commas, periods and quotation marks – according to strict rules that are not obvious in speech and are difficult to infer'. The MT is attuned to this. The medical record is also expected to exhibit an institutionally accountable/expected form. As doctors do not always dictate in an orderly manner, it often is up to the MT to group, separate and order entries to create form and clarity in the record. Doctors can be repetitive, add the wrong punctuation, speak in incomplete sentences, leave out information, and misspeak. In every event, the MT must decide what 'makes sense' and how it should appear. The SRT lacks this ability. The ASTM International Guide (2004: 4) to SRT products notes, 'SRT will not overcome dictation errors, improper grammar, incomplete or disorganised dictation, or incorrect punctuation'. As we have shown the problems that result are not small.

Healthcare professionals are beginning to recognise the limitations of systems such as SRTs, and the need for situated design and strategic applications of the technology that take the social properties of work and social expectations with regard to medical records into account. As Coiera (2000: 279) notes, 'To create processes and technologies that support the communication space, we first need to characterise the activities that occur within it and understand where improvement is needed'. Similarly, Shneiderman (2000: 65) observes that as SRT success stories start to increase, 'designers should conduct empirical studies to understand the reasons for their success, as well as their limitations, and their alternatives'. Or, as Greenbaum and Kyng (1991: 2) state, 'Computer systems are *tools*, and need to be designed to be under the control of the people using them'. While 'speech recognition is not, in and of itself, the final solution in clinical documentation' (AHIMA 2003: 1), it will have a place and function in creating medical records.

Our research has shown specific ways that the skilled work practices of MTs add value to the production of medical records. Furthermore, while MTs have typically been viewed as a cost and not revenue generating, the fact remains that in the US, with its profit-driven healthcare system, the work of healthcare professionals requires adequate documentation to generate revenue. In other words, it is not the work of the doctor (or other care giver) himself or herself that ultimately results in creating revenue; rather, the documents are the things through which procedures are represented and revenue generated. Medical coders base their billing codes on these documents, and auditors use them to determine if coding is supported by the documentation. In fact, in instances where documentation does not support the claims of medical practice, payment can be withheld or rescinded. While technology has a place in enhancing healthcare documentation production, it cannot be adopted as a replacement without significant risk not only to patient care, but also to the revenue cycle of healthcare organisations.

Based on this research, a number of recommendations can be made to those exploring the implementation of SRTs. First, the social competence and professional knowledge involved in the work of MTs is a critical link in the effort to reduce medical errors and mistakes in medical records. Any technology that integrates into that role needs to be designed to support that work. Procedural, staffing, and technological changes intended to improve the accuracy of medical records and reduce costs associated with that work should take the contribution of MTs into account as they design their systems. Secondly, SRTs can be a tool to facilitate as much as automate. As such, they may not 'save labour' as much as 'change labour' in terms of how work is done. Thirdly, understanding the medical record as a socially-constructed boundary object that is essential for collaboration across institutional domains creates a different sense of how errors should be identified and evaluated. Medical records and other socially construction information have essential social properties (Brown and Duguid 2002, Garfinkel 2008), and as such need to be considered within the context of their use.

As they currently exist, SRTs are not able to replace the skilled work done by MTs in making medical records. But, SRTs can effectively support the work done by MTs. In this way, SRT technology might be best suited to 'facilitate' rather than 'automate'. Of course, such general statements probably do not encapsulate all applications of SRTs in terms of their abilities and limitations. However, in recognising the ways in which medical records are and will be used, their creation becomes less about simply automating their production, and more about creating records that: (1) are accurate depictions of medical encounters, (2) provide relevant information for situated use, and (3) display competence of care. As tools, SRTs can be advantageous, but cannot construct records with such varied uses in mind. The issue then becomes what is the best way to design and implement SRT systems so that they can facilitate the work of MTs or other back-end editors.

Acknowledgement

The authors would like to thank the anonymous persons who gave their time to this project, as well as the editors and reviewers for their comments and recommendations. We also thank members of the medical transcription and speech recognition communities for their willingness to share their insights into their industries.

Notes

1   Training programs can range depending upon the provider. However, AHDI provides a guideline for a model curriculum, which includes approximately 400 transcription hours of practice

transcription, and 100 hours of actual transcription (AHDI 2008). Generally speaking, program completion can take approximately one year (depending on the program).

2   All HIPAA regulations regarding patient privacy were observed regarding removal of patient identification from the documents and audio used in this research. The Health Insurance Portability and Accountability Act (HIPAA) was enacted by the US Congress in 1996, and (among many other elements) stipulates regulations regarding the privacy of patient medical information.

3   The goal of conversation analysis is to discover the commonsense understandings and procedures people use to shape their conduct in particular interactional settings (Sacks 1984, Schegloff and Sacks 1973, West and Zimmerman 1982, Garfinkel 2006).

References

AHIMA (2003) *Speech Recognition in the Electronic Health Record Practice Brief*. http://library.ahima.org.

AHDI (2004) *A Survey of Error Trends*. http://www.ahdionline.org/scriptcontent/Downloads/AAMTQAReport.pdf

AHDI (2008) *The Model Curriculum for Medical Transcription* (4th Edition). Modesto, CA. http://www.ahdionline.org/scriptcontent/Downloads/ModelCurriculum.pdf.

ASTM International (2004) *Standard Guide to Speech Recognition Technology Products in Health Care*. http://www.astm.org/Standards/E2364.htm.

Atkinson, J. and Heritage, J. (1984) *Structures of Social Action*. Cambridge, UK: Cambridge University Press.

Berg, M. (1998) Medical work and the computer-based patient record: a sociological perspective, *Methods of Information in Medicine*, 37, 294–301.

Borowitz, S.M. (2001) Computer-based speech recognition as an alternative to medical transcription, *Journal of the American Medical Informatics Association*, 8, 101–2.

Braverman, H. (1955) Automation: promise and menace, American Sociologist, October. http://www.marxists.org/history/etol/newspape/amersocialist/amersoc_5510.htm

Braverman, H. (1974) *Labor and Monopoly Capital: the Degradation of Work in the Twentieth Century*. New York: Monthly Review Press.

Brown, J.S. and Duguid, P. (2002) *The Social Life of Information*. Cambridge, MA: Harvard Business School Press.

Castells, M. (1996) *The Rise of the Network Society*. Oxford, UK: Blackwell Publishers.

Clarke, K.M., Hartswood, M.J., Procter, R.N. and Rouncefield, M. (2001) The electronic medical record and everyday medical work, *Health Informatics Journal*, 7, 168–70.

Coiera, E. (2000) When conversation is better than computation, *Journal of the American Medical Informatics Association*, 7, 3.

Conn, J. (2005) Not dead yet. *Modern Healthcare*, 35, 38.

David, G., Chand, D. and Garcia, A. (2008) 2007 survey of medical transcriptionists: Preliminary findings. http://www.ahdionline.org/scriptcontent/Downloads/MTSurveyReport-Preliminary.pdf

Garcia, A., David, G. and Chand, D. (2008) The work of medical transcriptionists: sense-making and interactional competence in the production of medical records. Unpublished manuscript.

Garfinkel, H. (1967) *Studies in Ethnomethodology*. Oxford, UK: Polity Press.

Garfinkel, H. (1996) Ethnomethodology's program, *Social Psychology Quarterly*, 59, 1, 5–21.

Garfinkel, H. (2006) *Seeing Sociologically: the Routine Grounds of Social Action*. Boulder, CO: Paradigm Publishers.

Garfinkel, H. (2008) *Toward a Sociological Theory of Information*. Boulder, CO: Paradigm Publishers.

Garson, B. (1988) *The Electronic Sweatshop: How Computers are Transforming the Office of the Future into the Factory of the Past*. New York: Simon and Schuster.

Goedert, J. (2006) Is now the time for speech recognition? *Health Data Management*, 14, 44–50.

Greatbatch, D., Heath, C., Campion, P. and Luff, P. (1995) How do desk-top computers affect the doctor-patient interaction? *Family Practice*, 12, 32–6.

Greatbatch, D., Hanlon, G., Goode, J., O'Caithain, A., Strangleman, T. and Luff, D. (2005) Telephone triage, expert systems and clinical expertise, *Sociology of Health and Illness*, 27, 6, 802–30.

Greenbaum, J. and Kyng, M. (1991) Introduction: situated design. In Greenbaum, J. and Kyng, M. (eds) *Design at Work: Cooperative Design of Computer System*. Hillsdale, NJ: Lawrence Erlbaum Associates.

Harper, R.H., Randall, D. and Rouncefield, M. (2000) *Retail Finance and Organisational Change: an Ethnographic Perspective*. London: Routledge.

Heath, C. (1982) Preserving the consultation: medical record cards and professional conduct, *Sociology of Health and Illness*, 4, 1, 56–74.

Heath, C. and Luff, P. (2000) *Technology in Action*. Cambridge, UK: Cambridge University Press.

Hing, E.S., Burt, C.W. and Woodwell, D.A. (2007) Electronic medical record use by office-based physicians and their practices: United States 2006, *Advanced Data from Vital and Health Statistics*, no.393. Hyattsville, MD: National Center for Health Statistics.

Lynch, M. (1997) *Scientific Practice and Ordinary Action*. Cambridge, UK: Cambridge University Press.

Marx, L. (1987) Does technology mean progress? *Technology Review*, 90, 33–41.

Mohr, D.N., Turner, D.W., Pond, G.R., Kamath, J.S., De Vos, C.B. and Carpenter, P.C. (2003) Speech recognition as a transcription aid: a randomised comparison with standard transcription, *Journal of the American Medical Informatics Association*, 10, 85–93.

Orlikowski, W. (1992) The duality of technology: rethinking the concept of technology in organizations. *Organization Science*, 3, 3, 398–427.

Rawls, A.W. (2008) Harold Garfinkel, ethnomethodology, and workplace studies, *Organisation Studies*, 29, 5, 701–32.

Ritzer, G. and Walczak, D. (1988) Rationalization and the deprofessionalization of physicians, *Social Forces*, 67, 1, 1–22.

Roop, E.S. (2009) Healthcare technology – it's not foolproof, *For the Record*, 21, 5, 10–11.

Rose, M. (2004) *The Mind at Work: Valuing the Intelligence of the American Worker*. New York: Viking Press.

Sacks, H. (1984) Notes on methodology. In Atkinson, P and Heritage, J. (eds) *Structures in Social Action: Studies in Conversation Analysis*. Cambridge, UK: Cambridge University Press.

Schegloff, E.A. (1987) Analyzing single episodes of interaction: an exercise in conversation analysis, *Social Psychology Quarterly*, 50, 2, 101–14.

Schegloff, E.A. and Sacks, H. (1973) Opening up-closing, *Semiotica*, 7, 4, 289–327.

Schock, P. (2007) Less paper, less fuss, better patient care, *Health Management Technology*, 28, 62–3.

Shneiderman, B. (2000) The limits of speech recognition, *Communications of the ACM*, 43, 63–5.

Shriberg, E. (2001) To 'errr' is human: ecology and acoustics of speech disfluencies, *Journal of the International Phonetic Association*, 31, 1, 153–69.

Speech Recognition Adoption White Paper (forthcoming) Medical Transcription Industry Association and the Association for Healthcare Documentation Integrity. Unpublished Manuscript.

Star, S.L. (1999) *The ethnography of infrastructure, American Behavioral Scientist*, 43, 3, 377–91.

Star, S.L. and Griesemer, J.R. (1989) Institutional ecology, 'translations' and boundary objects: amateurs and professionals in Berkeley's Museum of Vertebrate Zoology, 1907–39, *Social Studies of Science*, 19, 4, 387–420.

Suchman, L. (2000) Making a case: knowledge and routine work in document production. In Luff, P., Hindmarsh, J. and Heath, C. (eds) *Workplace Studies: Recovering Work Practice and Informing System Design*. Cambridge: Cambridge University Press.

Timmermans, S. and Berg, M. (2003) *The Gold Standard: the Challenge of Evidence-based Medicine and Standardization in Health Care*. Philadelphia, PA: Temple University Press.

van Terheyden, N. (2005) Is speech recognition the Holy Grail? *Health Management Technology*, February, 42–5.

West, C. and Zimmerman, D.H. (1982) Conversation analysis. In Scherer, K.R. and Ekman, P. (eds) *Handbook of Methods in Nonverbal Behavior Research*. Cambridge, UK: Cambridge University Press.

Whalen, J. (1995) Expert systems versus systems for experts. In Thomas, P. (ed.) *Social and Interactional Dimensions of Human-Computer Interfaces*. Cambridge: Cambridge University Press.

Whalen, J. and Vinkhuyzen, E. (2000) Expert systems in (inter)action: diagnosing document machine problems over the telephone. In Luff, P., Hindmarsh, J. and Heath, C. (eds) *Workplace Studies: Recovering Work Practice and Information System Design*. Cambridge: Cambridge University Press.

Whalen, J., Whalen, M. and Henderson, K. (2002) Improvisational choreography in teleservice work, *British Journal of Sociology*, 53, 239–59.

Wright, G., Wiechert, S., Marshall, S., Merkle, S. and Dinsdale, V. (2007) Integrating ED with enterprise, *Health Management Technology*, 28, 38–9.

Zuboff, S. (1988) *In the Age of the Smart Machine: The Future of Work and Power*. New York: Basic Books.

Index

Note: an 'n' followed by a number after a page number denotes a note number on that page.

The Dada Reader
A Critical Anthology

Edited by Dawn Ades

Tate Publishing

First published 2006 by order
of the Tate Trustees
by Tate Publishing, a division
of Tate Enterprises Ltd, Millbank,
London SW1P 4RG
www.tate.org.uk/publishing

British Library Cataloguing in
Publication Data
A catalogue record for this book is
available from the British Library

ISBN-10: 1-85437-621-7
ISBN-13: 978-185437-621-3

Designed by
Matt Brown, DesignBranch
Printed by
T J International Ltd, Padstow

Front cover:
Raoul Hausmann
The Art Critic
1919–20
31.8 x 25.4 cm
© DACS 2006

This publication is a joint initiative
between Tate Publishing and the
AHRC Research Centre for Studies of
Surrealism and its Legacies.

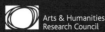

Arts & Humanities
Research Council

Contents

Contents

Contents

Contents

Contents

Contents

Dawn Ades
Introduction

The centrality of its little magazines to the many-headed phenomenon of Dada is well known, but relatively little of their contents has been available to an English-speaking audience.

These magazines tell the histories of this short-lived but prolific movement from within, charting its spread across Europe during and just after the First World War and revealing the international collaborations that defied cultural and political nationalisms. There was no common pattern to the reviews; they differ as radically from each other as Dada itself did in the various cities where it sprouted up. Even within a single review, issues vary widely from each other in size and style. Visually, they are among the most striking artefacts of the twentieth century, with their typographic innovations, startling photographs, overprinting, refusal to respect a normal reading order and intermixture of image and text.

The magazines were an explosive combination of manifestos, poems, verbal and visual experiments, theoretical statements, collages, reliefs, paintings, sculptures, drawings and objects, slogans, automatic writing, popular art and other indefinable contributions. And they also do their best to express the lost sounds of Dada, the recitals, readings and performances that were so central to it everywhere. Live performance had a special role in Dada and is recorded in the reviews from the very start. *Cabaret Voltaire* begins with Tristan Tzara's 'simultaneous poem' and public events of all kinds are registered throughout, from Hugo Ball's reading of his first phonetic poems to the tribunal set up by Paris Dada to try Maurice Barrès for crimes against the human spirit.

The Dada reviews belonged to an extraordinary moment of the avant-garde when the 'little review' became the primary medium of dissemination of new ideas across Europe. Although movements like Futurism had produced reviews before the war, the great explosion occurred during and just after the First World War. By the early 1920s these reviews had established an international network, advertising each other in long lists on the back pages. Tzara was in correspondence with numerous editors of little reviews all over Europe, from Seville to Moscow. While some were the mouthpieces of groups or even movements, others were one-man productions, like Francis Picabia's *391*. The same people contributed to a number of these reviews and the technique of photomontage, for example, became common currency.

Hugo Ball logged the discovery of the word 'Dada' to mid-April 1916. 'Tzara keeps on worrying about the periodical. My proposal to call it "Dada" is accepted ... Dada is "yes-yes" in Rumanian, "rocking-horse" and "hobbyhorse" in French.'[1] The virtue of the name 'Dada' for those who subscribed to it from so many different positions and places was its freedom from specific artistic programmes and its multilingual application. 'It is simply a meaningless little word thrown into circulation in Europe, a little word with which one can juggle *à l'aise*.'[2] For Ball, a phonic similarity to the name of the world-soul, 'O-Aha', in Frank Wedekind's eponymous satirical play, may have played a part in settling on this nonsense vocable.[3]

We had to make two difficult choices: which reviews and which texts? There is no hard-and-fast rule by which to sift the Dada reviews, and our decision was to keep largely to those that explicitly announce themselves as Dada. This has led to some inevitable omissions. In Berlin one wing of the group of writers and artists who produced *Der Dada* also published a clutch of satirical-political reviews: *Die Pleite*, *Der blutige Ernst* and *Jedermann sein eigner Fussball*. George

Grosz's drawings and John Heartfield's montages appear in all of them. However, in *Jedermann sein eigner Fussball* there is no mention of Dada. It is as though the participants had a double identity – the one Dadaist-anarchist, the other Communist. Whereas in the catalogue for the exhibition *Dada and Surrealism Reviewed* (Hayward Gallery, London, 1978) we took a relatively broad view and included *Die Pleite*, etc., in the German Dada section, here they have been left out. Nor are all reviews published under the Dada banner (such as Johannes Baargeld's *Freiland Dada* from Potsdam) represented. Yet we have included some that have become retrospectively annexed to Dada, like Marcel Duchamp and Henri-Pierre Roché's *The Blind Man*, which, although innocent of the name, share, as Duchamp said, the same spirit.

Narrowing the selection of reviews, however, helps to build a denser picture of core Dada ideas and practices, negative and positive. (All texts are published in their entirety – a decision that necessarily limited the number.) It also restores the specific histories of Dada movement in all their ambiguity and contradictions. Anthologies such as *Almanacco Dada* of 1976 and *Dada Global* of 1994 also focused on the reviews but took in virtually all avant-garde and modern art reviews of the time. To appropriate the entire avant-garde under the name Dada, while undeniably satisfying for a movement that was treated as a footnote for most of the twentieth century, distorts an intricate historical picture and obscures genuine and important differences. Although, for example, Dada and Constructivism are now understood to have overlapped, there were many causes of major divisions between their adherents. Indeed, one of the most extreme examples of double identity is that of Theo van Doesburg, editor of *De Stijl*, who was unmasked as the Dadaist I.K. Bonset and editor of *Mécano* to the horror of his Bauhaus comrades. In some quarters the two were definitely not seen as compatible.

Dada's brief life had overlapped with the utopian moment in the 1920s, which gave birth to Constructivism, before the rise of the totalitarian dictatorships in Europe, the grim struggle between Communism and Fascism, which crushed so many avant-garde artists and writers and which led inexorably to the Second World War. It is not so surprising that Dada should temporarily have been eclipsed, and it was virtually forgotten until the publication of the first major anthology of translations put together by the American Abstract Expressionist painter Robert Motherwell, *Dada Painters and Poets*, in 1951. This was the culmination of the series 'Documents of Modern Art' that had included a selection of Hans Arp's writings, *On My Way* (1948) and Max Ernst's *Beyond Painting* (1948). Motherwell had begun by translating Georges Hugnet's *The Dada Spirit in Painting*, but the project grew and Dadaists got involved; Duchamp was responsible for the inclusion of the pre-Dada section, claiming that 'dada had been "in the air" a long time before'[4] There is a notable Paris bias in *Dada Painters and Poets*, which from an historian's point of view seems to reinforce the Surrealist legacy, but Motherwell's purpose was to by-pass Surrealism and to make a connection between Dada and Abstract art: 'the works of dada appear more at home alongside abstract works than they do beside surrealist ones'.[5] However, the strong Dada-Constructivist axis, which would have added another dimension to this argument, is almost entirely lacking. Apart from Kurt Schwitters's important text 'Merz', there is little from the German and Dutch Dadaists, beside Richard Huelsenbeck's 'A History of Dadaism' (1920), which Motherwell nonetheless described as 'one of the most extraordinary expressions, not only of Dada but of the avant-garde mind in the strictest and narrowest sense'.[6]

The revival of interest in Dada in the 1960s, following Motherwell, was to an extent swept into the development of Anglo-American Pop art, but there has been an alternative historiography that valued Dada in terms of its active engagements in politics and culture. Dada became a kind of iconoclastic godparent of the 1960s revolutionary movements, absorbed into what became known as the 'historic avant-gardes' and emblematic of the attempt to re-engage art with life.

The role of the avant-garde reviews of the 1920s was recognised by the magazine *Form* in the mid-1960s, which paid homage to its own predecessors with a series on 'Great Little Magazines'. The magazines documented, with contents list, bibliography and selected translations, included *Ray, Mécano, De Stijl* and Hans Richter's *G*. It is interesting that, despite its Constructivist perspective, *Form* favoured, in its choice of translated texts from *Mécano* and *G*, Schwitters and van Doesburg, who straddled the Dada/Constructivist divide.

A series of 'Anti-classics of Dada' have been published in translation by Atlas Press, including *Blago Bung: The First Texts of German Dada* by Hugo Ball, Richard Huelsenbeck and Walter Serner (1995), Huelsenbeck's *Dada Almanach* of 1920 (1993) and *4 Dada Suicides: Writings by Arthur Cravan, Jacques Rigaut, Julien Torma and Jacques Vaché* (1995). While the Motherwell anthology, which incorporated much later texts and contemporary memoirs, became enmeshed in old quarrels such as the origin of the choice of the word 'dada', and had an explicit aesthetic agenda, the Atlas publications present primary texts as closely as possible to their original form.

The anonymous reviewer of Motherwell's anthology wrote in exasperation: 'How is one to define a movement that is not identified with any one person or place ... and is moreover intentionally negative, illogical, ephemeral and inconclusive?'[7] Despite such justifiable complaints, Dada remains fresh over eighty years later, and in the context of a manipulative global culture and economy its voice of protest non-conformity, irreverence and freedom to experiment is still relevant.

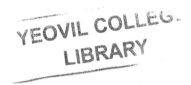

Cabaret Voltaire, Dada and Der Zeltweg

Dawn Ades

Cabaret Voltaire was the first of the 'Dada' reviews but bore the name of the literary and artistic cabaret opened by Hugo Ball in Zurich on 5 March 1916.[1] He hints at his reasons for choosing this title in his diary entry for 16 June 1916: 'The ideals of culture and of art as a program for a variety show – that is our kind of *Candide* against the times.'[2] The eponymous hero of Voltaire's novel *Candide* passed innocently through a world of horrors, war, torture and treachery, and Ball saw a parallel in the creative efforts that he and his fellow Dadaists, refugees in neutral Switzerland from the First World War, were making. As Hans Arp wrote in 'Dadaland': 'Losing interest in the slaughterhouses of world war, we turned to the Fine Arts. While the thunder of the batteries rumbled in the distance, we recited, we versified, we sang with all our soul.'[3]

Ball had issued an invitation to 'the young artists of Zurich whatever their orientation to come along with suggestions and contributions of all kinds'.[4] He was joined by Tristan Tzara, Hans Arp, Marcel Janco and soon by his Berlin friend Richard Huelsenbeck. Works by Arp, Janco and others hung on the walls. Every night there were poetry readings, music, songs and performances. It was soon evident that a new spirit had emerged, a spontaneous eruption that could not be pigeon-holed into existing 'modern schools'.

However, written and visual contributions from Futurists, Cubists and Expressionists appear in *Cabaret Voltaire* and in the first two issues of *Dada*, as well as work by the Dada group itself. One of the Italian Futurist F.T. Marinetti's *parole in libertà*, 'Dune', which combined visual, aural and written dimensions and was a significant influence on the development of the Dada phonetic poem, was printed in *Cabaret Voltaire*. Collages, woodcuts, a tapestry carpet (woven by Sophie Taueber after a painting by Arp) and drawings, by Janco, Arp, Emmy Hennings, Marcel Slodki and Otto van Rees, among others, are reproduced beside drawings by Pablo Picasso and Amedeo Modigliani.

Hugo Ball's editorial in *Cabaret Voltaire* had announced a new International Review to be published in Zurich that would bear the name 'DADA'. But by the time *Dada 1* appeared, in July 1917, Ball had withdrawn from Dada. Ball resisted organising a 'whim into an artistic school',[5] while Tristan Tzara was already flexing his impresario muscles. Ball's 'Dada Manifesto', read at the Dada soirée at the Waag Hall in Zurich on 14 July 1916, mocked the idea of a 'Dada movement' and was a 'thinly disguised break with friends ... Has the first manifesto of a newly founded cause ever been known to refute the cause itself to its supporters' face? And yet that is what happened'.[6]

Although Ball was no longer a participant by the time the review *Dada* appeared, his influence was long-lasting.

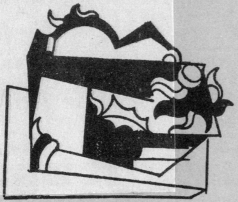

CABARET VOLTAIRE

1
Front cover
Cabaret Voltaire
1916

Performance, which was Zurich Dada's primary modus operandi, had its origins in Ball's ideal of theatre as a form of total expression. Belief in the *Gesamtkunstwerk* (the total work of art) was widespread at the time. But Dada's approach was novel. Dada's simultaneous poem, unlike Futurist simultaneity, which aimed to simulate the multiple stimuli of the modern city, was deliberate confusion designed to provoke. As the idea of 'total expression' disintegrated, so did the polite gap between performer/s and audience. Baiting the public became a feature of Dada events and at the same time there was the kernel of an attitude shared by other (future) Dadaists such as Marcel Duchamp: the audience was to be part of the 'work'. In his notes to 'The Admiral Seeks a House to Rent', Tzara suggested that the combination of unrelated 'simultaneous poems' would prompt different responses from individual members of the audience.

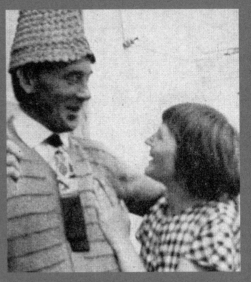

Abstraction was the cornerstone of Zurich Dada, both in the plastic arts and in Ball's experiments with words that destroyed rational syntax in the desire to rescue language from servitude to regimes responsible for the madness of the war. People had forfeited the right to be 'the measure of all things' and, as Arp wrote, 'Dada wanted to replace the logical nonsense of the men of today by the illogically senseless.' Arp's geometric collages 'arranged according to the laws of chance', his woodcuts and reliefs, together with Janco's plaster reliefs and constructions, rejected the principles of self-expression and aimed for a less egotistical and more spontaneous form of creation. Janco's *Construction 3*, reproduced in *Dada 1*, was a radical experiment in three-dimensional abstraction, using found materials such as

wire and cloth. With the appearance of a combusted machine, it follows no rules of composition or structure but those randomly conferred by the nature of the objects and fragments he has incorporated. Tzara responded with relish to the challenge of writing about such unprecedented works, in poem-texts that seem virtually automatic, spouting adjectives and verbs in unpunctuated succession. But here, as in his writing about Arp, he also articulates a new approach to art, which neither represents the world nor abstracts from it, but takes its place as another object in nature, creating 'directly' and often using unconventional materials such as wire, stone and textiles.

No editor was announced for the first two issues of *Dada*, which still had the by-line 'Literary and Artistic Review'; Marcel Janco and François Arp, Hans's brother, were respectively in charge of the administration. However, from the third issue, December 1918, which saw a

2
Hugo Ball and
Emmy Hennings
Zurich 1916

dramatic change of format and aggressive typographical inventions, Tzara was announced as editor, as well as director of the 'Dada Movement'. This issue opened with Tzara's famous 'Dada Manifesto 1918' and included contributions from Francis Picabia and the Paris-based writers Philippe Soupault and André Breton. The more nihilistic and ironic tone of *Dada 3* can be partly ascribed to direct contact between the Dadaists and Picabia, who was temporarily resident in Switzerland, where he published the eighth issue of *391* (with Dada's anarchist printer, Julius Heuberger, in Zurich) in February 1919. From this moment on Tzara's ambitions and organising talents ensured the rapid spread of Dada.

Despite the severe paper rationing, there were numbered de luxe editions with original woodcuts. The ordinary editions were on cheap, thin and often coloured papers. *Dada 4–5: Dada Anthology*, which appeared in May 1919, had orange, pink and blue pages. During the preparation of this issue the printer, Julius Heuberger, was sent to prison. In November 1919 the single issue of *Der Zeltweg* was published by 'Dada Movement editions'; edited by Otto Flake, Walter Serner and Tzara, the publication took its title from the Dada administration's address in Zurich: Zeltweg 83. In both French and German, it included texts by Huelsenbeck, now in Berlin, Tzara, Arp and Serner. Dr Serner, who joined the group towards the end of 1916, and published his own review, *Sirius*, was the author of some of the most nihilistic Dada texts and manifestos. He introduced his friend Christian Schad, one of whose 'Schadographs', cameraless photographs similar to Man Ray's Rayograms, was reproduced in *Dadaphone*.

In January 1920 Tzara followed Picabia to Paris; three more issues of his review appeared, all quite different in format. Numbers 6 and 7 (*Bulletin Dada* and *Dadaphone*) were published from Picabia's apartment. The Paris context is very marked; the reviews relate closely to the Paris Dada 'season' of 1920, and the only illustrations in *Dadaphone*, apart from the *Schadograph*, were photographs of the members of the Paris group. The final issue, No.8, *Dada intirol au grand air*, fruit of a holiday in Tarrenz, Austria (September 1921), prominently features Max Ernst, who shortly afterwards joined the Dadaists in Paris.

Hugo Ball
Cabaret Voltaire[1]

Translated from
the German by
Christina Mills

When I first set up the Cabaret Voltaire, I believed that there
might be a few young people in Switzerland who, just like me,
considered it important not only to enjoy their independence
but also to document it. I went to Mr Ephraim, the owner of the
Meierei and said: 'Please Mr Ephraim, let me use your hall. I
would like to put on a cabaret.' Mr Ephraim agreed and gave
me the hall. I went to see some acquaintances and asked them:
'Please could you give me a picture, a drawing, an engraving ... I
would like to organise an exhibition to go with my cabaret.' I went
to the friendly Zurich press and said: 'Give me some news
coverage. There's going to be an international cabaret. We want
to do beautiful things.' And they gave me pictures and news
coverage and on the 5 February we held our cabaret. Miss
Hennnings and Miss Leconte sang French and Danish songs. Mr
Tristan Tzara recited Rumanian verse. A balalaika orchestra
played delightful Russian folk songs and dances.

I had a lot of support and sympathy from Mr M. Slodki, who
designed the poster for the cabaret, and from Mr Hans Arp, who
obtained not only several works by Picasso but also pictures from
his friends O. van Rees and Artur Segall. I had a lot of support
from Messrs Tristan Tzara, Marcel Janco and Max Oppenheimer,
who all announced their intention to perform at the cabaret.
We organised a RUSSIAN and soon after a FRENCH soirée (with
works from Apollinaire, Max Jacob, André Salmon, A. Jarry,
Laforgue and Rimbaud). Richard Huelsenbeck came to Berlin on
26 February and on 30 March we set up a wonderful black music
session with constant big drum sound: boom boom boom boom –
drabatja mo gere drabatja mo bonoooooooooooo ... Mr Laban
was present at the performance and was enthusiastic. And, at
Mr Tristan Tzara's instigation, Messrs Tzara, Huelsenbeck and
Janco performed (for the very first time in Zurich and in the whole
world) simultaneous verses from Messrs Henri Barzun and
Fernand Divoire, as well as a simultaneous poem of his own
composition, which is reproduced on pages 6 and 7. The little
booklet we are giving you today owes its existence not only to our
own initiative but also to the help of our friends in France, ITALY
and Russia. The activity and interests of those involved in the
cabaret clearly show that it is aimed at the few independent
thinkers whose ideals extend beyond the war and their native
lands. The next goal of the artists assembled here is the
publication of an International Review. The review will
appear in Zurich and its name will be 'DADA' ('Dada') Dada
Dada Dada.

Zurich
15 May 1916

L'amiral cherche une maison à louer

Poème simultan par R. Huelsenbeck, M. Janko, Tr. Tzara

HUELSENBECK	Ahoi	ahoi	Des	Admirals	gwirktes	Beinkleid	schnell
JANKO, chant			Where	the	bonny	suckle	wine twines	itself
TZARA	Boum	boum boum	Il	déshabilla	sa chair	quand les	grenouilles

HUELSENBECK	und	der	Conciergenbuche	Klapperschlangengrün	sind	milde	ach
JANKO, chant	can	hear	the	weopour	will	arround	arround	the	hill
TZARA	serpent	à	Bucarest	on	dépendra	mes	amis	dorénavant	et

HUELSENBECK	prrrza	chrrza	prrrza	Wer	suchet	dem	wird
JANKO, chant	mine	admirably	confortably	Grandmother	said	
TZARA				Dimanche:	deux	éléphants

Intervalle rythmique

HUELSENBECK	hihi	Yabomm	hihi	Yabomm	hihi	hihi	hihiiii
TZARA			rouge bleu	rouge bleu	rouge bleu	rouge bleu rouge bleu rouge bleu
SIFFLET (Janko)						
CLIQUETTE (TZ)	rrrrrrrrr	rrrrrrrr	rrrrrrrrr	rrrrrrr	rrrrrrrrrr	rrrrrrrrr
GROSSE CAISE (Huels.)	O O O	O O O O O	O O O O O	O O O O	O O

HUELSENBECK	im	Kloset	zumeistens	war	nötig	hätt	aboi iuché aboi iuché
JANKO (chant)	I	love	the	ladies	I	love	to be among the girls
TZARA	la	concièrge	qui m'a	trompé	elle a vendu	l'appartement	que j'avais loué

HUELSENBECK	hätt'	O süss	gequollnes	Steildichein	des Admirals	im Abendschein	uru uru
JANKO (chant)	o'clock	and tea	is	set	I like	to have my tea	with some brunet	shai shai
TZARA		Le	train	traîne	la fumée	comme la fuite	de l'animal blessé	aux

HUELSENBECK	Der Affe	brüllt	die Seekuh	bellt	im Lindenbaum	der Schräg	zerscheilt	tara-
JANKO (chant)	doing it	doing	it	see	that	ragtime	coupple	over there	see
TZARA	Autour	du	phare	tourne	l'auréole	des oiseaux bleuilla	en moitiés	de lumière	vis-

HUELSENBECK		Peitschen	um die	Leaden	im Schlafsack	gröbit der
JANKO (chant)	oh	yes yes	yes yes	yes yes	yes yes	yes yes
TZARA	cher	c'est	si	difficile	La rue s'enfuit avec mon bagage à travers la ville	Un métro mêle

HUELSENBECK	zerfällt	the	door	a	swetheart	Teerpappe macht	Rowagen	in der Nacht
JANKO, chant	arround	commancèrent	à	broler	mine	is	waiting	patiently	hot	me	I
TZARA	humides				j'ai	mis	le	cheval	dans	l'âme	du

HUELSENBECK	verzerrt	in	der	Natur		chrza	prrrza	cherrza
JANKO, chant						my	great	room	is
TZARA	C'est	très	intéressant	les	grilles	des	morsures	équatoriales

HUELSENBECK	aufgetan	Der	Ceylonlö've	ist	kein	Schwan	Wer	Wasser	braucht	find
JANKO, chant							I	love	the	ladies
TZARA	Journal	de	Genève	au	restaurant	Le	télégraphiste	assassine

HUELSENBECK							Find	was	er	nötig
JANKO (chant)							And	when	it's	live
TZARA	Dans l'église après la messe le pécheur dit à la comtesse: Adieu Mathilde

HUELSENBECK	uro	uru	uru	uro	uru	uru	uru	uro	pataclan	putablan	pataglan	uri	uri	uro
JANKO (chant)	shai	shai	shai	shai	shai	shai	shai	Every body is doing it	doing it	doing it	Every body is
TZARA	intestins extrasés

HUELSENBECK	tata	taratata	taratata	im	Jonchiwara	drühnt der	Brand	und knallt	mit schnellen
JANKO (chant)	that	throw there	shoulders in the air	She said the	raising her heart	oh	dwelling	oh
TZARA	sant	la distance des bateaux	Tandis que les archanges chient et les	oiseaux	tombent	Oh!	non

HUELSENBECK	alte	Oberpriester	und	zeigt	der	Schenkel	volle	Tastatur	L'Amiral	n'a	rien	trouvé
JANKO (chant)	yes	yes yes yes	oh yes	oh yes	oh yes	yes yes	sir		L'Amiral	n'a	rien	trouvé
TZARA	son	cinéma la prore de	je vous adore	était au casino du sycomore		L'Amiral	n'a	rien	trouvé

NOTE POUR LES BOURGEOIS Les essays sur la transmutation des objets et des couleurs des premiers peintres cubistes (19 7) Picasso, Braque, Picabia, Duchamp-Villon, Delaunay, suscitaient l'envie d'appliquer en poésie les mêmes principes simultains. Villiers de l'Isle Adam eût des intentions pareilles dans le théâtre, où l'on remarque les tendances vers un simultanéisme schématique; Mallarmé essaya une reforme typographique dans son poème: Un coup de dés n'abolira jamais le hazard'; Marinetti qui popularisa cette subordination par ses „Paroles en liberté"; les intentions de Blaise Cendrars et de Jules Romains, dernièrement, amménèrent Mr Apollinaire aux idées qu'il développa en 1912 au „Sturm" dans une conférence.
Mais l'idée première, en son essence, fut exteriorisée par Mr H. Barzun dans un livre théoretique „Voix, Rythmes et chants Simultanés" où il cherchait une rélation plus étroite entre la symphonie polyrythmique et le poème. Il opposait aux principes successifs de la poésie lyrique une idée vaste et parallèle. Mais les intentions de compliquer en profondeur cette technique (avec le Drame Universel) en exagerant sa valeur au point de lui donner une idéologie nouvelle et la cloîtrer dans l'exclusivisme d'une école, — echouèrent.

En même temps Mr Apollinaire essayait un nouveau genre de poème visuel, qui est plus intéressant encore par son manque de système et par sa fantaisie tourmentée. Il accentue les images centrales, typographiquement, et donne la possibilité de commancer à lire un poème de tous les côtés à la fois. Les poèmes de Mrs Barzun et Divoire sont purement formels. Ils cherchent un effort musical, qu'on peut imaginer en faisant les mêmes abstractions que sur une partiture d'orchestre.
Je voulais réaliser un poème basé sur d'autres principes. Qui consistent dans la possibilité que je donne à chaque écoutant de lier les associations convenables. Il retient les éléments caractéristiques pour sa personalité, les entremêle, les fragmente etc, restant tout-de-même dans la direction que l'auteur a canal sé.
Le poème que j'ai arrangé (avec Huelsenbeck et Janko) ne donne pas une description musicale mais tente à individualiser l'impression du poème simultait auquel nous donnons par là une nouvelle portée.
La lecture parallèle que nous avons fait le 31 mars 1916, Huelsenbeck, Janko et moi, était la première réalisation scénique de cette esthétique moderne.

TRISTAN TZARA

6   7

Translated from the French by Dawn Ades

Tristan Tzara
Note for the Bourgeoise

The experiments in the transmutation of objects and colours by the first cubist painters (1907) Picasso, Braque, Picabia, Duchamp-Villon, Delaunay stimulated the desire to apply the same simultaneous principles in poetry.

Villiers de l'Isle Adam had parallel ideas in the theatre, with tendencies towards a schematic simultaneism; Mallarmé tried typographic reform in his poem 'A Throw of the Dice will never Abolish Chance'; Marinetti popularised this application in his 'Words in Liberty'; the intentions of Blaise Cendrars and of Jules Romain, most recently, directed Mr Apollinaire to the ideas he developed in his lecture published in *Sturm* in 1912. But the first idea, essentially, was exteriorised by Mr H. Barzun in a theoretical book *Voice, Rhythms and Simultaneous Songs* where he looked for a more direct relationship between the polyrhythmic symphony and the poem. To the principle of succession in lyrical poetry a parallel, vast idea. But the ambition to deepen this technique (with Universal Drama) by exaggerating its value to the point of conferring on it a new ideology and cloister it in the exclusivity of a school failed.

At the same time Mr Apollinaire experimented with a new genre of visual poem, which is even more interesting because of its lack of system and its tortured fantasy. It accentuates the central images typographically and offers the possibility of starting to read the poem from every side at once. The poems of Messrs Barzun and Divoire are purely formal. They seek a musical effect by making the same abstractions as a musical score.

I wanted to realise a poem based on other principles. Which consist in the possibility of letting each listener make links with appropriate associations. He retains the elements characteristic of his personality, mixes them, the fragments etc., remaining at the same time in the direction the author has channelled.

The poem that I arranged (with Huelsenbeck and Janco) does not provide a musical description, but tries to individualise the impression of the simultaneous poem to which we thereby give a new dimension.

The parallel reading we gave on 31 March 1916, Huelsenbeck, Janco and I, was the first staged performance of this modern aesthetic.

3
'The admiral seeks a house to rent',
(simultaneous poem)
Cabaret Voltaire
1916

Translated from
the French by
Susan de Muth

Guillaume Apollinaire
Tree

You sing with the others while the gramophones gallop
Where are the blind ones where did they go
The only leaf I gathered changed into mirages
Don't abandon me among this crowd of women in the
    market place
Ispahan has made itself a sky of blue enamel tiles
And I walk back up a path through the woods with you
    somewhere near Lyons

I haven't forgotten the long ago sound of the coconut-seller's bell
I can already hear the bitter sound of a voice that is to come
The friend who will wander with you in Europe while staying
In America
A child
A flayed calf hanging from the butcher's stall
A child
In this suburb of sand round a poor village in the heart of the East

A customs officer stood there like an angel
At the gates of some wretched paradise
And this epileptic traveller foamed in the waiting
    room of premieres

Nightjar Gurnard Badger
And the mole in the maze
We hired two berths on the Trans-Siberian
And took our turns at sleeping the traveller selling jewels and me
But the one who stayed awake never hid a beloved revolver

You strolled around Leipzig with a slim woman dressed as a man
A secret this as an intelligent woman should be
And legends must never be forgotten
Dame-Aboude on a streetcar at night in the heart
    of a deserted quarter
I saw a hunt as I followed the path
And the lift stopped at each level
Between stones
Between the multicoloured clothes of windows
Between the glowing coals of the chestnut seller
Between two Norwegian vessels moored at Rouen
Is your image

Growing between the silver birches of Finland

This beautiful black man in steel
The saddest thing

Is when you get a postcard from Coruna

The wind comes from the setting sun
Metal from the carob trees
Everything is sadder than it used to be
All the terrestrial gods are getting old
The universe uses your voice to complain
And new beings spring up
Three by three

Translated from
the German by
Christina Mills

Emmy Hennings
Song to the Dawn

For Hugo Ball

Octaves stagger through grey years with their echoes.
Days piled up high collapse.
I want to be yours.
My golden hair grows in the grave
And alien folk live in elderberry trees
A pale curtain whispers about a murder
Two eyes wander restlessly through the room
Ghosts stalk the kitchen shelves.
And small fir trees are dead children
Ancient oaks are the souls of weary old men
Who whisper the story of a failed life.
The Klintekongen lake sings an old melody.
I was not immune from the evil eye
and Negroes crawled out of the water jug,
The colourful picture in the story book, Red Hannah,[1]
Has bewitched me for all time.

Translated from
the German by
Timothy Adès

Morphine

We wait for a final adventure.
Who cares if it's sunny today?
Days teeter and fall – nights are restless –
In the purging fires we pray.

The post? We've given up reading it.
Into our cushions we quietly smile,
For we know it all by now. With guile
We flitter about in our shivering-fit.

Folk may have hustle and bustle and strife
The rain is more dismal today
We travel with never a pause through life
To our sleep we muddle our way …

Translated from
the French by
Michelle Owoo

Tristan Tzara
Dada Review No.2

For Marcel Janko
Five negresses in a motorcar
exploded their trajectories following the directions of my 5 fingers
when I put my hand to my bosom to pray to God (sometimes)
around my head there is a misty light from moonfaced fellows
the green halo of saints round flights of intelligence
tralalalalalalalalalala
which one sees now being pierced by shells

there is a young man who is eating his lungs
then has diarrhoea
then lets out a luminous fart
like a homing bird one sings about in poems
like death blasted from a cannon
his fart was so bright that the house became dark as midnight
the great sailing ships he opens his book like an angel though
    leaves have settled on it,
       spring, like a beautiful page in typography
zoumbaï zoumbaï zoumbaï di
your design in my intestines has devoured good and evil

above all evil like the joy of a general
because since I am scared of rats eating the church without
    servants I have
      transported the draperies and on each
        was our Lord and on each lord was my
      heart
I gave him my heart as a tip hihi

4
F.T. Marinetti
Dune (Words in Liberty)
Cabaret Voltaire
1916

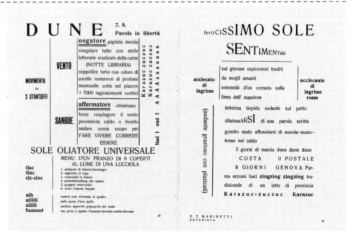

Translated from
the German by
Christina Mills

Wassily Kandinsky
Looking and Lightning

So that when he (the man) wanted to eat,
The thick white crest rid itself of the pink bird.
Now she is pushing up the damp window in its wooden sheets!
Not to the distant but to the crooked ones.
The chapel became empty – aye! aye!
Half-round pure circles are almost pressing down onto
    chessboards and! iron books!
Nuremberg wants to wants to be kneeling next to the jagged ox
… ghastly weight of eyebrows.
Heaven, Heaven, you can endure printed ribbons …
Out of my head too could grow the leg of a short-tailed horse with
    a pointed muzzle.
But the red jagger … the yellow hacker … at the North Pole lacquer
    … like a missile at midday!

Translated from
the German by
Timothy Adès

Hugo Ball
Cabaret

'3'   The Impresario struts round the curtain,
    Bewitched by Pimpronelle's red petticoats.
    Loud chatter in the stalls from green god Coco.
    Lust stirs in all the oldest Guilty-Goats.

    Tsingtara! blast from something long and brassy.
    Out comes a spittle-banner: 'Snake' – five letters.
    All pack their ladies in their fiddle-cases,
    Make themselves scarce. But then they get the jitters.

    Oily Miss Camodine sits at the entrance,
    Tinsels her thighs with the gold coins they've taken.
    Sadly, her eyes are poked out by an arc-lamp.
    The burning roof collapses on her grandson.

'4'   Flies from the donkey's pointed ear are quarried,
    Bagged by a man from somewhere else, a clown,
    Little green funnels, folded up and carried,
    Give him a link with noblemen in town.

    On the high platforms where the enharmonic
    Ropes intersect, where the flat walk dives off,
    A small-bore camel hazards a platonic
    Montage; and people hesitate to laugh.

    The Impresario, who manned the curtain
    Patient, alert for tips, aware of form,
    Forgets his good behaviour all of a sudden,
    Drives girls before him in a turgid swarm.

Translated from
the French by
Susan de Muth

Blaise Cendrars
Crepitations

The rainbowlike clashes of the tower in its wireless
　　telegraphy Midday

Midnight
People mutter 'shit' from all corners of the Universe
Like in the futurist manifesto signed by Apollinaire.
Sparks
Chrome yellow
We're in contact
Transatlantic liners come in from all directions
Head off again
Every watch set to the right time
And bells clang.
PARIS-MIDI reveals that a german teacher has been eaten
　　by cannibals in the Congo
A good thing too.

L'INTRANSIGEANT tonight publishes verses for postcards
Idiotic, when all the astrologers are looting the stars.
You can't see there any more.
I'm interrogating the sky
The Meteorological Institute warns of bad weather
There is no futurism
There is no simultaneism
Bodin burned all the witches
There is nothing
There are no more horoscopes and I have to work
I'm worried
The Mind
I'm going on a journey
And I'm sending this poem flayed to my friend R.

Translated from
the German by
Christina Mills

Emmy Hennings
Maybe the Last Flight

Deep in the night. Quiet. A room with sloping ceiling in a foreign
　　town. Cosy.
A candle flickers with a feeble flame.
A door opens demonically.
Two beings sit opposite each other. A man and woman.
The man (sinking in the two grey and turbulent lakes) speaks:
　　'I would like to look at you. Keep looking at you … take a good
　　　　look at you …'

The woman (slowly and with drawn-out voice): 'I think one
should never look closely. Not look closely at all. I think ...'
The man: 'What is it that you think?'
The woman (hesitantly): 'Yes. Everything seems doubtful to me.
    Everything is questionable. Maybe ...'
He (as though drinking): 'Oh speak to me ... I'm listening!'
She (consumed with passion, moving jerkily):
    'Take me! Take me!'
They fall upon one another. She runs to him ...

Later he immediately grabbed a cigarette.
She smiled gently (a smile all the sweeter for being rare):
    'Ah! You are one of them.' Hmm. She is immediately struck by
        these new charms.
He: 'Another subject.'
His eyes stared coolly ahead. A cruel smile played around his lips.
The smile of a murderer.
Aghast, she looked at his open mouth. His eyes narrowed in a
    cynical manner. Then it struck her. Their eyes burned into
    each other. Sucked each other in. Because she recognised him.
        A secret sign for sure.
He: 'Yes. Yes. I'm one of them ...'
She trembled. She fell blushing into his arms. And then, looking
    at him and stretching herself out on the floor:
        'I will live for you ... I will die for you.'
And again that cruel murderer's smile on his narrow lips.
.......The next day they met again. He asked: 'How are you?'
And she died because she felt watched.

Translated from
the German/French
by Christina Mills

Richard Huelsenbeck and Tristan Tzara
DADA – Dialogue Between a Coachman and a Swallow

Characters
Huelsenbeck – **German-speaking coachman.**
Tzara – **French-speaking swallow.**

Huelsenbeck **(coachman):** Hüho hüho. Greetings, oh lark.
Tzara **(swallow):** Bonjour Mr Huelsenbeck!
Huelsenbeck **(coachman):** What does your song tell me about
the Dada newspaper?
Tzara **(swallow):** Aha aha aha aha (f.) aha aha (decrescendo)
cri cri
Huelsenbeck **(coachman):** A cow? A horse? A street cleaning
machine? A piano?
Tzara **(swallow):** The heavenly hedgehog has melted into the

earth which has spewed up the mud from its core I turn shining halo of the continents I turn I turn comforter.

Huelsenbeck **(coachman):** The sky is bursting open into little scraps of cotton wool. The trees are walking about with swollen bellies.

Tzara **(swallow):** Because the first edition of the Dada Review comes out on 1 August 1916. Cost: 1 Fr. Editorial and administration: Spiegelgasse 1, Zurich. It has nothing to do with the war and is an attempt at a modern international activity hi hi hi hi.

Huelsenbeck **(coachman):** Oh yes, I saw that ... Dada emerged from the body of a horse as a basket of flowers. Dada burst like a boil from the chimney of a skyscraper, oh yes, I saw Dada ... as the embryo of the purple crocodile flew his cinnabar tail.

Tzara **(swallow):** That smells bad so I'm off into the sonorous antipyrine blue I hear the liquid call of the hippopotamuses.

Huelsenbeck **(coachman):** Olulu Olulu Dada is great Dada is beautiful. Olulu pette pette pette pette ...

Tzara **(swallow):** Why are you petting so enthusiastically?

Huelsenbeck (taking a book written by the poet Däubler out of his pocket): Pfffft pette pfffft pette pfffft pette pfffft pette ...

O Tzara o!

O embryo!

O sacred head sore wounded.

Your belly hair roars

Your coccyx soars

And is entwined with straw ...

Oh oh oh that's not how you usually look!

Tzara **(swallow):** Oh Huelsenbeck, oh Huelsenbeck

What is that flower you wear round your neck?

Is it your talent they say is so great

Little poo-poo swallow?

What is that flower you wear round your neck?

And there you go with your pette pette pette ...

Like a German poet.

Dada
Zurich
July 1917–May 1919

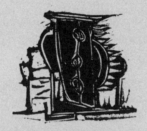

Translated from
the French by
Ian Monk

Alberto Savino
A Musical Puking

Although brought up to be gallant
'*signor jocundo, e
sempre de le donne ... perfecto amicho
savio e cortese più che belle dama*',
I have never been able to hold back the spasms of the most pressing
nausea each time I find myself face to face with Euterpe[1]. My
stomach is still refractory to the company of this artistic figurative
representation of sounds, the very presence of which sets off in my
intestines the same effects and consequences as the most swaying
heave of our childhood's swung vertigo.

We have often been wrong about painting and poetry; we
have always been wrong about music.

Its tardy development will later operate on that of the other
two. Despite this considerable handicap, it will overtake the leaders
of the race and arrive, as though in a bath chair, at the finishing post
of utter stupidity and huge misunderstanding.

Among the music-makers there has never been a single
clairvoyant mind. *Senza il menomo madore d'affettazione* –
I must confess a natural aversion for anything touching the
chromatic world.

Thanks to intense training, I now easily resist any titillation
that comes from harmony or melody.

Everything to do with this decrepit and malevolent art
plunges me into the meanest sadness.

I take to all sorts of reading: a 'History of Music' demands a
painful effort from me. I blush when I see myself placed in the
shady tableau of makers of sharps and flats.

One evening, before going to bed, having imprudently opened
a book of music, it disturbed that sort of serene mood which is vital
to me at this solitary and, above all, precious hour of the day, and it
gave me, during my succeeding sleep, a series of obscene dreams
and harrowing miseries. I thus learnt from experience and, since
then, if I have to devote myself to sharps, I do so in the middle
hours of the day; I then have time to repair my palate with some
entertaining occupation and reparative thoughts.

In its current state, music is a demented and immoral art; an
example of bourgeois perversity; an art open to all the vices.

More odious and sticky than pity, it welcomes in its arms not
only widows and orphans, but also entire crowds of renegades and
the accursed.

Deceitful consolation for the degenerate, for all those with a
weight on their consciences, with cancer in their souls, for all the
vile, the submissive, the born-cursed.

Art that flatters and encourages the crowd's basest instincts;
shameless mirror of all the obscenity of a world without laws or
morals.

I emphasise two moments in my life that gave me the most intense and most inexpressible disgust: the first took place in my childhood, one day, at the instigation of a blood-thirsty kitchen boy, I sawed the head off a nestling; the second happened in my adolescence, one evening when I was pushed by a music-loving German into attending a sort of theatrical orgy where the sonorous turpitudes of Richard Strauss provided a scene of debauchery.

Above all, in its current state, music is an insult to the dignity of all citizens, be they aristocrat, bourgeois or proletariat, rather lacking in honesty or clean in their linen and business.

The charm of harmony is the greatest threat to the honour of free men. Among the primary causes of criminality due to degeneracy we must place - in first position - music, well in front of alcoholism!

Dense populations of idiotic, ignorant, filthy, sick, degenerate people enter into the Temple of Music as if they were at home there. And they are - indeed - perfectly at home there, because here there is celebrated a devotion within the reach of all the most repugnant baseness of the mind: it is a publicly funded hospice for all of humanity's rejects.

At the time when, unprejudiced, I abandoned myself foolishly to the embrace of this rabble-rousing vice - alas, so few years separate me from that woeful era! - I constantly experienced distasteful reactions. Remorse gripped me - and I had not even slept with Aspasia! - I loathed myself, I felt guilty, I groaned under the weight of my sins. When the grin of libidinous bestiality had been wiped from my face, I sunk into desperation, I bent my head and doubled over, like a brute who has just reached orgasm.

Post coitum animal triste est!

Translated from the French by Dawn Ades

Tristan Tzara
Marcel Janco

nerves zigzag like a cosmic harmonica pull pull the line through foliage and pauses
in the black light the warm and sick-happy egg elongates the netting for him:
art is stabile[1] sensibility serious time reckoning leaves and points
seriousness of unalterable needs in the tidy fantasy
grand rule
ruled action
he has made sculptures with surfaces up till now people superposed
bodies and he used wire as drawing in space (for the first time)
the upper part of *Construction 3* offers matter the possibility of
showing its life wire tremble felt moon sun sea horse sea-depth blue
he makes reliefs to be constructed in the wall architectural totality
productive protest against the frame and the baroque

6
Marcel Janco
Construction 3
Dada 1
July 1917

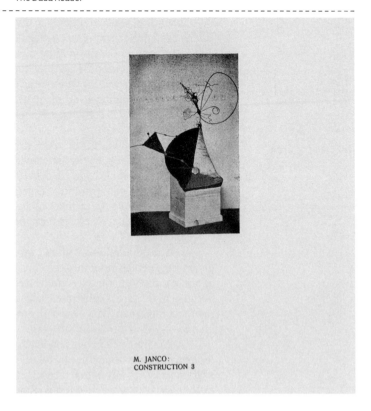

M. JANCO:
CONSTRUCTION 3

he pursues the tradition of pure art after 5 centuries of sugary
dreaming
direct reality specialisation with neither external influence nor
compromise
vertical joy I call naivety the sight of the object even in the sad soul
and blood memory of iron of sickness of stone of stuff of rain of
violins of soldiers of fire furniture
which grew during centuries past
rusty religious bitter
light order in the whole rich complex
without transformation, without decomposition: direct light
order reality
pictures: with pure elements: colours in the form line point
surface
necessity
in his order: struggle against his temperament
skeleton-tree-matches rubs humanity
divided in planes large wide bands
there where the soundings and smoke are brush strokes and the
crystal dissolves as it moves

1.3

Dada 2
Zurich
December 1917

Translated from
the French by
Michelle Owoo

Tristan Tzara
Note 2 on Art. H. Arp

The summit sings what is spoken of in the depths.
Nature is organised in her totality, the rigging of great ships
pointing up towards the convergence of sunrays, by principles
which rank crystals and insects in hierarchy like the branches of a
tree.
In nature all things have this imperceptible clarity of
organisation, united in kinship, bound together like children of
lunar light, the axis of a wheel infinitely turning, its freedom, its
ultimate, absolute existence, bound to these innumerable laws of
progression.
My sister is root, flower, stone.
The organism is complete in the voiceless intelligence of the veins
of plants and insects and their appearance.
Man is filthy, he slays animals, plants, his brothers, he quarrels,
he is clever, he talks too much, he is incapable of expressing his
thoughts.
But the artist is a creator: he knows how to work the organic form.
He makes decisions. He improves men. He tends the garden of
the mind, watches over it.

The purity of an idea makes me happy, to see beyond the horizon
which stretches out tending the new plant life of distant lands;
blossoms of ice.
The vertical: in solemn contemplation before the infinite sensing
the depth of a moment before the animal in us.
H. Arp
symmetry
midnight meeting flower
where bird and summit are embraced by the halo of the sun
and the hop vine climbs
the flower becomes crystal or scarab, magnet or star
the wish to lead a simple life

If we can live the miracle we will have reached the heights where
our blood will join the order of archangels, medicine for
stargazing, reader – a belief clearly held in simple hearts –
wisdom and knowledge.

Translated from
the French by
Susan de Muth

Pierre Albert-Birot
Mechanical Razor

Lie on your back and count the leaves on the trees
        IN THE FOREST ONE BY ONE
        THE YOUNG GIRLS WENT PAST
The splendour of green worlds united with blue worlds
     ii   iiiiiiiii   i
Forest of elephantslionstigressessnakesjaguars
You're in foreign parts
Yet I dream of Clamart
Forest of Asia A NUT and the two Americas
       PIGEON FLYING
       AIRPLANE FLYING
       LEAD WEIGHT FLYING
    HEE HEE HEE HEE HEE   HA HA HA HA HA
Incommensurability
Of our eternity
Blankness and blueity
       MARY COME SEE

Of insonority
Our iron-horsity
Off to a port-city
       HE WENT THIS AWAY
       LADIES THE FOREST FERRET
       HE WENT THIS AWAY
Boats trains
Carriages voyages
Oceans terrains
       IT RAINS

Off to see

FOR DADA
AN AN AN AN AN AN AN AN
AN AN AN
IIII I I
POUH-POUH POUH-POUH   RRRA
sl   sl   sl
drrrrr   oum   oum
AN AN AN AN
aaa aaaa aaa   tzinn
Ul llll
HA HA HA HA HA HA HA
rrrrrrrrrrrrrrrrrrrrrrrrr

Dada 3
Zurich
December 1918

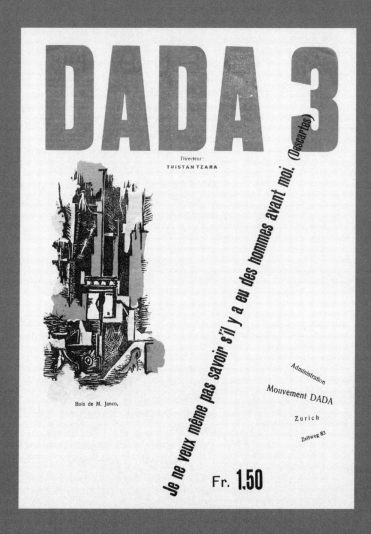

Translated from
the French by
Ralph Manheim

Tristan Tzara
Dada Manifesto 1918[1]

The magic of a word - Dada - which has brought journalists to the gates of a world unforeseen, is of no importance to us.

To put out a manifesto you must want: ABC
to fulminate against 1, 2, 3,
to fly into a rage and sharpen your wings to conquer and disseminate little abcs and big abcs, to sign, shout, swear, to organise prose into a form of absolute and irrefutable evidence, to prove your non plus ultra and maintain that novelty resembles life just as the latest appearance of some whore proves the essence of God. His existence was previously proved by the accordion, the landscape, the wheedling word. To impose your ABC is a natural thing - hence deplorable. Everybody does it in the form of crystalbluffmadonna, monetary system, pharmaceutical product, or a bare leg advertising the ardent sterile spring. The love of novelty is the cross of sympathy, demonstrates a naive je m'enfoutisme, it is a transitory, positive sign without a cause.

But this need itself is obsolete. In documenting art on the basis of the supreme simplicity: novelty, we are human and true for the sake of amusement, impulsive, vibrant to crucify boredom. At the crossroads of the lights, alert, attentively awaiting the years, in the forest. I write a manifesto and I want nothing, yet I say certain things, and in principle I am against manifestos, as I am also against principles (half-pints to measure the moral value of every phrase too too convenient; approximation was invented by the impressionists). I write this manifesto to show that people can perform contrary actions together while taking one fresh gulp of air; I am against action; for continuous contradiction, for affirmation too, I am neither for nor against and I do not explain because I hate common sense.

Dada - there you have a word that leads ideas to the hunt: every bourgeois is a little dramatist, he invents all sorts of speeches instead of putting the characters suitable to the quality of his intelligence, chrysalises, on chairs, seeks causes or aims (according to the psychoanalytic method he practises) to cement his plot, a story that speaks and defines itself. Every spectator is a plotter if he tries to explain a word: (to know)! Safe in the cottony refuge of serpentine complications he manipulates his instincts. Hence the mishaps of conjugal life.

To explain: the amusement of redbellies in the mills of empty skulls.

DADA MEANS NOTHING

If you find it futile and don't want to waste your time on a word that means nothing ... The first thought that comes to these people is bacteriological in character: to find its etymological, or at least its historical or psychological origin. We see by the papers

that the Kru Negroes call the tail of a holy cow Dada. The cube
and the mother in a certain district of Italy are called: Dada. A
hobby horse, a nurse both in Russian and Rumanian: Dada. Some
learned journalists regard it as an art for babies, other holy
jesusescallingthelittlechildren of our day, as a relapse into a dry
and noisy, noisy and monotonous primitivism. Sensibility is not
constructed on the basis of a word; all constructions converge on
perfection which is boring, the stagnant idea of a gilded swamp, a
relative human product. A work of art should not be beauty in
itself, for beauty is dead; it should be neither gay nor sad, neither
light nor dark to rejoice or torture the individual by serving him
the cakes of sacred aureoles or the sweets of a vaulted race
through the atmospheres. A work of art is never beautiful by
decree, objectively and for all. Hence criticism is useless, it exists
only subjectively, for each man separately, without the slightest
character of universality. Does anyone think he has found a
psychic base common to all mankind? The attempt of Jesus and
the Bible covers with their broad benevolent wings: shit, animals,
days. How can one expect to put order into the chaos that
constitutes that infinite and shapeless variation: man? The
principle: 'love thy neighbour' is a hypocrisy. 'Know thyself' is
utopian but more acceptable, for it embraces wickedness. No
pity. After the carnage we still retain the hope of a purified
mankind. I speak only of myself since I do not wish to convince, I
have no right to drag others into my river, I oblige no one to follow
me and everybody practises his art in his own way, if he knows the
joy that rises like arrows to the astral layers, or that other joy that
goes down into the mines of corpse-flowers and fertile spasms.
Stalactites: seek them everywhere, in mangers magnified by pain,
eyes white as the hares of the angels.

And so Dada[1] was born of a need for independence, of a
distrust towards unity. Those who are with us preserve their
freedom. We recognise no theory. We have enough Cubist and
Futurist academies: laboratories for formal ideas. Is the aim of art
to make money and cajole the nice nice bourgeois? Rhymes ring
with the assonance of the currencies and the inflection slips along
the line of the belly in profile. All groups of artists have arrived at
this trust company after riding their steeds on various comets.
While the door remains open to the possibility of wallowing in
cushions and good things to eat.

Here we cast anchor in rich ground. Here we have a right to
do some proclaiming, for we have known cold shudders and
awakenings. Ghosts drunk on energy, we dig the trident into
unsuspecting flesh. We are a downpour of maledictions as
tropically abundant as vertiginous vegetation, resin and rain are
our sweat, we bleed and burn with thirst, our blood is vigour.

Cubism was born out of the simple way of looking at an
object: Cézanne painted a cup 20 centimetres below his eyes, the
Cubists look at it from above, others complicate appearance by
making a perpendicular section and arranging it conscientiously
on the side. (I do not forget the creative artists and the profound

1 In 1916, at the Cabaret Voltaire, Zurich.

laws of matter which they established once and for all.) The Futurist sees the same cup in movement, a succession of objects one beside the other, and maliciously adds a few force lines. This does not prevent the canvas from being a good or bad painting suitable for the investment of intellectual capital.

The new painter creates a world, the elements of which are also its implements, a sober, definite work without argument. The new artist protests: he no longer paints (symbolic and illusionist reproduction) but creates – directly in stone, wood, iron, tin, boulders – locomotive organisms capable of being turned in all directions by the limpid wind of momentary sensation. All pictorial or plastic work is useless: let it then be a monstrosity that frightens servile minds, and not sweetening to decorate the refectories of animals in human costume, illustrating the sad fable of mankind.

Painting is the art of making two lines geometrically established as parallel meet on a canvas before our eyes in a reality which transposes other conditions and possibilities into a world. This world is not specified or defined in the work, it belongs in its innumerable variations to the spectator. For its creator it is without cause and without theory. *Order=disorder; ego=non-ego; affirmation=negation*: the supreme radiations of an absolute art. Absolute in the purity of a cosmic ordered chaos, eternal in the globule of a second without duration, without breath without control. I love an ancient work for its novelty. It is only contrast that connects us with the past. The writers who teach morality and discuss or improve psychological foundations have, aside from a hidden desire to make money, an absurd view of life, which they have classified, cut into sections, channelised: they insist on waving the baton as the categories dance. Their readers snicker and go on: what for?

There is a literature that does not reach the voracious mass. It is the work of creators, issued from a real necessity in the author, produced for himself. It expresses the knowledge of a supreme egoism, in which laws wither away. Every page must explode, either by profound heavy seriousness, the whirlwind, poetic frenzy, the new, the eternal, the crushing joke, enthusiasm for principles, or by the way in which it is printed. On the one hand a tottering world in flight, betrothed to the glockenspiel of hell, on the other hand: new men. Rough, bouncing, riding on hiccups. Behind them a crippled world and literary quacks with a mania for improvement.

I say unto you: there is no beginning and we do not tremble, we are not sentimental. We are a furious wind, tearing the dirty linen of clouds and prayers, preparing the great spectacle of disaster, fire, decomposition. We will put an end to mourning and replace tears by sirens screeching from one continent to another. Pavilions of intense joy and widowers with the sadness of poison. Dada is the signboard of abstraction; advertising and business are also elements of poetry.

I destroy the drawers of the brain and of social organisation:

spread demoralisation wherever I go and cast my hand from heaven to hell, my eyes from hell to heaven, restore the fecund wheel of a universal circus to objective forces and the imagination of every individual.

Philosophy is the question: from which side shall we look at life, God, the idea or other phenomena. Everything one looks at is false. I do not consider the relative result more important than the choice between cake and cherries after dinner. The system of quickly looking at the other side of a thing in order to impose your opinion indirectly is called dialectics, in other words, haggling over the spirit of fried potatoes while dancing method around it.

If I cry out:

Ideal, ideal, ideal,
Knowledge, knowledge, knowledge,
Boomboom, boomboom, boomboom,

I have given a pretty faithful version of progress, law, morality and all other fine qualities that various highly intelligent men have discussed in so many books, only to conclude that after all everyone dances to his own personal boomboom, and that the writer is entitled to his boomboom: the satisfaction of pathological curiosity; a private bell for inexplicable needs; a bath; pecuniary difficulties; a stomach with repercussions in life; the authority of the mystic wand formulated as the bouquet of a phantom orchestra made up of silent fiddle bows greased with philtres made of chicken manure. With the blue eye-glasses of an angel they have excavated the inner life for a dime's worth of unanimous gratitude. If all of them are right and if all pills are Pink Pills, let us try for once not to be right. Some people think they can explain rationally, by thought, what they think. But that is extremely relative. Psychoanalysis is a dangerous disease, it puts to sleep the anti-objective impulses of men and systematises the bourgeoisie. There is no ultimate Truth. The dialectic is an amusing mechanism which guides us/in a banal kind of way/to the opinions we had in the first place. Does anyone think that, by a minute refinement of logic, he has demonstrated the truth and established the correctness of these opinions? Logic imprisoned by the senses is an organic disease. To this element philosophers always like to add: the power of observation. But actually this magnificent quality of the mind is the proof of its impotence. We observe, we regard from one or more points of view, we choose them among the millions that exist. Experience is also a product of chance and individual faculties. Science disgusts me as soon as it becomes a speculative system, loses its character of utility – that is so useless but is at least individual. I detest greasy objectivity, and harmony, the science that finds everything in order. Carry on, my children, humanity ... Science says we are the servants of nature: everything is in order, make love and bash your brains in. Carry on, my children, humanity, kind bourgeois and journalist virgins ... I am against systems, the most acceptable system is on principle to have none. To complete oneself, to perfect oneself in one's own littleness, to fill the vessel with one's individuality, to have the courage to fight for and against thought, the mystery of bread, the sudden burst of an infernal propeller into economic lilies:

DADAIST SPONTANEITY

I call *je m'enfoutisme* the kind of like in which everyone retains his own conditions, though respecting other individualisms, except when the need arises to defend oneself, in which the two-step becomes national anthem, curiosity shop, a radio transmitting Bach fugues, electric signs and posters for whorehouses, an organ broadcasting carnations for God, all this together physically replacing photography and the universal catechism.

ACTIVE SIMPLICITY

Inability to distinguish between degrees of clarity: to lick the penumbra and float in the big mouth filled with honey and excrement. Measured by the scale of eternity, all activity is vain – (if we allow thought to engage in an adventure the result of which would be infinitely grotesque and add significantly to our knowledge of human impotence). But supposing life to be a poor farce, without aim or initial parturition, and because we think it our duty to extricate ourselves as fresh and clean as washed chrysanthemums, we have proclaimed as the sole basis for agreement: art. It is not as important as we, mercenaries of the spirit, have been proclaiming for centuries. Art afflicts no one and those who manage to take an interest in it will harvest caresses and a fine opportunity to populate the country with their conversation. Art is a private affair, the artist produces it for himself; an intelligible work is the product of a journalist, and because at this moment it strikes my fancy to combine this monstrosity with oil paints; a paper tube simulating the metal that is automatically pressed and poured hatred cowardice villainy. The artist, the poet rejoice at the venom of the masses condensed into a section chief of this industry, he is happy to be insulted: it is a proof of his immutability. When a writer or artist is praised by the newspapers, it is proof of the intelligibility of his work: wretched lining of a coat for public use; tatters covering brutality, piss contributing to the warmth of an animal brooding vile instincts. Flabby, insipid flesh reproducing with the help of typographical microbes.

We have thrown out the cry-baby in us. Any infiltration of this kind is candied diarrhoea. To encourage this act is to digest it. What we need is works that are strong straight precise and forever beyond understanding. Logic is a complication. Logic is always wrong. It draws the threads of notions, words, in their formal exterior, towards illusory ends and centres. Its chains kill, it is an enormous centipede stifling independence. Married to logic, art would live in incest, swallowing, engulfing its own tail, still part of its own body, fornicating within itself, and passion would become a nightmare tarred with Protestantism, a monument, a heap of ponderous grey entrails. But the suppleness, enthusiasm, even the joy of injustice, this little truth which we practise innocently and which makes us beautiful: we are subtle and our fingers are malleable and slippery as the branches of that sinuous, almost liquid plant; it defines our soul, say the cynics. That too is a point of view; but all flowers are not sacred, fortunately, and the divine thing in us is our call to anti-human action. I am speaking of a paper flower for the buttonholes of the gentlemen who frequent the ball of masked life, the kitchen of grace, white cousins lithe or fat. They traffic with whatever we have selected. The contradiction and unity of poles in a single toss can be the truth. If one absolutely insists on uttering this platitude, the appendix of libidinous, malodorous morality. Morality creates atrophy like every plague produced by intelligence. The control of morality and logic has inflicted us with impassivity in the presence of policemen – who are the cause of slavery, putrid rats infecting the bowels of the bourgeoisie which have infected the only luminous clean corridors of glass that remained open to artists.

Let each man proclaim: there is a great negative work of destruction to be accomplished. We must sweep and clean. Affirm the cleanliness of the individual after the state of madness, aggressive complete madness of a world abandoned to the hands of bandits, who rend one another and destroy the centuries. Without aim or design, without organisation: indomitable madness, decomposition. Those who are strong in words or force will survive, for they are quick in defence, the agility of limbs and sentiments flames on their faceted flanks.

Morality has determined charity and pity, two balls of fat that have grown like elephants, like planets, and are called good. There is nothing good about them. Goodness is lucid, clear and decided, pitiless towards compromise and politics. Morality is an injection of chocolate into the veins of all men. This task is not ordered by a supernatural force but by the trust of idea brokers and grasping academicians. Sentimentality: at the sight of a group of men quarrelling and bored, they invented the calendar and the medicament wisdom. With a sticking of labels the battle of philosophers was set off (mercantilism, scales, meticulous and petty measures) and for the second time it was understood that pity is a sentiment like diarrhoea in relation to the disgust that destroys health, a foul attempt by carrion corpses to compromise the sun. I proclaim the opposition of all cosmic faculties to this gonorrhoea of a putrid sun issued from the factories of philosophical thought, I proclaim bitter struggle with all the weapons of

DADAIST DISGUST

Every product of disgust capable of becoming a negation of the family is *Dada*; a protest with the fists of its whole being engaged in destructive action:

Dada; knowledge of all the means rejected up until now by the shamefaced sex of comfortable compromise and good manners: Dada; abolition of logic, which is the dance of those impotent to create: Dada; of every social hierarchy and equation set up for the sake of values by our valets: Dada: every object, all objects, sentiments, obscurities, apparitions and the precise clash of parallel lines are weapons for the fight: Dada; abolition of memory: Dada: abolition of archaeology: Dada; abolition of prophets: Dada; abolition of the future: Dada; absolute and unquestionable faith in every god that is the immediate product of spontaneity:

Dada: elegant and unprejudiced leap from a harmony to the other sphere; trajectory of a word tossed like a screeching phonograph record; to respect all individuals in their folly of the moment: whether it be serious, fearful, timid, ardent, vigorous, determined, enthusiastic; to divest one's church of every useless cumbersome accessory; to spit out disagreeable or amorous ideas like a luminous waterfall, or coddle them – with the extreme satisfaction that it doesn't matter in the least – with the same intensity in the thicket of one's soul-pure of insects for blood well-born, and gilded with bodies of archangels. Freedom: DADA DADA DADA, a roaring of tense colours, and interlacing of opposites and of all contradictions, grotesques, inconsistencies: LIFE

Translated from
the French by
Michelle Owoo

Tristan Tzara
Guillaume Apollinaire

is dead – he fell like the feverish 'rain' which he composed so carefully for a Parisian journal;/; will the trains, dreadnoughts, variety theatres and factories muster the winds of mourning for the most vivacious, the most agile-minded, the most enthusiastic French poets? – ? mist will not suffice, nor the greatest commotion; – ; the joy of victory should have been his, our own, that of new practitioners working in the darkness, of language, the essence : – : he knew the mechanism of the stars, the exact balance of tumult and quiet, what it must be. His mind coursed with clarity and the hail of cool words guided him from their crystalline clusters, those of angels.

He will meet Henri Rousseau – is Apollinaire dead?

Translated from
the German by
Christina Mills

Richard Huelsenbeck
The Work of Hans Arp

It is clear that knowledge of the new viewpoint and an extensive
understanding of the latest developments in the visual arts are
today regarded as essential. The old perspective has vanished
with Picasso and the Cubists. Gone are the models ... gone are the
beautiful easels and the top hats have made their exit from the
world. The picture, having lost its illusory moral values, now
attempts to have multiple meanings. It seeks a new audience, a
society of enthusiastic and devout people. It is being singled out
and plucked in all its shapes and colours from its wedge frame. It
acquires hands and arms; it wishes to offer itself heart and soul to
the Buddhist idols under which huge fragrant fires burn. It wants
to devour the souls of men just as those idols devoured the bodies
of little children.

The subject loses all philosophical reality so that no attempt
is made via these pictures to explain the world or to represent a
'for or against' view of any sort through art. The abstraction is so
serious and worthy that, in the final analysis, what is important is
the vertical, the 'normal' position. Following the change of values
brought about by the Cubists, Hans Arp's art is the first to have
found a dogma in which all difficulties are relieved, just as cramps
and spasms are relieved.

The world is huge and full of miracles. Those miracles may
be the strangest of abstractions ... the spiritual essences of which
will lurk beneath the surface of things. God spoke and so created
the first day from evening and morning. A new will for spirituality
has returned to us, the prophets. It is fantastic, pulsating,
burning with zeal. We could liken this zeal to that displayed by
the Inquisition when it distributed posters simultaneously
threatening both death and public excommunication.

Anyone could stand in front of these pictures and reel off
the following fantastical litany: the idols are red-hot frying pans
on the freestones, which start off the strongly rhythmical dance.
The Spherical is as compact as the villas of the well-heeled
landowners – *mirabile dictum* – and who would doubt that
elephants glide over these curves with a sense of inner joy. On
their heads they carry great sacks of sugar, kaleidoscopes and
barrel organs. Farmers turn somersaults from the top of their
tiled roofs (Cinnabar! a thousand times Cinnabar! and then, with
a bang on the big bass drum, what more lovely than a good
Prussian blue sky) ... oh the farmers, who spread their celluloid
buttocks over the tulip beds. Oh *furor rusticus* and cotillion of
crocodiles. But beyond the rivers you will see, dear enchanted
onlooker, a rock face, cylinder-shaped and made of papier mâché,
pieced together from the beauty of the *Berliner Tageblatt*,
postcards and cigarette papers. The two-dimensional widows are
already stretched out on the washing line – which church has no

à Kisling

Etoile qui brille

Regard humide

Fil de la vierge

Pitié

flotte au vent

Cette compresse sur mon cœur

Trop vite   trop vite et quel délire

Quelque chose vient de se casser

dans la MÉCANIQUE DE MA VIE

Paul Dermée

M. Janco

TRISTAN TZARA:

BULLETIN

à Francis Picabia   qui saute avec
de grandes et de petites idées de New-York à Bex
A. B. — spectacle
POUR L'ANÉANTISSEMENT DE L'ANCIENNE BEAUTÉ & Co.
sur le sommet de cet irradiateur inévitable
La Nuit Est Amère — 32 HP de sentiments isomères

Sons aigus à Montevidéo âme dégonflée dans les annonces offerte
Le vent parmi les téléscopes a remplacé les arbres des boulevards

nuit étiquetée à travers les gradations du vitriol

vient de paraître :

à l'odeur de cendre froide vanille sueur ménagerie

craquement des arcs

on tapisse les parcs avec des cartes géographiques

l'étendard cravatte

perce les vallées de gutta-percha

54 83 14:4 formule la réflexion

renferme le pouls laboratoire du courage à toute heure

santé stilisée au sang inanimé de cigarette éteinte

cavalcade de miracles à surpasser tout langage

de Bornéo on communique le bilan des étoiles

à ton profit

morne cortège o mécanique du calendrier

où tombent les photos synthétique des journées

„*La poupée dans le le tombeau*" (Jon Vinea œil de chlorophylle)

5ème crime à l'horizon 2 accidents chanson pour violon

le viol sous l'eau

et les traits de la dernière création de l'être

fouettent le cri

tristan tzara - 25 poèmes
h arp - 10 gravures sur bois
collection dada - 3. fr.
édition nummérotée - 15 fr.
édition sur hollande - 60 fr.

H. Arp

8
Hans Arp
Page from *Dada 3* with
woodcuts by Janco and Arp
Dada 3
December 1918

chimney – and which chimney would not (should the case arise) serve as a megaphone for the lustful screams of beautiful Negroes.

Philosophies have both quickly and slowly found a deep and happy ending. The frescos are as vivid to the eyes of the completely refined man as they are to his nearest relative, the completely primitive man. Can we be in any doubt about the malign and witty superiority of geometry? Music hall has died and the motor car is extinct. The Great Vertical has come in all its glory to the besieged century. It is the law of gravity, the law of statics ... divided surfaces race from it, parabolas and ellipses whirr from it (boomerang! boomerang!)

We hold the pig's bladder in our hands and catch the burning waste with our ears. We old priests, we are so solemn and so melancholy. In the valley they are beating the big kettledrum and the Cinnabar tide is rising. The porcelain stars are falling to earth ... eioay eioay ... we are so solemn and so serious at this hour. We have forgotten the little things we learned, we have torn the hyacinths from our heads, lifted the earth from our stomachs. So we are serious then. Have we ever had more reason to behave in a more marvellous, crazier, more beautiful, more serious fashion? Have we ever had more reason to blow the red-hot smoke from our noses and be prouder? We have killed a quarter-century, we have killed several centuries dead for the good of what is passing through us. You can call it what you wish ... surgery, kleptomania, callography [sic] – because it all means the same thing: we are here ... we have worked towards something ... revolution ... reaction ... Extra! Extra! We are ... we are ... the very first Dada ... the very first word ... whose fantastical nature cannot be invented.

Translated from the French by Susan de Muth

Francis Picabia
Guillaume Apollinaire

I still find it impossible to believe that he's dead. Guillaume Apollinaire is one of those rare people who followed and completely understood the whole evolution of modern art; he defended it valiantly and sincerely because he loved it, as he loved life, and all new forms of activity. His mind was rich, sumptuous even, flexible, sensitive, proud and childlike. His work is full of variety, spirit and invention.

1.5

Dada 4–5
Edited by Tristan Tzara
Zurich
May 1919

Translated from
the French by
Dawn Ades

Tristan Tzara
Zurich Chronicle

shit was born for the first time Zurich in cheese – but the people
have their art it's nice even the theories an explosion is feared,
huge exhibition at the Kunsthaus: Picabia, Arp, Guillaume's
mountains and suchlike by Bauman, etc. other religiosities,
cubism in matchboxes. Tr. gives a lecture on Tz. professors etc.
projections declaimed poem big box office takings stresses sleigh
bells left a break interruption dry sober scientific static repeat
arrangement chemical explanation of à a o, a o i, i i e, image of
some starry snapshots fibres unite again in a major festival to the
hint of two-step and bowie between the legs well nourished by
our olympic partners gramophone for wisdom of each insect in its
mortal chirping and biological penetration in the spheres of
magic and tranquillity – Dr Jung having eaten the feet of his wife
the products are called psycho-banalysis, and the famous futurist
Rubiner is preparing a work about Jesus on holiday

Rebirth of 391 no.8 travelling review founded in New York printed
in Barcelona appears in Zurich ...

Translated from
the German by
Jean Boase-Beier

Hans Arp
From the cloud-pump

saint jigjag jack jumps out of the egg
tararaboom the dandy man
forget-me-not rolls around the chair
all the clocks strike one and two

abyss opens up with might
stars roll right to the lovely mouth
dewdrop hare hangs on the hill
down in the stones it is lovely night

saint graspandgape jumps out of the egg
tararaboom a house and land
forget-me-not rolls around the chair
all the clocks strike one and two

alas good old jack is dead and who will carry the burning flag in his
pigtail now who will wind the coffee-mill who will entice the idyllic
hind on the sea he confounded the ships with the little word
umbrella and the winds he called father of bees alas alas our good
old jack is dead holy bells jack is dead the hayfish rattle in the bells
when you say his first name out loud so I just sigh jack oh jack why
did you turn into a star or a chain of water on a hot whirlwind or an
udder of black light or a colourless brick on the groaning drum of
rocky being now we are drying out from the top of our heads to the
soles of our feet and the fairies lie half-charred on the funeral pyres
now the black bowling run thunders beyond the sun and no one
now will wind up the compass or the wheels of a barrow who will eat
now with the rat at the lonely table who will drive out the devil when
he tries to seduce the horses who will tell us of the monograms in
the stars his bust will grace the mantelpieces of all who are truly
noble but what snuff and comfort is that for a death's head

Translated from
the German by
Christina Mills

Raoul Hausmann
Latest News from Germany

Berlin is the football of traditional youth which plays its hypothetical
match (Groß-Herzfelde-Ruest-Mynona) every Saturday with the
appearance of a senile, pop-eyed old man. Theodor Däubler has gone
into the People's Marine Division. Maximilian Harden and Herwarth
Walden are highly recommended as the young lovers. The 'Oberdada'
proclaims the Nikolassee World Republic. Weimar no longer exists.
In its place is a huge loudspeaker for spreading the word of Schiller
and Goethe. Munich is now the region of Ararat and the folk art of
Schrimpf. Not like this, like that! Goltz is a depot for Dada
publications though he would like to keep that a secret. Landauer and
Toller go to a great deal of trouble to stage Abel in the Soldiers' and
Workers' Theatre. Dresden is actually called Hellerau, after its
founder and owner Paul Nämlich, known as Adler Elohim. This
master of world literature got laid in the most republican manner at a
committee meeting on the subject of the intellectual Manasse. A
democrat Pharisee-changeling has been born who will no doubt be
quite at home in the area of society responsible for the preservation of
1914 wine and the church. Hugo Zehder is sweating it out with his
newspaper. Young Felixmüller was born in Klotzsche, near Hellerau
... he considers himself human but he is only a Monday newspaper.
Spreewald. The junior doctor Richard Huelsenbeck of Roland Meyer
Publications has, through his wet nurse Kurt Hillier, been awarded a
fabulous sum of money for his achievements on behalf of the
Association of Intelligent Headworkers but has modestly declined to
accept because his own active intelligence cannot be located.

As regards the rest of Germany, the Communist movement is
now almost fully under control and every German is busy publishing
his own newspaper. Food is no longer necessary as everyone is
downing printers' ink.

Translated from
the German by
Christina Mills

Hans Richter
Against Without For Dada

**This piece was first communicated orally at the
eighth Dada gathering**

?!Dada!! – Does anybody belong to it!? –
Oh yes, we belong.

We have your 'social system' (oh state!), your so-called
'community' to thank for our lack of belief in any form of solidarity
... a society which forces us to *differ* from it in any way we can and
which is, at the same time, the driving force behind this
moonstone-coloured Dada –
   The duty we undertook in opposition to them the belief in the
importance of 'belonging to something' is a mistake, for which you
have only yourselves to blame.
   Our solidarity (unlike the solidarity of those groups which
hold themselves in such high regard), is steeped in an acid bath of
slightly pathetic or cruel desperation ... this is a true position ... and
one that is completely separate from the group, from the Dada
newspaper movement. Juggling with one's own bones and
intestines is the normal means of attaining a world-view.
   Those gentlemen DA ... there ... are in motion DA ... this is
DADA ... the soul's means of defence against the **unpredictable** ...
   We are riding the curves of a melody and love to swing to the
beat, to and fro, wide and long and in rhythm, or else in politics (oh
beautiful seriousness – incomparable admiration for your changing
facial expressions).
   Umst, Umst (?) it was never there, impossible for it to be
there. It is *Dada*. It is as clear as the stars and comes to me as I fall
asleep at night – Oh much-compromised Dada! While the
associations watch through bars, business is bad for us (Glory to
Dada).
   Let's consider the miracle! Dada? – Dada! ... Each time we are
undone, we try to spring back into shape, we compose railway
tickets out of easily digestible salad and as a last-minute response,
we compose a melody with the irregular beat of all voyages of the
soul.
   Let me ask you do you *want* to be happy?
   Voilà, but do you want it for real, without stealing it from
anyone? Take this mixture (salad, railway, response – come on,
you already know!)
   If you want the miracle instead – Do you want to see it? We
rent out the miracle. Only (excuse us) we require a bit more than
your 'seriousness' (applause). Make no mistake! You can make
many things out of this 'seriousness' business, war, children,
cruelty. What else? Tzara Dada, hasn't got the miracle in *training*
(we have no sense of our own superiority either); it isn't as though

he had it on a leash – the miracles would be astonished at themselves if he did – but there, he pelts everything that is not a miracle with his honourably moulded conviction that rubbish must be taken out, so that the miracle does not escape a certain personal relationship with him (oh, dearest cloud-thumper).

A curse on Dada. (We'll give you the formula) a curse on Dada for standing in our way, for not letting us make direct contact with the miracle. A moment's unbelief ... in the one to come, already born. Serner's head like a flower-bulb within the fully matured womb of the brain, in a pus-filled air balloon which he, in his rising despair, has punctured. Insure yourselves on your word of honour with your world-view insurance-company against the trickery, against the pus. Otherwise, everything in you will break out *imperceptibly*. Let me come to no good here, mid-gesture, *in* the gesture and then let me crawl away from you with it.

No need to be suspicious! Something must finally succeed that suits you and makes it easier for you to form an opinion, on what you **must not** approve at any price.

Cheap! Fate has bought us so **cheaply** that we are now paying off the interest with our beautiful rights (Hurrah!). We will make it expensive for you to stand.

Der Zeltweg
Zurich
November 1919

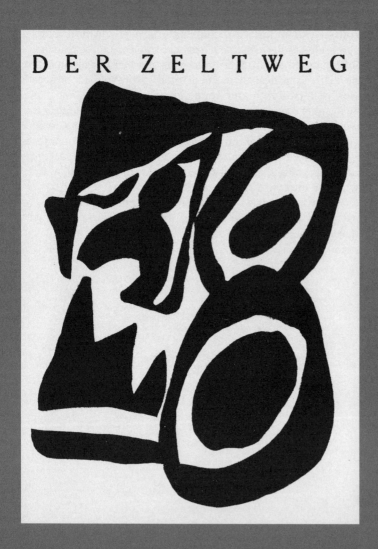

Translated from
the German by
Jane Ennis

Otto Flake
Thoughts

No church door is necessary as it was to the monk, and things can be expressed more concisely.

Art is dying, as religion has died.

What issues from the human brain is mortal. Nothing that proceeds from the human brain is immortal. It is sentimental, if not indeed an act of despair, to make art the exception to this mortality.

Art is dying, but not because we are becoming weaker or more rational; it is dying because we are stepping up on to a higher plane of intellectual activity where aids like this are no longer enough.

It is not a question of enlightenment, but of recognition.

Like religion, art was a perceptual means of making the life force visible, a projection of darkness into light. There are no more gods, saints, dogmas or churches in the higher reaches of religious feeling; similarly, landscapes, bodies, lines, representations, themes, dramatic subjects no longer exist in the higher realms of art.

The prerequisite of art and religion is dualism; on the one side, the creature and its longing; on the other, infinity and consummation. If the creature no longer feels separate from God, if it conceives of God as the totality of all existence, and if the metaphysical is no longer located in the 'beyond' but in the brain, then a state of monism (unity) is achieved.

God is a mode of perception, like time and space, the mode of perception of causality. God is the concept of sexuality transferred into philosophy – just as a son has a father, an object must have a cause. Art is a mode of perception based on causality; its subject matter is the disjointed world, the line that goes backwards and forwards but does not make a circle.

The circle is a higher level of our intellect. Perception becomes a viewpoint. At the same time it surmounts the linear progression that we call human history, or successive generations. As long as we are moving along this line, every generation leaps into the fray with naïve energy, and the incredible body of knowledge stored in the brain of the dying Goethe is lost to younger generations; the quest begins anew.

This quest is becoming tedious. Some minds that draw increasing energy from the work of previous generations are beginning to manifest themselves. The human brain, previously a subsidiary organ with dull forebodings, is becoming an independent organ with an imperious will. One day it will become identical with the totality of all phenomena. Today an artist's mind suffers from everything that confronts it – ideas, feelings, passions – but then it will no longer suffer, it will be stronger than them.

The prerequisite for all art is devotion and humility. These are feminine qualities. Poets are those who experience the occurrences in their minds as new and breathtaking. Poets are not superior personalities. Superior natures are stronger than what occurs within them. The artist's pathos is the eloquence of one who is overwhelmed. Such a one is a beginner. One who knows is wise.

This wisdom is not the triumph of reason over feeling, but feeling that has reached its culmination, the result of which is a pantheistic clarity.

Just as the masculine spirit is stronger than the feminine, so a state of superiority will make art unnecessary.

There will be Buddhas of art; they will stop producing.

The conflicts between superiority and the femininity of devotion will take the form of *disgust* with art, *irony* towards pathos, *laughter* at the seriousness of problem-solving. The greater the artist, the more problematic art will appear to him.

The soul is an intermediate condition, a larval stage. Its final state will be complete identity with the sensuality of the universe. While it is still developing, it considers itself to be a thing in itself, and the criterion by which things are to be measured – it considers itself to be the summit of humanity; which is a wretched delusion of grandeur. Nothing is less to be trusted than the soul.

How they pester us with the moods, agitation and self-importance of their souls – their art becomes a burden. If they have found an idea or a feeling, they start cackling like a hen who has laid an egg. Could you not just wait and see, be neat and practical?

The word 'humanity' is nonsense. Previously it was said that art dealt with the Divine; now, Humanity, which concerns us all. Certainly it concerns us all, but it is puerile to run next door to announce this discovery. How could we be other than human? It is as trivial as democracy.

The favourite expression of the bourgeoisie is 'be positive'. To be positive means saying yes to life. But there is a higher level: on this level, one is not negative, denying life, but one has transcended enthusiastic acceptance, one is unsentimental, clear-sighted, sceptical about pathos.

It is sentimental to seek an idea to which one can surrender, or a God to confront. Either an idea has me, or I have an idea. It is more comfortable to set a master over oneself than to be the ruler of one's own inner world. The former creates illusions, the latter destroys illusions but creates honesty. If people are stripped of their illusions, they will at last show what they are capable of.

Pathos is eloquence; eloquence is prattle. Art creates too many words about things. Cinema is purer than theatre: cinema is sentimental and stupid; theatre is presumptuous and deceitful.

Artists pretend to create a beautiful character that doesn't exist. They start from the assumption of the unity of humanity, which doesn't exist. We learn nothing from them of basic laws of feeling, of things cancelling each other out. As soon as we have conceived of an idea, a feeling or a mood, we put it to one side and turn to its opposite, which is just as valid. Art is doctrinaire, this is why it is inferior.

There has already been an intellectual period which preceded this cancelling out: German Romanticism; Romantic irony was the cancelling out of the banal seriousness of Positivism. But irony soon became *Weltschmerz*, again a fickle feeling, enjoyment of suffering.

The great final battle for art is under way. All mediocre and naive artists, everything feminine, which cannot cope without suffering, will unite in order to protect art under threat. Their livelihood will be in danger when there is a general conviction that there can be nothing more idiotic than repeatedly painting asparagus, orphan girls, cows in landscapes and Lake Engadin.

Nature has made people sentimental so that they can be creative and say 'Yes' to existence. We have reached the stage of liberating ourselves from Nature and seeking the limits of this 'Yes', just as Kant sought the limits of knowledge.

Translated from the German by Jean Boase-Beier

Arp, Serner, Tzara
Hyperbola of the crocodile hairdresser and the walking stick

(Public company for the cultivation of Dadaist vocabulary)
St Elmo's fire rushes round the beards of anabaptists
from out of their warts they conjure drinking-lamps
sticking their behinds in puddles
who sang the nail-dumpling of the ice-floes
and whistled it well round the corner of decay
till a castiron grid slid
4 eugens on a scandinavian tour millovitsch's blue box
a rampaging success
down in the haircream of a canaltrotter
the lagladdest bird lays the bushbeaten ways
of a buttersack in the tin feathers
terror-ride up a steep wall
while father shatters neatly
a skull with his tomahawk
and mother yells completely
her onceforever squawk
the children go cavorting
into the evening sun
father bows low while boarding
a boat that fires a gun
the jammy belts bear gymnasts
into the evening bun

ape-glitter sillyboots
viennese rear customsvowels of malevolent bent
circusphobe keel
hanging their profile
in international
channels
suppermarshells
foursomephistoffles
scansion scandeals

Translated from
the German by
Jean Boase-Beier [1]

Tristan Tzara
In-between – Painting (as we approach the point de tangence) [1]

The new art can be seen as the result of a normal, pure outpouring – those who have once made the effort to grasp intuitively the inner logic of forms will be able, in the future, to rely on gentle, precise terms. Clarity will become the essence of an ice-landscape, geometrical simplicity the fairytale to which we all aspire. Anaemia stays in the glass, ideas plough the air like dogs. In diamonds. With the strength of a waterfall Picasso throws up problems. With the wisdom of an archangel he thrust his experiences into an atmosphere shot through with electricity and his ascetic temperament right into the innermost flesh of organisms. In his experiments he was, in the primitive sense of Rembrandt, the painter confronting nature. He didn't philosophise.

Views of painting are relative and personal. I love crystals as I do old furniture and modern art. The different relations between height and tension were discovered, which allowed different materials to become the painted canvas, and opened up the collective mouth of the respected public, stuck closed as it was, right across the board.

And still that application of an idea to the material was one of the most important discoveries of aesthetics. I find in its realisation an echo, which does not break, a flight/*sans prétention*/on the horse of the equinox, with the typography of the soul.

The artist brings to objective reality a truth that he alone sees; for me, the distance between these two things measures the height which the artist's conception of the object means to him; this region of the brain, where ideas become metal and the entrails of the poet become little flowers on the arc of night jewels. Instead of the steps of a staircase you can use a ladder without the uprights between the steps. The sound of a piano is different from the same sound played on a 'cello and different again when a tenor sings it. In a series of differences I constantly change the vibrations / the symphony. I am not making analogies./The density of materials means weights, which I distribute, in order to make constructions possible. Tooth bites material. Like the teeth of a zip, the hour slots in between blood-vessel and phosphor.

In addition to all these new problems we filtered the value of development, simultaneity, movement/futurists/of new materials/carpets, embroidery, paper pictures/of depth, line, colour.

To be dangerous is the most pointed probe.

A small segment of an old painting is well made, stable; the main joint. Colour and line determine dimension and frame. The modern painter compresses, centralises and achieves a synthesis and the measure he uses is order. His art must hold up mandarins, comb flowers, be stiffly ordered, clean.

In ARP I see: vegetation in explosion, things thrown together, burgeoning asymmetry, freed from any rules of organisation, a bursting out from asceticism, theories, tradition, the future. A hatred of oil painting, oily. A mad bird rushes into the slippery-fingered system of the ear. I feel hairs on stone, hermacoitus of animal and car, aphrodisiac for the natural growth of archaeological bonbons.

In CHIRICO: line staccato. The world of his mind covers the gazer with greenish ice. He abstracts things then leads them down the path of poisoned mystical scorn. Deepsea-Hamlet-patina. Yes.

LÜTHY: leads through corridors of gold and blood from sensibility into fantastical peace. Deepsea-riches grounded in astronomical exactness. A bible myth in which two parallels cross.

VAN REES: peaceful thrust of lines, living side by side; x-rayed cleanliness.

The mathematical purity of Mrs VAN REES' embroidery sends fountain rays into infinity. Clear colours have the sonorous swing of nights that circle the milky ways.

RICHTER: vision realised as a musical score. Things formed apart and obsessively wasted.

To collect the coloured fibres of vitality and function in a phial: thus a world could be made. These sentences would be in the depths of a shaft that would come into being: the cup of a sunflower. Cold waters would circle, cables bark, calendars snow under. Waypieces of flaking ifnamely mean the end of the negro's stylus/ expressionist-softened painting/the most relative. The stiffest most burst. The most arbitrary-intensive. Wild.

As the angels provisionally drip from the Christmas tree.

[1] Written in 1916 for the first Dada exhibition, Zurich, Switzerland [2]

Translated from
the German by
Jean Boase-Beier

Hans Arp
The cloud-pump

Laughing animals foam from iron cans the cloud-rollers squeeze
the animals out of their cores and stones naked hooves stand on
stoneage stones mouse-still in twigs and bones antlers prong
snowballs on chairs kings gallop into the mountains and preach
the horn of december lets straw-bridges down brings iron letters
silently and with clear sounds on the icesurface the turtledoves
freeze

never has the he the sweat-breaking mountain forest climb
through black resin and are quiet in fine air-steps in stalks in the
iron armoury of the bird the child turns above a fire-red **troika**
nor the corpses of angels harrowed with golden harrows nor the
bushes soaked in burning birds nor driven over the cooling
summer ice with the wax sledge nor pulled closed the curtains of
black fish nor carried air in small glasses in to the castles nor
knitted birds out of water and least of all on stilts above the clouds
on pillars above the seas

surely no one break the birdless stone of sharp swans in the
moneyrumpstump the dead milked in the wind stood at a slant
the silver ribs of the bent man ring beside peacocks in arabian
coats this scolding of dragons cockadoodledoo who knit
industriously in the abyss of light like the built-in bride in a
wooden salad around the feathered towers calorie-rocking
droning of mind-roses out of pods roll the seven suns passion the
huge bird dances thunder on the drum throws shadow-hands on
the porcelain who has opened the springs now the birds flow out
of the cool pipes earth-chains chain the water beds

in january it snows graphite into goatskins in february the
chalk ostrich appears to white light and white stars in march the
chokeangel is courting and the bricks and moths flutter off and
the stars swing in their rings and the windtunnel-flowers rattle on
their chains and the princesses sing in their fog bowls who goes
hurrying by on little fingers and wings chasing the morning wind

if you unroll from your spool
your redbrick plait will break
and the winds will gather
the flames from your beak

and out of your tube
the black star-fish will fly
and reach out his claws
and the first-born will die

10
Double page spread
Der Zeltweg
November 1919

in the sea black snow will start to fall
an udder sing out from the waternest
the fishes' wheel will borrow someone's pipe
go with painted-on hair as an unenlightened guest

the water-stewards will anchor to the dying stars
the lighthouse in a sack drift off in the wind
amber creatures will disappear unmilked
childwreck and a leaking dwarf will float behind

and nothing will stop the drums and thuds and bangs
the sea's hard work nor the sponges' cry
the wind will whet its claws all over again
hang captains out on its antlers to dry

the dwarfs' thin horn will sing out
the lightning mate with lice
the harp will sound from rivet and crack
and on the rats the ships will ride

the air will dry to black stone
so bride and rose and beak can be ground
into the pit the circus will fall
and the stars fly up and dance around

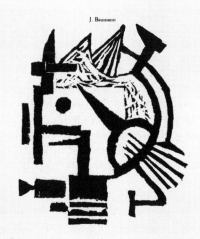

J. Baumann

Voilà
Et se purifie entièrement au dépôt général en gros.

Ici les antennes brûlent l'impatience des agences télégr. les rayures appellent les scorpions.
qui règlent le lavage automate des urinoirs, envoie gratuitement des cigarettes à ceux qui
en désirent avant le suicide. peach Brandy auréole de tes yeux. Les scorpions enfoncés
dans les organes y circulent librement. les cadrans annoncent l'intoxication voilà les saints qui
jouent la ronde parmi les chaînes, et le saut qui se prépare chez les modèles des peintres,
dans les pavillons — voilà le fer menace sa chute liquide, la grêle, les dents. Voilà le re-
mède. Extra-fin.
Voilà

Sophie Taeuber

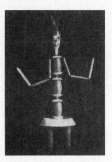

W. Serner

Dada-Park

Ad Aktion. Man spreche nicht von Realismus . . . Revolutionsliedchen im Kaiser-Ge-
burtstags-Stil. Nach stattgehabter Konsumation des vorrätigen Klischee-Zeugs bleibt es,
Herr Pfemfert, erstaunlich gar sehr, mit welcher Vehe(wehe!)menz Sie und Konsequenz
unentwegt Stiljünglinge, deren Expressionsmöglichkeiten allenfalls hinter Ohrfeigen lie-
gen mögen, zu lancieren sich nicht entbrechen können. Und jedennoch: Allwo bleiben
Ihre vorkriegerischen Spezial-Trottel-Sonder-Extra-Nummern (Mangold, das Gollchen,
Chajim Hirsch!!)? Noch zur Belebung: In Zürich, wo in großen Zeiten jeder Alleinerich
hastenichtjesehn sowas wiene Aura (Au!) rund um sich herum zu spinnen imstande ist,
blies ein Arri- und Auravist, ansonsten in der Mitte ganz hervorragender Dinierer (Rubiner),
auf seiner mit nachtschweißtriefenden Warmwichsbriefen gepflegten Beziehungsschalmei
und — schwupps quetschten Sie, Herr Pfemfert, jeden Ohres har, eine Vonzurmühlen-
Extra-Sonder-Gans-Spezial-Nummer aus. Dieses war fürwahr sehr schlimm . . . Man
spreche jedoch nicht von Realismus. Man spreche von einer Aktion . . .

2 5

Translated from the
German by Caitríona
Ní Dhubhghaill

Walter Serner
The Swig about the Axis

Manifesto

1 It's a long way to Tipperary. For sure. Because properly
considered: psychology is a handicap. Every rule has its exception,
without a doubt. In fact as a rule. Therefore take extra care: every
rule is to be applied as an exception, for the rule is the exception.
(An important rule, that!) ... You can only relatively establish
relative interrelations. And not even that. Psychiatrists and
examining magistrates are, at bottom, ticketsellers manqué
(wandering circus), as every (oh well!) – psychological judgement is
an exercise directed by the one who is judged, the results of which
so seldom please merely for the reason that the exercise is
inaccurately commissioned owing to the deficient self-knowledge
of the one who is judged. As has been proven, the best judgements
are posed in the worst way, the worst ones in the best way. (The
seedless fruits are the sweetest. Oh the dear idle physogs!) As has
been proven: the quite terrific variety of judgements about (ha!) –
bad people. (The ones about good people are always right.) Sub-
proof: judgements only interest the lads, when they hear them; but
the toffs already care even before anything's been – (down boy!)
given in ... Every piece of advice is a downright lethal affair; but just
in passing: administering bad judgements about yourself is
nonetheless the most honest way of avoiding good judgements
that are also false. *Tant de bruit pour une – occasion perdue?* ... But
sometimes nothing helps: neither grinning for nor grinning
against. They trust you anyway. Oh, where is the audience for *really*
heavy fellows? I have become so narrow and sprattish ...
2 The ultimate disappointment? When the illusion that one is free
of illusion reveals itself as such. (The most oppressive manoeuvre
of vanity: making oneself out to be more stupid and bad than one
would like to be in order to indulge the vanity of not being vain.
Fails miserably.) ... The height of *naïveté?* When someone wants all
at once to find out the (ogodogodo) – truth. (A clout on the ear is
after all only a desperate approximation. Also, false tears often
seem more genuine than – false ones.) ... Two joke questions? Not
at all. Two bracelets.
3 An excellent cigarette definitely required ... Various symptoms of
bad conscience (ding!), of guilt (dong!) such as deep blushing, going
pale, stuttering, unsteady gaze, the compulsion to speak of that
which will reveal all etc. pp. rubbish, appear when sensitivity
(deficient mastery of the high idiom) has reached a very great level,
merely by virtue of this sensitivity, which so quickly anticipates
them at the instantly realised possibilities, that it is no longer
factually capable of fending them off (or no longer even wants to do
so: THE condition ...) ... This overlong sentence formation is so
lightly spat out after the in any case overly magnificent bankruptcy
of psychology!

4 As is notorious, Descartes and Swift loved squinting. *Chapeau bas!* (All the same ...)

5 The greatest certainty in his doings is projected by the one who has convinced himself of the restless uncertainty of all and who is therefore sick of it. The broadest self-awareness (*Patent Oil Urinoir*) is merely the ultimate uncertainty, which presents to the penultimate the impression of certainty. The ultimate certainty, tasted as such absolutely: THE certainty (the keen whoomph). Thus all is play-acting, as all is uncertain (*rastaquouèresque*). Furthermore, who has not felt, when he cried, as if he were lying, when he smiled, as if he were concealing himself, and when he forgot his face, as if he were betraying himself, eh? All mimicry (the little muddle): – acting a part ... Camels believe in their masks. Those who notice them discover that they are already acting a part as soon as they open their mouths. Well observed: it is best to act a part when one keeps to silence AND mimicry (the great muddle) ... Naturalness (chuck chuck pre pre) falls sadly into the heroic ranks of unconsciousness: it has nonetheless become a criterion for senior schoolteachers, who extol as a virtue that which may be natural; otherwise: a little baby son is natural today if he does not notice that his manufacturer is a camel ... folding edge: the seemingly certain become undeniably uncertain, when they appear in a bad light; if the light falls on that which speaks for the other, while that remains in darkness which would speak against the other and often also against that which now speaks for the other (SHUT UP!) ... But there where there is neither light nor certainty the only proven means that remains not to become uncertain is: not to become certain in the first place ... Thumb on shoulder, one should fix on the location of the left nipple (or thereabouts) of one's opponent, the nasal bone or the shoulder area and should not give up in any case. Under no circumstances. That suffices!

6 Seriousness can be so fiercely laid down that the victim (who does not whinny) is not capable of noticing how the rogue opposite has for quite some time been inwardly rubbing his hands together with tenderness. At this moment, the victim feels most moistly the need to leap out of his current state (claustrophobia + syllable-rumble) and into his proper one (to some extent dicky-bird). This prettily proves how (well!) – one can attain to oneself in a roundabout way if one has not yet held total interior raids with any success. For, initially, every flâneur overestimates himself, and a sharper fellow (whoomph) always takes himself for THE genius as long as he hasn't cracked it that this is only the talent for becoming famous. Thereupon, however, he swiftly debauches (*raté*), limits his speed of making fructifiable sums from In-Dications (talent) to his private business (Bryant 1098), becomes, if he is unfortunate, famous anyway and fills his idle hours in front of a hand-mirror – whinnying ...

7 'What do the little angels do, when they are not singing?' Dear

Jakob Böhme, they surely bemoan themselves, when they are not.
8 But now the middle deck would very much like to know what one is to do with one's health (which continues to exist, after all). As one only notices it insofar as one loses it where possible, this joker's suggestion would be worth discussing: 'Give yourself up all at once!' (Capisco?) Impressive! ... Nothing doing! Frigidity is nothing but a very low level of (well) – *béguin*. An absolutely frigid person is – dead. Simply dead. But in the end one is always disappointed by oneself and it is as if one took a clotheshorse and placed it on the same spot. At twenty one has to spit out the monocle, at thirty to remove the cigarette from behind the ear and to know once and for all that one will only get rid of Madame by suddenly beginning to – love her (to become jealous, if that is more difficult) ...

9 In the final track ... one becomes malicious out of boredom. Then it becomes boring to be malicious. And finally one begins collecting little pictures made of chocolate. Idealism still is criminal realism. A braggart who has remained gentle is a little less gruesome (as he is an Idealist) than an Imagist gone wild (as he is a Realist). Whoever invented the ampulla 'soul'! Perhaps the somewhat disappointing sight of the naked man ... But this disappointment: one should take oneself by the ear, build up one's courage and admit to oneself, that one has, as opportunities no longer earn, what others used to get off danger – a secret admiration for one's own legs ... Yes, one goes so far as ALMOST to feign one's *tabula rasta* to the totality, in order to deliver one's most devastating blow with the apparently unapparent remains of the 'almost'. A blow which admittedly strikes one's own flesh: ... last little pleasure ... last little rage ...

10 You can stare into space so expressionlessly, that it gives the impression of assurance of victory. Oh, it is difficult. Concerning the scale: hate jumps onto distrust, distrust onto hate, until you can stand it no longer and convince yourselves that you love each other. The last psychic belly-upswing of (sure, sure) – unconsciousness. But if you are staring ... you must constantly work with a bow in your gaze (or your voice). Provided that it is technically possible to execute from the point of view of communication, it would surely lead to verbal injury (or to damaging inner secretions). Oh, it is difficult ... (Theoretically the global one has long been banned; that he is effectively still grazing, is just as inexplicable as that ban.)

11 There are days when everyone makes a stupid face. And nights when the most stupid still looks too significant. And there are weeks and months and years and ... The most blown-through vocabulary, the slackest pauses, the tongue stuck out, the long nose, etc. are therefore communicative gestures that afford great relief; the more so, the more every situation is actually intolerable in every respect. One should let these dear gestures become tenderly tinged with madness (THIS the high idiom!), and one will be amazed how excellently everything turns out ... And as one can, by merely passionately (so to speak) talking away, demolish

ALL relations between people (they are ALWAYS constructions!), it offers moreover a healthy palliative. Speaking of which: one lives together, as is known (as long as one doesn't) … always in a mostly self-spun and often very finely spun net (conjugal paranoia: Juan Suvarin and his Marva); only in a yet far more finely (as long as one doesn't) … One should begin at long last to speak out against oneself! One should begin!! One!! (For a long time now I have, in quiet hours, been spitting on my own head … Oh, I don't give a damn about … Yes, about what? …)

12 The swig about the axis: not giving a damn about anything.

Translated from the German by Jean Boase-Beier

Kurt Schwitters
World of Madness

I
You
He she it
We you they
a graveyard,
Living trout-sauce far-too-loud.
I over you
Over-loud
Troutgrave yard over
He you trout fishing
Living still
You!

A graveyard over-still
We live
We –
Trout lives graveyard
Living trout plays
We play life
I play you.
Still!
Will we play?
Will we live?
We
You
They.

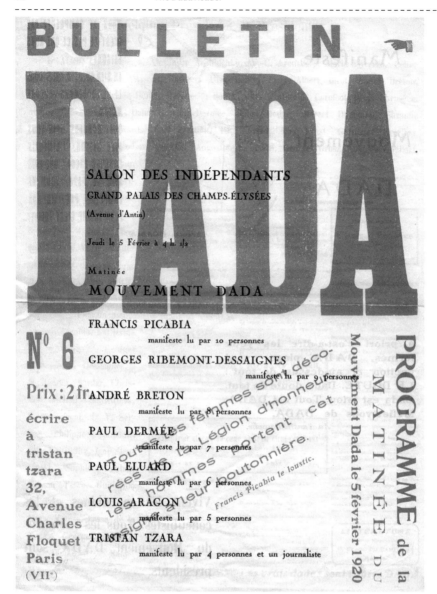

11
Front cover
Bulletin Dada, (no. 6)
5 February 1920

Dadaphone No. 7
Paris
March 1920

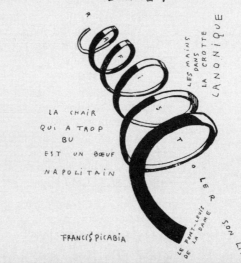

Front cover
Dadaphone, (no. 7)
March 1920

Translated from
the French
by Ian Monk

Georges Ribemont-Dessaignes
Artichokes

As Dada has only a few more years, or months, or days to live,
find a lawyer to make its will and testament.

Dada mathematics has not yet been cultivated. So far, the
study of numbers makes people idiotic. Idiocy is the lead
poisoning of the mathematician.

There is also something that is unknown: Dada Dadaism.
But Dada's breasts hang down to its toes.

Dada has doubts about everything. It is said that this, too, is
a principle. No, doubt is not *in principio*. But when that is, if Dada
believes in doubt, it will prove that it has no principles.

When Dada sees castrated pigs begin to have the voices of
jaguars, it will react like iodine, it will become sublimated. And it
will live again in the air breathed by the castrated pigs and in their
wallow. And the saveloys served at the family table will despite
everything be possessed by Dada.

Dada, oh Dada, what countenance? So sad? So merry? Look
at yourself in the mirror. No, no, don't look at yourself.

What is beautiful? What is ugly? What is big, strong, weak?
What is Carpentier, Renan, Foch? Dunno. What is I? Dunno.
Dunno, dunno, dunno.

Looking at the stars or the inside of a stomach with a
theatrical eyeglass is an artistic occupation. Finally, man's only
occupation. And they weep, they weep as if onions were entering
the composition of the glass.

It is interesting to observe to which parts the smiles of
alliances offered to Dada are directed. Politics and marriage.
Dada has a large dowry for the devouring. But Dada is difficult to
deflower. Strait is the virgin.

Translated from the
French
by Ian Monk

André Breton
and Philippe Soupault
Barrier

'I have been told of a luxurious restaurant where the most varied
foods are served. There are musical place mats, double-spouted
carafes, stemmed glasses and a magnificent front door.'

'The most magnificent doors are those behind which one
says: "Open, in the name of the law".'

'To such dramas, I prefer the silent flight of bustards and
family tragedies: the son leaves for the colonies, the mother
weeps and the little sister thinks of the necklace her brother will
bring back for her. And the father inwardly rejoices because he
thinks that his son has just earned himself a position.'

13
From top left to bottom right:
Philippe Soupault, Georges Ribemont-Dessaignes, Francis Picabia, Tristan Tzara, Céline Arnauld, André Breton, Paul Dermée, Louis Aragon, Paul Eluard
Dadaphone
March 1920

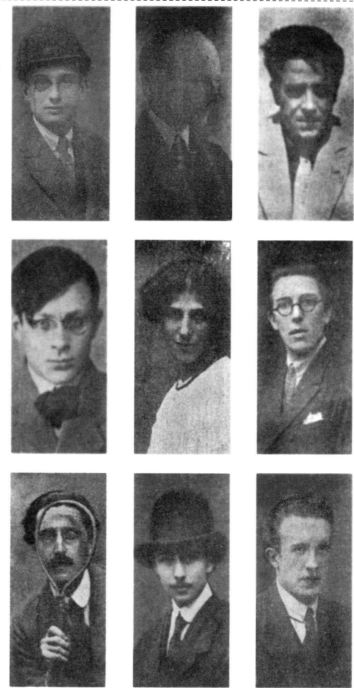

'From my earliest youth I was given over to a pet, and yet I always preferred a little tale of times past to the warmth of his tongue on my cheek.'

'With pursed lips you can drink that green liquor, but it is considered better to order a tonic.'

'Convicts make an enormous effort to remain serious. Do not talk to them of these supernatural kidnappings, the young girl still has hair down her back.'

'There are thus only brown cars that favour escapes. Every day, at noon, someone runs away.'

'May he watch out for those ladders that are thrown horizontally over avenues and which are made of all those "stop hims".'

'He does not care. Look, here is a person running towards us at full tilt. Not a cry will fly from his lips. He is moving faster than the shortest words. I know that behind us we can only blanch with fear.'

Translated from
the French
by Ian Monk

Tristan Tzara
Dada is a Virgin Germ

Dada is against an expensive life
Dada
limited company for the exploitation of ideas
Dada has 391 different attitudes and colours, depending on
the sex of the president
It transforms itself – affirms – says at the same time the
opposite – without importance – cries – fishes with a rod
Dada is the chameleon of rapid and interested change
Dada is against the future, Dada is dead, Dead is idiotic
Long live Dada, Dada is not a literary school scream

Translated from
the French
by Ian Monk

Ezra Pound
Dada No. 1

A few intelligent young men stranded in Zurich want to correspond with other unfortunates similarly situated in other godforsaken corners of the earth.DADA: Bulletin 5 Feb. They have escaped. They have got to Paris. A bomb!! The DAMN-excelsior!! London.

1.8

Dada Intirol
Au grand air
Tarrenz, Austria
September 1921

Translated from
the German
by Christina Mills

Max Ernst
The Unbeaten Fustanella

As requested, I herewith give my permission for you to fill up the
fifty-six weathering steps of fresh stone to make a six-petalled
relief rose with goethe's mineral estate. The transverse and
longitudinal lines of your parallelogram will then run
synchronously. Crochet a round metre of air first as a
replacement for the stem then as a slot for your porphyry lapis
lazuli and you will be able to deal with any orders concerning your
PT director's unbroken heart. Repeat the third and fourth rows
twice more so that the petals can marvel at their beauty. The
masterpieces of your confectionery will have to be neatly
upholstered. So give them another careful spray of gneiss, mica
schist and grey slack and on no account forget to sew up your
arches with stalactite as puff pastry.

14
Front cover
Dada intirol au grand air, (no. 8)
September 1921

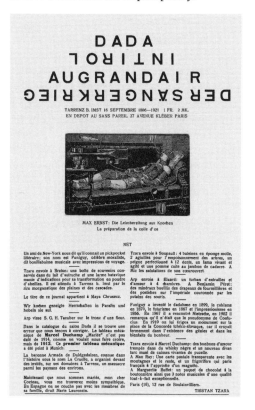

Translated from
the French
by Ian Monk

Hans Arp
Declaration

I declare that Tristan Tzara coined the word DADA on 8 February
1916 at 6 o'clock in the evening; I was there with my twelve
children when for the first time Tzara uttered this word that
raised an understandable enthusiasm among us. This was in the
Café Terrasse in Zurich and I was wearing a bun in my left nostril.
I am certain that this word has no importance, and that only
imbeciles and Spanish teachers bother about dates. What
interests us is the spirit of Dada and we were all Dada before
Dadas existence. The first Holy Virgins that I painted date back to
1886 when I was a few months old and enjoyed pissing graphic
impressions. The morality of idiots and their belief in geniuses
pisses me off.
6 August 1921

Translated from
the German
by Christina Mills

Max Ernst
The Old Vivisectionist

Tarrenz bei Imst, Austria
Over there on that hill, shouted the general, I see dense lines of
soldiers. Why haven't they reported to me?
They are puppet thieves and inflorescences, replied the adjutant.
And those artillery observation points over there?
Those are incubation buds on their ladders.
Half left there is a huge battery of men of apparently good calibre,
said the leader once more ... those are not the sort we lead.
Your Excellency is quite right. Those are the entrails of egg cells,
the top dogs of the future whose limbs are buried in the snow.
They far surpass the spores in beauty and clarity. They are thickly
coated in rooted hair. Their throats are lined with fine cilia. They
hide their poisoned fangs in their women's soft parts. Opening
breath and threads of assimilation a thousand times over.
Dew on the floor of the jug.
Forward, he answered. The shrinking of the cell wall. The
germination of spores. The incorrigible drinking woman.

Club Dada
Emily Hage

In April 1918, Richard Huelsenbeck, who had recently returned to Berlin from Zurich, where he had carried out Dada activities, collaborated with Raoul Hausmann and Franz Jung to produce *Club Dada*, the first official Dada journal in Berlin.[1] The journal featured two long texts by Huelsenbeck, 'Foreword to the History of the Age' and a fragment from his novel, *The Ruin of Dr Billig*, as well as an essay by Jung, 'American Parade'. These three pieces are marked by a disjointed style and a nihilistic tone, and they are filled with references to modern urban life. Although printed in a conventional, two-column format, they are intersected by words printed diagonally in red ink, advertising the Dada movement and Dada publications such as Huelsenbeck's *Fantastic Prayers*, and nonsensical statements about current political concerns.

The two illustrations in *Club Dada*, Hausmann's cover design and his advertisement for Jung's novel, *The Leap from the World* (1918), exhibit his innovative tactics for integrating texts and images, as well as his continued proclivity towards Expressionism. On the cover, the letters of the review's title are jumbled within an abstracted woodcut shape that looks like a hen. Hausmann's design for the advertisement for *The Leap from the World* centres around an abstracted woodcut showing a man surrounded by trees and buildings. *Club Dada* includes two pages entirely devoted to advertisements: one page promotes *Club Dada*, while the back cover features announcements for *The Ruin of Dr Billig*, drawings by Grosz and a 'Great Propaganda Evening' for *Club Dada* in May 1918, featuring simultaneous poetry, bruitistic music and Cubist dances. However, this event never took place. One of the first Dada reviews, *Club Dada* anticipated the aggressive, propagandistic and jingoistic language of the Dadaists, as well as their inventive approach to graphic design, both of which came to be defining characteristics of the Dada movement.

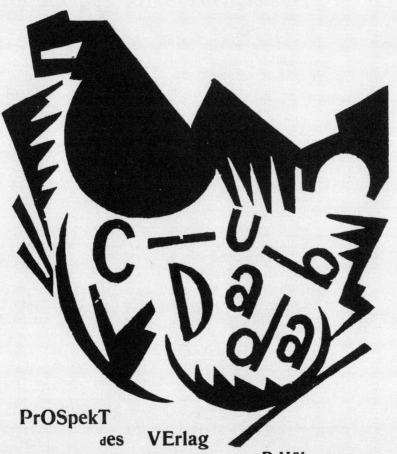

**15
Front cover**
Club Dada
1918

Richard Huelsenbeck
Foreword to the History of the Age

Translated from
the German
by Michael Kane

An at best crazy moment, the world in its lethargic, opossum-like breadth to be glimpsed through a gaping hole in the stage backdrop, volcanoes to be perceived as the nostrils of sub-tellurian beasts of prey – oh, oh, my darling, oh, oh, my dear Dr Rubiner[1] – sea, wind and towns, towns, women (women, women, women – as unchaste as possible, as false as possible, as instinctively whorish as possible) women and carnival (xylophone, banjo and kettle drum for the blasé) in their dance, in order to make sense of oneself. But later you sit, Old Billy or munificent Don, but later you sit with your long legs on the terrace of the Café Imperial where once the great Napoleon played cards with Mr Pfemfert[2]. The scene is Biarritz or Ostend, it is San Sebastian or Hoboken, but it certainly must not be Heringsdorf. Gloves made of goat's leather specially tanned for you render you unapproachable – spiritually unapproachable, intellectually unapproachable, *mon dieu!* morally unapproachable. Whole philosophies are exhausted even in the short forewords and responses. You are unapproachable – Kitty sends you three messenger boys daily to no avail, you kicked the Russian Princess in her softest parts, red-haired women were slapped in the face. Your mind is completely preoccupied with itself, you make the history of the time as one makes a baby – you experience the crazy moment (see above!) – your peace is hyper-exclusive, beyond the reach of your admirers.

We recall that we were always utterly cold, even on the day when we discovered the first signs of infection. Utterly cold, player and opponent, ice and counter-ice, polar opposites through the iciest calculation. This observation shrinks one's stomach, whips the obese out of the poets' armchairs and turns the Gothic upside down. To live without principles will be almost impossible – we slave-owners have our slaves. But the principles of sentimentality – oh, oh, Dr Rubiner, oh, oh, Dr Panhaas – now they have discovered that the logic of one's own soul is far too childish a phantasm. He who makes himself a religion will be the bonze of his catechism, the exegete of his spiritual excrement. He who lives his logic is a liar. We have our coldness, we have our elasticity. You are orientated either towards the West or towards the East. America has eaten you up, or perhaps it was the Negroes of St Domingo – our composure remains nevertheless admirable. Your religion does not impress me, Jung. I have sat on the terrace of the Café Imperial – shoes from Paris, underwear from London, lecherousness from Berlin. I am an international act. I hear the pessimists and the connoisseurs of human nature shouting: he has mocked the Sacrament, he has derided our most sacred moment (when the stage backdrop is torn apart etc.), to him the soul is business, to him women are business, he stuck a knitting needle in his grandmother's navel – this cur, this blackguard, this sensationalist and unpolitical person. Now – in a moment of total desolation and happy imbecility – I get up on my tiptoes: But business is soul and when you buy a woman, you communicate. In the end everything will depend on how nimble you are, whether you can go to dine with your last bit of sentimentality. However, everything has to touch you more deeply, delight you stupendously. Thoughts would have to be capable of tearing your skin apart, capable of smashing your jaws and, if need be, bring your heart to a complete standstill. For example, there are thirty nuns sitting around a table in the Esplanade playing skat. They are sitting there in their blouses enjoying themselves. There is an English horn, which Mr Johnson is blowing into, a triangle played by Weiss and a guitar being swung around by Mr Hallensleben. Three women have absented themselves. Whisky is more important than the card game. Look – now they are lying in the porter's lodge – not a single person has given them a blanket to keep warm. Not even you, Master Panhaas, and not even you, little rascal, purveyor of spices and seller of shit. Ah, how weak and frail you've become since you've had to play the revolutionary all the time. What a miserable state of affairs! And think of the three nuns, three nuns in their blouses drinking schnapps. That would have reminded you of your best days, of your circus and bicycle days, when you still had strength in your legs and not in your head. Everything has been distorted upwards – that is truly a rheumatism of the soul and of the mind. The good is sprayed like fog around our heads (yes, yes, that is what I call constructing a nice aphorism).

Under these circumstances – and who would have thought it – it is a matter of extraordinary fortune and a divine coincidence that one found the gentleman, who, in a fit of genuine enthusiasm, dropped his trousers on the Potsdamerplatz. This explains everything. Our attitude will be clear and unambivalent – one can then appreciate the differences between us and our enemies. Our crazy moment (see above) will be the central and middle moment of all people. For this – and let it be said without reservation – we have Dr Billig to thank, the same who, in a fit of genuine enthusiasm, dropped his trousers on the Potsdamerplatz. He had already been observed for a few days in Heidelberg; then a policeman in Mannheim found him talking gibberish, the charitable chairwoman of the *Froebeheim* gave him a glass of milk and a copy of the *Kölnische Zeitung*. The story is, as you see, very involved and complicated.

On the squares of the large towns numerous lunatics sit behind the flower-boxes moaning aloud. One notices them instantly and one realises that one must punish them with one's contempt.

However, this Dr Billig – here the tissue of lies of decades of scholarly work is torn asunder. Here, gentlemen, a ray of light in the benighted realms of psychological bewilderment, here the Freudians' mestizo dance is eminent. It is one of the outrageous facts which grumble out of back-street apartments, rise from the sewers and hum down at us from the electric wires of the high-voltage cables. Dr Billig – *The Stars and Stripes* by Philippe Sousa[3] – *revue* in the brightly lit Folies Bergère – sensational arrest in Whitechapel. The novels of Mr Wells come nowhere near this wondrous fantasy. No Goethe, no Dostoevsky could have helped in this case; here the spectators stood more naked than Dr Billig, their souls, their legs and their jaws were trembling. Not the least scintilla of sentimentality could now be justified. You see – there you would have had an opportunity to sharpen your wits, to arrive at a more precise expression of your views.

The facts are beginning to rise again, to become more complicated. Everything is spinning around. The man had a sweetheart by the name of Rosa or Kathy (women usually called Catty or Rosie at home). This woman for her part had an uncle, who was said to pursue the lowest kinds of passions and who was reputed to have been alarmingly foolish even in his youth. This uncle is glowing and handsome – I am attached to the uncle, whatever one may like to say. One sees them in their hundreds going up on the facades of houses with amazing speed, in the Indian summer or on bright, frosty days. The electrical railway rings out shrilly and little, white, rolled-up clouds fall and burst on the houses.

Dr Billig might have had a vulgar (to avoid a bon mot) desire to participate in the carousing of the thirty nuns in the Esplanade. He would only have had to hire a black suit for 7.50 marks. The Ten Commandments are quickly recalled and Catholic ritual would be the most fitting at one of Trimalchio's banquets.

It is scandalous that one must omit so much of a sensational nature in order to arrive at one's destination. Meanwhile, the destination has become the most sensational of all. Life is cruel. The uncle probably says to you: 'Listen Billig – it's important for your future. Nature has given you some fine talents – learn an "honest trade". Go to a tailor's workshop and sew on trouser buttons, become a tram driver so that with your 125 marks a month you can get your wife respectably pregnant.' The uncle has been sitting in the Piccadilly Bar for quite a while. Kitty has laid her hand on his temperament. Manhatttan is trumps. Hennessy or Grand Marnier. George Grosz is tearing his cigar to shreds in his mouth – Cadoza – Cadoza – that's what I call leading a good and noble life. Messrs Kölsch and Seiffert, Messrs Grosse-Schmittmann and Vogler, and even the master painter Borchert are wiping the tables with their bellies. It is a great day for us underwear fetishists. Now Kitty has laid her leg on the uncle's lap. The uncle has spilt his red wine on his cravat.

One day someone says to you: 'Billig, you are a decent sort!' You realise how things have turned out and weep bitterly.

The uncle is sitting with Rosa or Kathy, for example, and says to her: 'Listen, that fellow Billig.' Or he says: 'Hm – as I see it, there's quite a difference.' Then Kathy or Rosa realises that she has always got a raw deal. There were nights when Billig was full of energy. That was simply a pose or a repression complex. There were nights when Billig was melancholy, he could have spared us that. But there were also nights when Billig simply wasn't up to it – and he will never be forgiven for that.

At this moment, perhaps, Billig comes into the room with his tie slipping over his collar. Billig has his grey trousers on again with the soup stains of the last few weeks. In front the trousers form a kind of nest from which many small, comical creases radiate. That is enough to make one blush, but the rear is a catastrophe. The rear has the soul of tired hackney-carriage horses, it is a cheese, a toy for old men, a corpse in a tree, a pornographic cinema.

A defeat is now unavoidable for Billig and all he can do (now that he knows everything) is look for sympathy. This strategy is dangerous, calculated to appeal to Kathy's maternal instincts, but the uncle is coincidentally – it is unspeakable – wearing green silk stockings. This is the end of the world.

The desperate individual is a sign of the time, in his heart one reads the history of the time. He sits in the lavatories as a blind man and smokes a pipe with a picture of one-time champion Hindenburg on it. He is to be seen as a tattooed marvel in Kastan's waxworks. His stomach has folds like the stomach of a woman who has borne six children and on his arm (which has already lain many a time on the anatomists' dissecting table) one may read a beautifully entwined legend: God with us. One sees the desperate individual here and there as a stuffed bird, especially in the windows of small music halls and brothels. One does not require much knowledge of life to find him. Billy found Dr Billig immediately and indeed at a time when the latter had already given up his profession – he was a qualified engineer. The signs were becoming more numerous. Sometimes someone brushes past your coat with paint, apparently by accident, but you can still see by the movement of his hand that it was intended as an attempt on your life. In the restaurant the waitress pours the greasy soup on your trousers – they are conspiring to ruin one item of your clothing after another. They want to have you naked when they kill you. Daily now at around twenty minutes to nine one may see the old bulldog bitch behind Kormein's coffin shop. She puts her front paws up on the picket fence and it is quite apparent to a keen observer that she has been trained to attack people, so that one day she may be used against Billig. Yes – not to omit anything – even that artificial moon was seen, the one Wissmann claims to have observed as he was crossing the Zambezi.

On the first evening Billy stole a pair of well-lined gloves from Billig's overcoat and Billig scornfully placed a stink bomb under Billy's posterior. Then they knew that they were friends. As we averred earlier, there is no doubt that Billig could have participated in the carousing of the thirty nuns in the Esplanade under such altogether favourable circumstances. The time is ripe for such things, it gives birth to them, spits them out and is pleased with them. Billig could have acquired a deep insight into the nature of things, the basis of many philosophies would have become clear to him. Three had absented themselves – Cordelia, Margot and Loulou. The whisky was more important to them than the card game. They found themselves in the porter's lodge, which one had unfortunately neglected to heat. This was a case simply made for Billig. If only his character had contained the slightest aesthetic leaning, if only he had had to mourn ever so slightly the death of a relative, then he would have been compelled to partake in this carousing. But he did not succumb. Desperate people have an objective – they see their objective through the dancing houses and the screaming bridges, they hope for deliverance – and thus the advent of the catastrophe could not be delayed, a catastrophe which has become such a liberating deed for so many here. Billig decided on that course of action mentioned at the beginning and above as a result of the deep crisis in his soul and in order to find speedy deliverance from an army of ghosts.

The liberating deed plays a most particular role in the history of the time. Billig's eastern orientation became his undoing. In this regard I still consider a strictly meteorological method of observation to be the most correct. Facts have always kept the world in suspense, but everything depends on the kind of suspense, this is, so to speak, the heart of the matter. For example, somebody could come along and say: With Schopenhauer I am of the opinion. Now all would be lost: if one had not kept oneself busy thus and for so long with the strength of one's own arm muscles. In the meantime, the effect of the liberating deed is not to be sought only in an attempted murder. 'Panta rhei,' said the old philosopher and I believe all will agree when we say: he is quite right.

Billig, whose person we consider so exceedingly important for the history of the time, would have responded to all this by saying something along the following lines:

Move along, ladies, in here, place your foot in the soul seller, permit the savage to take the shirt off his back before you purse your lips for a kiss. Come on, ladies and gentlemen – they're giving the local cleric a thrashing with neon signs, the full moon is rising out of the jaws of the paralytic with a whirring noise and a great general din. Hurry up, hurry up, lift your legs, your hearts, get those trousers going, let the engine of the women's blouses rattle – damn it, look, look, the lasso is flying, life is rising out of the sewer, the old man is shaking the moss wig – *eilomen, eilomen*[4] – here you see Cyra, the beautiful compatriot performing the dances of her homeland. Lights! Music! Leporello, the crazed – Labero as a man without a soul – the man with soul – ah you, you priest of all Bavarian births and archangel of ill-temper. The stallions have broken free long ago and the laurel wreath has been hung up on the mantelpiece. Yes – yes, that is the meaning of life; that is the subterranean gramophone. Aztecs upon Aztecs, bearded vultures upon bearded vultures. Aah, aah, no, no – now do come in, ladies and gentlemen, place your hearts in your hats and let your teeth be watched over by this dog, compliments of the company.

What do you want from Siberia? Did you not see Siberia in the train, in the goat pen, on a flowery meadow, in the morning, when the first sun shines on the first signs of infection. What? Have you no sense of honour? Generation after generation sent their children to the cinema, and not one of them has become a councillor yet. Oh – shame and flute playing – oh, horror behind the wallpaper. What good are passions, Governors, lashes from the cossack's knout – *eilomen, eilomen*. A nod from my friend Purzel and the apparatus collapses on itself. Already the prima donna is buttoning on to her wire. What mishap has happened in this Protestant church? A woman, ladies, a mother of her son, I'm appealing to your sympathy, ladies, a son of her mother, a poor washerwoman, comes to grief. The fantastic devils come out of her ears – madness, madness, daylight robbery and murder, Siberia, Siberia I say, Siberia, lashes of the knout on the posterior, yeah, lashes of the posterior on the knout – to nouns that cannot be declined, the neuter gender is assigned – yes, sir, come on in – Siberia, Siberia. Here Meidner, the painter, is writing his librettos with a peacock feather, here you can see the meliorist dancing bear practise the scales of his limitations. Here one may see Eleonara Duse, Agnes Sorel, and Minnehaha, getting along nicely, here you see Becher, the genius of Berlin, and Däubler, the mighty, in a casual pose. What is Siberia, ladies and gentlemen? Bring the lyre, Elfriede, and pluck a tail feather out of the parrot. My pupils are dislocated, strained by too much seeing. Bring me blue spectacles, so that I can live and stay awake. For all too long have I looked into the icy wastes and murder fields where Arctic foxes are suspended as hanging lamps among the stars, where the ecstatic Father towers up as a porphyry-coloured glacier, where, apart from all other horrors, one's heart dries up in one's body. Oh – how far I am then from the silk stockings of my girlfriend Irene. Why can I not let myself be lied to by her, why can I not call her virgin: Siberia, what? – Well, give us an answer then, have you no tongue, no lung – no? Are you a clay doll, perhaps only a figment of yourself, a thought that wants to become flesh? One has come across so many afterbirths. Pssst ... Emil, a bowl of gold – out, I say, out, not another image, no street lamp, no Japanese General.

Should I slowly become myself again – should I drive the somnambulists out of my skull, take the little flag from my nose? Perhaps one can do the impossible. For three long years one has lain under the date-palms and been led by the nose by the Prince of Thebes. Out with him, out with the polka prince, down with the scribbling females. Opening one's eyes, one saw the castle with battlements in bright air, one saw the leopards, the tigers and the circus elephants. And the evening and morning were the fifth day. The prayers drone on from the minarets, the doors of the good-time houses are open, the pennants are hoisted on all the ships.

Look, look at the Dadaist dance around the lion on Bürkliplatz. They have made a lion out of *papier maché* – he is making a tremendous sound like thunder and shooting fireworks out of his ears. That is a fine conspiracy – it has been set up nicely, good snares have been laid – but we have rubbed our feet with the fat of carcasses – *eilomen, eilomen* – we have dipped our arms in the blood of pygmies. How long will this state of affairs last? For how long, I ask, is one to balance the clouds on one's fingers? Not long, ladies and gentlemen, permit your hearts to beat for another minute, give your lungs one more push forwards, allow this mummy its eternal sleep – deliverance is coming ever nearer, the din is coming closer, the heavenly racket begins. Place your hands on the cold steel – who knows what good it may do. Do not ask – no, no – oh no; I hear you whistling, Levisohn, put your whistle in your trouser pocket. This is not a business undertaking – you see, did I not tell you, you are already below par, and the sparrows are sitting on your top hat.

The tightrope walker was struck by a flash of lightning. His scream awoke us out of the most pleasant thoughts – we were thinking of the birth of the young devils, the bottom of the sea and the embers of all dispensable things – we were thinking of far-off meadows. Dome-shaped moon, hoofbeats, witches' dance. We were thinking of the earth's maternal scream – clouds of commotion around our ears. Ah, we are closely related to those gaunt priests who whip their bodies with chains, those harlequins all over the world, sailors and explorers of the soul. Hourly we are roused by the cry of those dying from heavy lethargy – where – where is the railway, the witches' coven, the Brocken[5] and Gaurisankar[6] of the abstract fantasists? Where is the forest of shadows, the blue forest, the moon forest of the solitary dancers? Without a sound they turn their supple limbs, without a sound or a cry is their language which reaches the stars. They dance the perfume and the innocence of the May evening. Oh plants, how you proliferate over the drowned dogs on the edges of forest lakes. The valley is dreaming. Towns rise up in the dream, towns lean against mountains in the dream, flutter their eyelashes like little girls. Ah – ah, look, look my twin brother, kneel, kneel down, laugh at the moon, pray to chastity, sprinkle earth on your hair, tear your garments. Take fullness into your heart, let stillness rise in your soul. The fat devils are already raising their burning heads over the side of the well, the dragon and the bat make the air fibrous. What has happened to the air, what has happened to the mountain? The river becomes a river of tar, the moon becomes a moon of blood. Plants and trees are turned to stone – shout, my twin brother, shout – eternal up and down, eternal to and fro. The heavenly slapstick begins, the celestial racket is on. Baggy, baggy, baggy! Three steps are one step forward, one step back and a fall. Head up means off with their heads, fantastically fast, white woman empties out the castle, but don't catch her. Fairy hand, flower chalice, leprosy and consumption – ochone! – ochone! – hospital, house for the sick, morgue, house for the dead. Come all ye bloated, ye prematurely dead and ye suicides. Open your mouth, the gong has sounded, be a witness, be a martyr. Ah, my twin brother, listen, listen, do not look, do not look, press your lips together, listen to the misery of ten thousand years. They all died for the sake of justice, and lo! the devil got them in the end. They all died for the sake of paradise, and hell gobbled them up. No explanation for such suffering, no one can say why. Ah, power, my twin brother, power. Knock the sorcerer's apprentice out of his chair – see, this banker was on the Children's Crusade. This horse collapsed under him and he shoots foxes dead with these rifles. Why do you not knock his teeth out, slit his trousers open? Are you he? Is he you? His lips are blue, lust sits in his belly. Where is the revolutionary who would force him to his knees before an image of the Virgin Mary? There is no one there – no one is listening. At least take his beer from him, take, take, I say, steal from him, whore him, slander him – my God, what am I saying? Steal from him, slander him? Out, I want out of this hell. Air, air – to see God, to see angels, images, rosaries. Let us go quickly to the old priest who confirmed us – a living person must have compassion, the door must open somewhere. A bomb can explode; he can throw me out too – what? He is not there? Why? Why not? Is he fearful for his nakedness? Why is nobody there when the soul needs him? Are people all quacks, clowns, curs? You do this, you do that. Do me, I say to you – do me – your twin brother is crying for his life. I am a carpenter and I have no wood, I am a blacksmith and I have no iron. Have pity on me, my fellow man. Rattle your stomach, empty out your pockets. You riff-raff and carrion flies, you soul sellers and hangmen – throw your children behind you, they're good for nothing. Tear your eyes out of your heads, they have seen falsely. What's that all for, what's the purpose of all the chatter, why this interest in beautiful things? You bibliophiles and literature traders, you string puppets, you student teachers and medical students – you lawyers of injustice, all you distorters of existence – hey there! – come out of your holes, you hedgehogs and fieldmice, the great trumpet has been raised, they are beating the drum and the prisoners are free. This is the Day of Judgement. *Lux tenebris lucet* – the apple does not fall far from the trunk of the tree.

Yes, yes, now your bones are knocking together – now you are whistling through your hollow teeth – *eilomen, eilomen* – the time has reached fulfilment – the storm has broken.

Translated from
the German
by Michael Kane

Franz Jung[1]
American Parade

Wind sails a curve. Open road – crescendo – plains, houses, a
lamp-post, an engine. Note the rum – tum – tiddle – dance. Spirit
– fluttering – ceases to haunt. Legs, belt on trousers, allied with a
sensible shoe, hat at a diagonal, smiling slightly lightly. Coolies,
Japanese as schoolteachers join in the general motion, rather
reluctantly. Chewing-gum triumphs, followed by Havana cigars,
and later whisky, then a chopped-up tangled knot squeezes
together philosophy, the methods of life, religion, in so far as one
brings the tottering sense of self into contact with it, and the so-
called great gestures, such as prayer, revolution and singsong.
Love is the prayer of human beings to and with each other – it is
important to me that I remain comprehensible to the general
public.

Nevertheless, what we are concerned with here is
unhappiness. I want unhappiness to march. Merrymaker's
Dance. I myself am unhappy (want to be). If not completely so – to
write that kind of thing here is already bad luck. It's known that I
resist it. Unhappiness will open the floodgates. God Unhappiness
– I am now in the territory of childhood memory. Unhappiness,
which rears up against the light.

Unhappiness which feeds on limbs and intestines.
Unhappiness – sorrow is merely a weak presentiment of it. Pain
like absinthe, cocaine, malaria and the guillotine during the great
revolution – unhappiness is fabulously first-rate and long-
lasting. To trade in unhappiness for happiness – not a chance. A
woman buries the child clinging to her, a man, besieged by love,
chews a dynamite cartridge, not to have to keep up in the
responsible rhythm of longing, like the child that still clings, in a
word: living, that is unhappiness.

Well shouted! The pedlars of the notion of simply bad luck,
starry-eyed idealists, so-called sexual practitioners puff away in
vain at the clouds of the law. Bad luck, more and more of it. The
bad luck specialists are lucky devils. Between misfortune and
happiness lies a point of equilibrium so subtly specific to each
individual in a thousand different ways, each of which is further
subdivided into ten more ways. Followed by choral singing for the
Lord's mercy, then cheque. Rrum – tum. Masses! Masses – It is
not enough to have contempt for the Japanese, formerly to smile
at and currently to fear them. Conquer, become yellower. Edge
sheets and keep taut.

The individual grows younger with it. Young, Franz Jung.
Democracy like free beer. He who drops out, drops out. The sects
are becoming more powerful.

It is a wretched swindle when they say this or that is to be
restricted, when it is simply cleared away. All they need for it is a
syndicate, the rubber-stamped. The law still governs – one could

hang a tirade on it: weighing heavily over high and low, enticing to gentle rest, reviled, feared and dearly longed for through bitter tears of doubt, from one's human best, for the best: the law of happiness, which Contradiction (on the march) has not yet learned to balance sufficiently – still governs unhappiness. Please excuse me: unhappiness is more like happiness – although that is already in the Bible. But I do not mean bad luck. The people moaning today have bad luck. Bad luck means: the law above you.

To experience oneself: happiness. To experience bad luck: to experience unhappiness. To experience experience – Because he who calls for help – perhaps not even the author – because he who is still wriggling somewhere, the sheet of paper, the thought, the crowd turns the corner – Alexander's Ragtime Band – the Party, the author. That is why the smithereens of our being will still march on.

Conquest, fixated in foreign tensions. The whistle!!

Fifty copies of this pamphlet signed by the editors are available at a price of 5 marks per copy. Ten signed copies, including a handwritten poem by Richard Huelsenbeck are for sale at 10 marks a copy. Orders may be sent to R. Huelsenbeck, Charlottenburg Kantstrasse 118 III.

Der Dada
Emily Hage

As the main organ of the Dadaists in Berlin, *Der Dada* articulated many of the group's political and artistic convictions. It also served as a venue for some of its members' first experiments with typography and collage. Raoul Hausmann edited *Der Dada 1* in June 1919, *Der Dada 2* in September 1919 and *Der Dada 3*, published by Der Malik Verlag, in April 1920, with George Grosz and John Heartfield. While *Der Dada 1* is illustrated primarily with abstract woodcuts by Hausmann, the second and third issues feature some of the Berlin Dadaists' first collages, or 'glued pictures'. The cover of *Der Dada 2*, for example, presents a collage by Hausmann made up of cut-outs from publications of his own writings, making it a self-portrait of sorts. Johannes Baader's collage, *The Vision of the Big Dada in the Clouds of Heaven*, shows a photograph of the artist surrounded by letters, words and excerpts from newspapers and Dada ephemera. For his collage portrait of poet Paul Gurk, Hausmann arranged newspaper and magazine cut-outs, including fragments from Tristan Tzara's *Dada 3* in Zurich and earlier Berlin Dada publications, to create the shape of a face. Heartfield's collage, *The Pneuma Travels around the World*, dominates the cover of *Der Dada 3*. In addition to cut-outs of the word 'Dada' from Dada publications, this busy composition is made up of texts and images from entertainment and news media that situate the movement within a wider context.

Der Dada features many long essays in which the Berlin Dadaists promote themselves using language borrowed from advertising, war propaganda, as well as bureaucratic and religious institutions. Each issue of *Der Dada* is peppered with satirical and even perverse statements. Many of them are signed by the 'Central Office of Dadaism', reflecting the Berlin Dadaists' sense of independence from Zurich. In his manifesto, 'Dada in Europe,' Hausmann emphasises the Berlin Dadaists' anti-bourgeois stance, asserting that Dada is both a bluff and the truth. Textual contributions to *Der Dada* came from outside Berlin as well. The third issue, for instance, includes Erwin Bloomfield's poem, 'Atze', Francis Picabia's 'Dada Cannibal Manifesto' and various epigrams and gossip about Dada members, which had appeared in *Dadaphone No.7*. *Der Dada* served as a major source of inspiration and information about the movement for Dada enthusiasts internationally. It exhibits the Berlin Dadaists' international reach, offering a valuable record of their relationship with the Zurich Dadaists as the Dada movement developed in Berlin.

Der Dada 1
Edited by Raoul Hausmann
Berlin
June 1919

Translated from
the German by
Jean Boase-Beier

Contributors: Baader, Hausmann, Huelsenbeck, Tristan Tzara
Year 1 of World Peace

Dada Statement
Hirsch Copper and Brass weaker than ever. Will Germany starve?
Then it must sign. Attractive young lady with 38:22:38 figure for
Herman Loeb. If Germany does not sign, then it will
probably sign. In a marketplace of unit values, prices
tend to fall. If Germany signs it will probably be
signing so as not to have to sign. Lovehalls.
Latenightextratheskywhizzingalong. From Viktorhahn. Lloyd
George thinks it was possible that Clemenceau is of the opinion
that Wilson believes Germany must sign, for she won't be able
not to sign. As a result club dada declares itself in favour of
total freedom of the press-ure because the press-ure is the
cultural weapon
without which we would never learn that Germany really
will not sign simply in order to sign.
(Club dada, Dept. for Freedom of the Press, in so far as good form
allows.)

The new age begins with the year of Chief Dada's death Ad[1]

Translated from
the German by
Kathryn Woodham
and Timothy Adès

Raoul Hausmann
Alitterel [1]

Tooth roots are to be removed by hand grenades. Property and
Intellect are the economy of the latrine. How else would the
intellect-dregs exist but by taking control of the world-intellect in
their minds. Every swine of a writer is already independent,
communist. Communism as boot polish, ten pence a litre, that's
how you write good references for yourself. The masses coerce
these cowards, who were already manipedicuring self-discipline.
Without a doubt, the masses are unintellectual. We are anti-
intellectual. Thanks for the flea in the ear. The masses are on the
move, the intellectual has had the same Buddho as a backside for
the last 10,000 years. The masses couldn't care less about art or
intellect. Neither could we. But that doesn't make us a society in
transition to communism. The atmosphere of shady horse-
trading (German Revolution) is not ours. The masses do well to
destroy (themselves instinctively and other things). We rip down
the intellectual junk shop. We demand forced labour for these
theatre-spectators of Schiller's mercy. We want to go further, and
raise the destruction of all reason to absolute idiocy. We demand
the manufacture of intellect and art in factories.

Delitterel

Have a care. We can see through you. We've already sicked up your mangled futility, the day before yesterday. (I demand of the German spirit an organ. It can only be a chamber pot.) The writing in *Aktion* is worse than blue murder. Haven't they sawn up that Johannes Becher alive yet, between boards? He spews over people and things with his revolting poet-snout. But the proletariat say nothing about it. And Mr Pfemfert accepts any scribble, so long as it's daft enough. I demand the literature factory. Or German poets from Schiller to Werfel and from Goethe to Hasenclever to be dunked in the latrine.

Sublitterel

Wilhelm II was the peace-German incarnate. Ebert and Scheidemann are the true face of the German revolutionary. A sleepy backside with neat beard edging. (Yes, the masses are marching even so. But those who see it can't hold out in this stifling fug.) Even the bourgeois is armed, he is superior to Dada, so we give the wretched Dada a kick. (He'll see you get it. You've no cause to laugh.) The World Revolution runs from 2 August 1914. We don't need to take a position for or against Versailles. This peace is the second stage of the inevitable. But people cluelessly go out to war, peace, work, pleasure, whatever, only to drop off to sleep. It comes of sleeping together in the dark. Candles would make more difference than condoms. The wretched Jesus said: look at the lilies of the field. I say: look at the dogs in the street. Although tragic culture doesn't touch them. (Daemonidal mynonania is in the end what all these senile idiots concoct with a Stirnered heaven as an ethical law.) But, heck, the intellectuals love to hold out their hand to be spat on, and the bourgeois rakes in the pennies. We are going to prepare your doom. Communist vitality against the bourgeois, and intellectuals into the art factory for intellectual break-up. Why is the communist manifesto silent about the intellectual bourgeois, who uses his secretions to secure the perimeter of his property. So the world goes on as a sewer of the ceremonious. Compulsory servitude and the whip are the only recourse. We demand discipline! Against free art! Against free thought!

dada cordial
The dada club has established a bureau for breakaway states. States founded, any size, according to tariff. Round and about.

Sell your corpse towards settlement of the German

Fat Supply!

Translated from
the German by
Kathryn Woodham

Central Office of Dadaism
Put Your Money in dada!

dada is the only savings bank that pays interest for eternity.
The Chinese has his tao and the Indian his brahma.
dada is more than tao and brahma. dada doubles your income.

dada is the secret black market and protects against currency depreciation and malnutrition. dada is the war loan of eternal life; dada is solace for the dying. dada is something that every citizen must have in his will. Why should I reveal dada? dada is as effective in the small and the large brains of apes as it is in the backsides of statesmen. Whoever invests his money in the dada savings bank doesn't need to worry about it being confiscated, for anyone who touches dada is taboo-dada. Every 100-mark note increases at a rate of 1,327 times a minute in accordance with the rules of cell division. dada is the only salvation from the slavery of the Entente. All transfers in the dada savings bank are valid anywhere in the world. When you are dead, dada is your only nourishment; the Ancient Egyptians were already feeding their dead on dada. Gautama thought he was going to nirvana and when he died he found himself not in nirvana but in dada. Dada was hovering over the waters before the dear Lord created the world, and when he spoke: let there be light! there was not light, but dada. And when the twilight of the gods dawned, the only survivor was dada. Put your money in dada. Dada is not subordinate to the sovereignty of the inter-allied economic commission. Even the DEUTSCHE TAGESZEITUNG lives and dies with dada. If you want to accept our invitation, go to the Siegesallee, to the place between Joachim the Lazy and Otto the Milksop, between 11 a.m. and 2 a.m. and ask the bobby about the secret dada depot. Then take a 100-mark note and stick it to the golden H of Hindenburg and shout three times, the first time piano, the second time forte and the third time fortissimo: dada. Then the Kaiser (who doesn't live, as is claimed for tactical reasons, in Amerongen but between Hindenburg's feet), will rise up from the trapdoor through a secret passage with a loud dada, dada, dada and give you our receipt. Make sure that behind the 'W.II.' it doesn't say 'I.R.' but 'dada'. I.R. won't be honoured by the savings bank. You can also pay money into your dada account at any deposit counter of the DEUTSCHE BANK, the DRESDNER BANK, the DARMSTÄDTER BANK or the DISKONTOGESELLSCHAFT. These four banks are called the 'D' or the dada-banks and the Kaiser of China and the Kaiser of Japan and the new Kaiser Kolchak of Russia have their royal dada in every bank (they used to be called 'Gold-shitters', now we call them 'dada'; there's one in the left corner-tower of Notre-Dame). All the money is collected and sent via Versailles to the Vatican, where the holy dada blesses it and pushes it into the lap of the holy mama. Yes, yes, dada cannot be revealed. Dada multiplies everything in the hundreth and thousandth part. Tao and brahma are dada. Dada creates children and grandchildren. Dada will be fruitful and multiply you. Dada alone is the redeemer from adversity and affliction. Put your money in Dada!

Der Dada 2
Edited by Raoul Hausmann
Berlin
December 1919

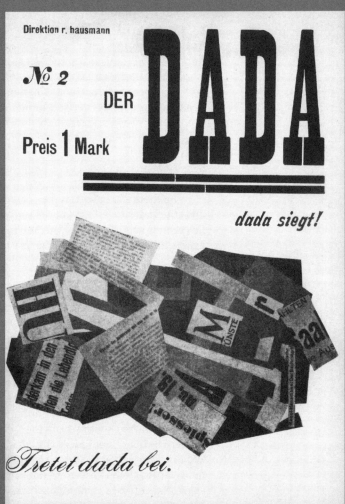

Translated from
the German
by Rebecca Beard

Raoul Hausmann
The German Petit Bourgeois is Cross

Why? Who is the German petit bourgeois to be getting cross about Dada? It's the German poet, the German intellectual bursting with rage because the perfect form of his lardy sandwich-soul has been left stewing in the sun of laughter, raging because he was hit right in the middle of his brain, which is what he is sitting upon - and now he has nothing anymore to sit on! No, don't attack us, gentlemen, we are already our own enemies and are better at getting at ourselves than you. You must understand that your positions are a matter of sheer indifference to us, we've got other limbs on our bodies. Just stir the drum of your intellectual pursuit with all your might, just beat around firmly on your belly until a god has mercy on the noise - we tossed this old drum aside ages ago. We tootle, squeak, curse, laugh out the irony: Dada! For we are - **ANTI-DADAISTS!**

So there you have it! Have a care for your scratched old bones and stitch back together your torn-up gob, everything you've done has been in vain! Seeing as you didn't manage to have us put up against the wall, well that puts us in a festive mood. And so we're going to rinse out your entrails and present you with the balance sheet of your festive values.

After the sense of life had been monstrously watered down into aesthetic abstractions and moral-ethical farces, out of the European sausage pot emerged the Expressionism of the German patriot, who, in ceaseless lip-smacking enthusiasm, took the honest movement that came from the French, Russians and Italians and fashioned it into a small, profitable wartime business. The barrel organ of pure poetry, painting and music was played in Germany on the level of an extremely efficient business venture. But this pseudo-theosophical Germanic tea party that made it as far as gaining recognition from the East Prussian Junkers need not concern us here - nor indeed the commercial machinations of Mr Walden who, a typical German petit bourgeois, believes it necessary to clothe his transactions in a pretentious little Buddhist cloak. Hats off to his flair for business, but his aesthetic and his arty Prussianism back to where they belong please: the shady lawyer's office. If Walden and his school of poetry were the slightest bit revolutionary then they would have to grasp at least this one thing, namely that art cannot be an aesthetic harmonisation of bourgeois ideas of ownership.

Oh, dear petit bourgeois gentlemen, you say that art is in danger? Yes, well don't you know that art is a fair female figure, no clothes, and that she reckons on being taken to bed or inciting this to be done? No, gentlemen, art is not in danger - for art no longer exists! She is dead. She was the development of all things, she still shrouded Sebastian Müller's great bulbous nose and piggy lips with beauty. She was a beauteous appearance, emanating from a bright and sunny sense of life – and now there is nothing more to elevate us, nothing more! Give up the romance of the sexes, my dear poets – we don't fancy that any more; show your prettily tattooed bellies instead, spew out words, adulterate geometry in colours and call it Abstract art – we don't give more of a hoot for that than we do for your tightrope shenanigans with Expressionism. **THE COMPLETE INCAPACITY** to say anything, grasp something, play with it – **THIS IS EXPRESSIONISM**, an intellectual compress for rotten innards, a slimy meal that was ruined from the start and gave you pretty festive stomach pains. The petit bourgeois who writes or paints was able to think himself properly holy here, somehow he finally rose above himself into an indefinite, general swooning about the world – oh, Expressionism, you world-turn of Romantic deceitfulness! But this farce only really became unbearable when those activists came along who wanted to bring to the people the intellectual and artistic elements they were copying from Expressionism. These airheads, who somehow once read Tolstoy and, it goes without saying, failed to understand him, are now dripping with an ethics only to be approached with a dung-fork. These clots, incapable of political involvement, invented the activist eternity marmalade in order to triumph and reach their audience, here the proletariat. But no proletarian is so – pardon me – thick as not to notice the sheer hollowness in which the petit bourgeois so fruitlessly rages. Art to him is something that comes from the petit bourgeois. And we are Anti-Dadaists to this extent that if one of us still wants to propound something beautiful, aesthetic, a safely bounded little feeling of well-being – Abstract art, for example – we will throw his nicely filled sandwich into the muck. For us there is no profound sense to the world today other than that of the most unfathomable nonsense, we don't want to hear any prattle about intellect and art. Academic enquiry is foolish – the sun is probably still spinning around the earth today. We are not propagating any type of ethics that always remains ideal (a swindle) – but this doesn't mean we're going to tolerate the bourgeois who has capped man's possible existence with his sack of money just like Gessler hung up his hat. We wish to regulate the economy and sexuality in a sensible manner and we couldn't care less about culture, which was never anything tangible anyway. We wish to put an end to it, and with that also to the petit bourgeois poet, the producer of ideals that were only ever his own excrement. We wish for the world to be moved and moveable, for unrest instead of rest – may all chairs be flung away and all feelings and noble gestures banished! And we are Anti-Dadaists, because for us the Dadaist still possesses too much feeling and aesthetic. We have the right to all sorts of amusement, be it in words, forms, colours, noises; but all of this is a fantastic nonsense that we consciously love and produce – a monstrous irony, like life itself, and completely true to the workings of nonsense finally recognised as the sense of the world!!

Down with the German petit bourgeois!

Translated from
the German
by Rebecca Beard

Dada club
Join Dada

Dada has so far resisted taking on members, but, in view of the strains of bustling city life in our time, we can no longer turn a blind eye to the exceeding gravity of the situation that called our movement into existence, and the notion of providing, within the bosom of the Dadaist society, comfort to the uncertain and support to the weak rose up most forcefully before us. Only several weeks ago one could gather from the *Berliner Tageblatt* newspaper that the enlightened intellects from abroad, together with the enlightened intellects here at home, publicly announced that they were embarking on the intention of calling into existence an alliance for the reconciliation of nations on an intellectual-activist basis. This undertaking cannot meet with our approval. For even in the best of cases of active reality, where does it lead – as we can indisputably prove from all examples offered up by history's tale? The Dadaist intellect begins differently. We intrigue the individual through the discreet form of unobtrusive advertising, which, passing from mouth to mouth and from body to body, whirls people around the electro-magnetic pole of social rotation and thereby gives them a possible counterbalance to those adversities that make life into a hellish inferno, that is to say, we move what is immediate into the foreground and automatically trigger off distance through the telescopic effect of anatomic relations. For this reason we have decided to build upon the esoteric Dadaist club an exoteric Dadaist club with social relevance that will meet twice monthly on an informal basis in order to bestow upon the Dadaist structure within the Reich's capital a more vital consistency. This exoteric club embraces members from all echelons of society; every adult over the age of sixteen can take part in its internal events. To this end he must obtain a membership card that is available for purchase in all bookshops or may be ordered on written request from the Central Office of Dadaism, Charlottenburg, Kantstrasse 118, where information concerning all benefits associated with the membership card can be obtained, namely 10, 20 and 50 per cent reduction on all Dadaist publications; 10, 20 and 50 per cent reduction on all non-public club events; access to club rooms; advantageous rates when using the Dada Graphology Institute, the Dada Medicinal Department, the Dada Detective Institute, the Publicity Department, the Central Bureau for Private Male and Female Welfare, the Dada School for the Renewal of Psycho-Therapeutic Life Relations Between Children and Parents, Spouses and Those Who Once Were or Intend to Become Such. It is impossible for us to enumerate all of the advantages that the acquisition of this membership card entails. No one should fail to capitalise on this offer: join Dada directly. Each person must decide for himself whether to take advantage of a saving to the degree of ten, twenty or fifty per cent. We are offering cards to the value of 10, 20 and 50 marks that are valid for a whole year, beginning on 1 January, Year B of the Dadaist calendar, which starts in four weeks. The colour of the 10 mark card is yellow, the 20 mark card red and the 50 mark card green. The cards are only valid when they carry the personal signature of one of the six Ur-Dadas (Baader, Grosz, Hausmann, Heartfield, Huelsenbeck, Mehring[1]). Honorary Dadas can only be accepted from a minimum yearly contribution of 100 marks, but otherwise there are no restrictions for entry into the
Dada club

Der Dada 3
Berlin
April 1920

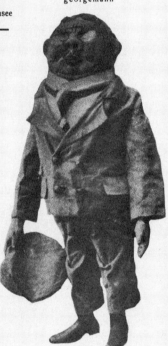

Translated from
the German
by Timothy Adès

Richard Huelsenbeck
Dada Reed-Pipe

Fluting strong and straight, no frills,
Onward plays the dada fluter:
By the stream the cricket trills,
Night has moonlight for her suitor.
Tra-diddle-da.

Ah, the soul is parched and rotting
And the head's in disarray.
Up above where clouds are squatting
Flit the grisly birds of prey.
Tra-diddle-da.

Yes, I'm playing an adagio
For the bride who now is dead,
Call it sorrow, call it trash – Oh
Lost, we eat our daily bread.
Tra-diddle-da.
Nearing daybreak's glowing fountains,
To the world of spirits wafted,
It adheres to icy mountains
Like a couplet Goethe crafted.
Tra-diddle-da.

May this dada song I'm singing
Come to you with compliments,
May it fly on two wings winging
Like a fly in slow suspense.
Tra-diddle-da.
Think of Arp and think of Tzara,
Think of mighty Huelsenbeck!

R. HUEL+SEN+BAG

Translated from
the German by
Jean Boase-Beier

Raoul Hausmann
DADA in Europe

Now understand, dear reader – it's the dadactic who knows best
what DADA is. You see, dada was invented by three men:
Huelsenbeck, Ball and Tzara. At first dada meant nothing, just four
letters, and they decided its international character. But once people
had considered the actual meaning and publicity potential of the
word DADA the 'Cabaret Voltaire' was founded (Zurich, 1916)
where, amid music, dance, Montmartre *chansons*, Cubism and
Futurism were satirised, and new types of poetry were advertised.

At first DADA was a declaration of basic primitiveness, greeted by the Zurich public partly with incomprehension, partly with amusement. But DADA developed into the vast elasticity of the time, which took its measure from the citizens: as they grew stiffer and more senile, so DADA grew more mobile, until today it has spread across the whole world. Because, as you must know, DADA is the truth, the only proper practice of real people, as they are today, always in motion because of the immediacy of events, of adverts, markets, sexuality, community affairs, politics, the economy; with no room for superfluous thoughts that lead nowhere. Indeed, if I may make so bold, DADA is (and this annoys most people beyond all bounds) against the life of the mind; DADA is the total absence of what is called mind. What's the point of a mind in a world that just goes on mechanically? What is a human being in all this? By turns a silly, a sad thing, sung and played by its own products. You see, you imagine that you think and make decisions. You imagine you are original – and what happens? Your surroundings, this rather dusty atmosphere, have set the soul's motor in motion and it all runs of itself: murder, adultery, war, peace, death, shady dealings, values – it all slips from your hands, it isn't possible to stop it: you are simply being played on. You are the victim of your views, your so-called education, which your whole generation gets in great chunks from the history books, the book of civil law and a few classics. You fall victim to your own presuppositions ... the dada person recognises no past which might tie him down, he is held up by the living present, by his existence ... DaDa organises the world according to its own criteria, it uses all the existing forms and habits in order to beat the moralistic, self-righteous bourgeois world at its own game. I hear you argue: DADA is just a bluff. But human beings crave sensation, they love to be horrified; the Dada gets over his own need for sensation and his own gravity by bluffing. Bluffing is not an ethical principle but a practical means of detoxification; because DADA and bluff are the same, bluff is truth – for DADA is the exact truth. And so DADA is more of a way of life, more the form of one's inner state than an artistic movement. DADA is insight into the hypocritical world of poetic tragedy and ceremony. It is insight into the shamelessness of science. For the Dada the sun still revolves round the earth ... but if it didn't, this would not be a major cause for concern. If you consider that after six thousand years of useless mental strife philosophy still fails you dismally and that the natural sciences are equally unable to put forward an agenda, then you'll surely see that DADA, born as it was of the unfathomableness of a happy moment, is the only practical religion for our time. **Free yourself from all restraint, forget your card games and the familiar warmth of your family** – and you will see through the tricks played on you by artists and poets. You will learn to see these things for what they are: problems caused by the system, which needs a particular technical know-how to keep it going, but which will be exposed through DADA in all its boastfulness and false ambition. Become a Dada and you will start to share our delight in the attack and in the unconquerable power of irony.

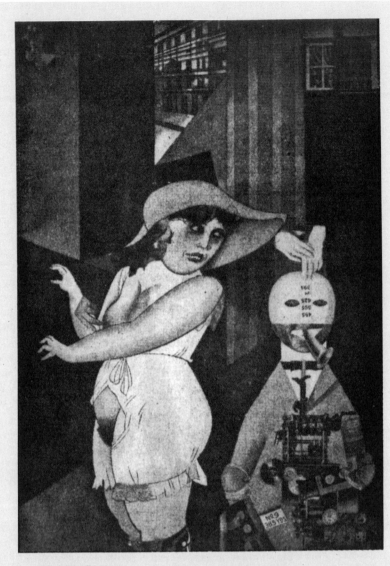

GEORGE GROSZ:

„Daum" marries her pedantic automaton „George" in May 1920, John Heartfield is very glad of it. (Meta=Mech. constr. nach Prof. R. Hausmann.)

254 km

18
George Grosz
Daum marries her
pedantic automaton...
Der Dada 3
April 1919

DADA in Europa.

Begreifen Sie, bester Leser — was DADA ist, weiß am genauesten der Dadasoph. Dada, sehen Sie, Dada wurde erfunden von drei Männern: Huelsenbeck, Ball und Tzara. Zunächst bedeutete Dada nichts, als vier Buchstaben, und damit war sein internationaler Charakter gegeben. Nachdem man also den eigentlichen Gehalt und die Reklamemöglichkeiten dieses Wortes, DADA, erfaßt hatte, das „Cabaret Voltaire" (Zürich 1916), in dem zwischen ontmartre-Chansons, Kubismus und Futurismus ironisiert der Dichtung propagiert wurden. DADA war ekenntnis zur unbedingten Primitivität, er Publikum teils verständnis- ert begrüßt. DADA große Elasti- ie ihren m

ROSZ

Dada-Company, Berlin sendet
Charlie Chaplin,
Künstler der Welt und guten Dadaisten, Sympathie-proteftieren gegen die Ausschließung der Chaplin-eutschland.

HEARTFIELD HUELSENBECK HAUSMANN BLOOMFELD
GUTTMANN ARP TZARA SERNER SWITTERS ERNST
E HERZFELDE ARCHIPENKO CHIRICO HUSTÆDT
NOLDAN PISCATOR

je seniler und steifer dieser wurde, um so beweglicher wurde DADA, das heute über den ganzen Erdball ver- breitet ist. Denn, , müssen Sie wissen, ist die Wahrheit, die de Praxis des realen er heute ist, stets in ch die Simultanität der eklame, des Marktes, , der Gemeinschafts- itik, der Oekonomie; ige Gedanken, die zu Ja, erlauben Sie, (und dies ärgert die en gr nzenlos) sogar eden Geist; DADA ige Abwesenheit

Der Monteurdada JOHN HEARTFIELD lehrt den intellektuellen Eseln Dada

20. Juni:
Beginn der großen DADA-
AUSSTELLUNG BERLIN
Kunstsalon Dr. Otto Burchard
Lützowufer

437 I

Translated from
the German
by Jane Ennis

Raoul Hausmann
Instant Wit or a Dadalogy

(The stage is ominously dark; bread rolls rain down by moonlight. Previously there was a house on the left. Enter from the past, first the Dada-Fitter, then the DadaSage.)[1]

FITTER: I feel so abandoned – my eyes are indeed newly minted, but in the current revolutionary atmosphere ... I believe something has to happen. Something with a loose collar and radical poetry. Otherwise things will get worse. Let's sing a song. A bit of art (he sings).

Herr Hölz he plays the gramophone,
Herr Ebert's quite ecstatic,
Herr Seeckt is waiting till he's done,
To give his rear a kick.

A good song, a beautiful song. And then people claim I've got bad teeth. These Dadas are idiots; when I think of the oafs who know nothing about photography! For instance the DadaSage, who imagines he's something special. He's just a ... hush, here he comes!

DADASAGE: Oh, good morning, Fitter, I'm glad I've caught you. Could you just open up my left ear – I have to compose something for Dada 3 this evening, but I've sprained my hand and can't get into my head.

FITTER: You're an ugly individual. You require things from me that you won't do yourself. I'll get Georg Grosz to draw you, so you can see how ugly you are. Just exert your brain for 5.75 marks – no Freikorps soldier from the Baltic gets that, it's too much – and compose a political couplet. You can't do this on your own, I have to fit you up, you Prague servant.

DADASAGE: I – I just need a sheet of paper – and then my chamber pot of a brain starts spinning like a humming top. Just give me a kick, you wage slave of capital, that'll do my stomach good, and then you'll see.

Heels ra-a-a-aise,
Lo-o-o-ower!
If Hausmann has dadaism's ugliest mug,
Picabia has the prettiest dada face.
George Grosz
We advise you: Pour out your heart before Dada!
There is not one wheel that moves
If my fat HANS ARP dis-ARP-proves
The Dada-Fitter
No work till fat Hans
Grows out of his pants!
All I've ever managed is to put water in my water.
The most learned and
complete picture
grazes the grass
of my garden.

19
Der Dada 3
April 1919

"Buy the books of
Malik publishing and
don't forget: DADA
conquers!!!"

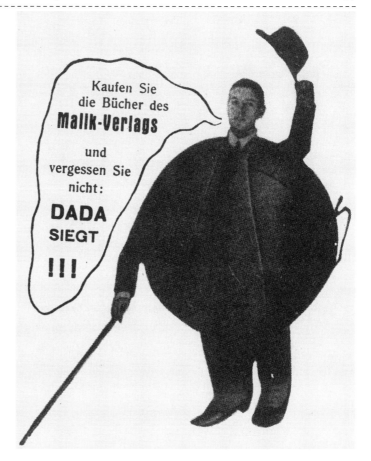

Translated from
the French
by Timothy Adès

Francis Picabia
[Charivari]

Tristan Tzara adores
his friends. The
newspapers are the
panorama of his life.

Francis Picabia
is always
attacking himself.

Erik Satie has
invented
furniture music;

----

a way to become
known in the world.
(Hire for soirées.)

Archipenko is a man
as closed-up as a
private establishment.

Marcel Duchamp
continues to give
love lessons.

Scandinavians delight in
evening strolls, when they can
contemplate the moon. And in
foggy weather, Matisse's
'moonlike' pictures take its
place in the apartment.

DADA is against pricey living.

Dadaco
Unpublished anthology
Munich
1920

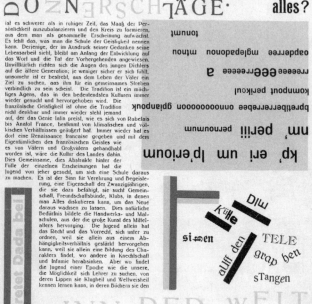

The first issue of *Der Dada* (Berlin, June 1919) announces *Dadaco*, an ambitious collection of Dada poems, essays, collages and drawings, promoted as a 'Dadaist Handatlas', edited by Richard Huelsenbeck and published by Kurt Wolff in Munich in January 1920. This project was never finally realised, probably for financial reasons, but it was well advanced before it was abandoned, and a number of sources allow us to reconstruct it partially. Wolff sent Huelsenbeck a booklet of sixteen trial sheets of *Dadaco* in February 1920, and reproductions of these pages indicate that Huelsenbeck was planning an inventive, dynamic publication featuring Dadas worldwide.

2.5

Dada

What is **dada**?

An Art? A Philosophy? **A Politics?**

A Fire Insurance?

Or: *State Religion?*

is **dada** real **ENERGY?**

or is it **Nothing,** i.e. **everything?**

Translated from the German by Kathryn Woodham and Timothy Adès

The intellects of an unimportant era face a large and difficult task. All the life of the mind stands in the closest relationship to Reality, and draws from it the strongest part of its impulses. When reality is torn apart in an extreme frenzy, when events tumble over one another like

T H U N D E R C L A P S

it is harder than in quieter times to balance out the measure of personality and establish the orbit from which one can grow up as a self-possessed presence. What may be called the school of the intellect is missing. The individual who sees the expression of his thoughts as his life's work remains, at the outset of his development, directed to the words and actions of his predecessors. The young writer's eyes turn unwillingly towards the older generation; the more insecure he feels, the more he struggles to find in the life of his forerunners a goal which seems to bind him to a shared endeavour. Tradition is a mighty force, which in the major cultures is repeatedly sought out and brought to the fore. French culture is unthinkable without tradition. Again and again someone stands up to praise the *génie latin*, as it has expressed itself from Rabelais to Anatole France, shaped by the circumstances of climate and people. Again and again there has been a *renaissance française*, and if the qualities of the French spirit were left in the care of fathers and grandfathers, the country's culture would be lost. This shared abstraction behind the mass of individual phenomena is what the young have always looked for, so as to build themselves an education from it. It is the feeling for reverence and excitement, a feature of twenty-year-olds, that gives them that ability: that looks for community, friendly groups, clubs, where the old can be talked about, so that from it the new can grow. This natural requirement was met by the schools of craft and painting which produced the great art of the Middle Ages. Youth

21
Page from Dadaco
1920

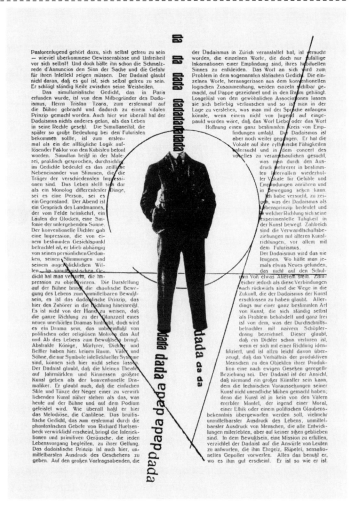

alone has the right and privilege of subordinating itself, because youth alone can emerge strengthened from a dependent relationship, can build up its character while others sink into subservience and disgrace. But where is the youth of an age like ours to get the chance of finding teachers from whose lips they can learn good sense and worldly wisdom, in whose books they can seek and find the

MEANING OF THE WORLD?

The insight that it is not possible to grasp the meaning of phenomena through objectivity has been exploited by them, as a cloak for their hysteria and nervous weakness. The fact that there were people who scoured the world in vain and at the end of their journey despairingly admitted to ignorance has now been turned into a philosophy that regards contact with the outside world as corrupting. Tired people have called themselves visionaries. Tenors from the salons cried themselves up as prophets. What kind of children's firework display is this, being staged here by grown-up people, what kind of a minuet is this, being danced under the pretext of a saraband. The cautious newspapers of the big publishing houses are still counting them on the fingers of one hand, but they are already seeing themselves as a movement like Classicism or Romanticism, always bearing in mind that a later literary historian might say: This was what the cultural Germany looked like at the time of the world war. And the dear public that admires its young Germany, its young generation, its risng youth, races along behind, claps its hands together in astonishment, is more delighted than ever before: what will they think of next? They sit in the lecture theatres as if they were in church, notebook in hand, ears blocked, so that not a sound is lost. The newspapers pray their most beautiful prayer, there are leaders and little sheep and the young poet is now born with Expressionist pathos. Expressionism could have become a movement like the Gothic in the Middle Ages, but it was slaughtered by this younger generation before it had really begun to develop. Now it is smudged in its goals like a gloomy fog painting, dangling before our eyes like a rich idyll, a chat over a cup of coffee filled with witty exchanges. Expressionism originated in the picturesque. It was a struggle against the impressionistic realisation of the world, against the child of materialism that had torn the eye's field of vision apart into a thousand small shreds, as if it were being viewed through several microscopes. It was a struggle against the realistic logic of the scientific person, who, with his atlases in his head and scalpel and chronometer in hand, wanted to observe phenomena and through his observations, explain. A fight against the machine age, in which humans were forced like bugs into the vast gear system of pistons, boilers and connecting rods. The division of work into the tiniest parts deprived them of the vision to grasp things as a unity, created serfdom, slavery, as against objects and human beings. An objection to the view of Darwin and his followers, that no-one lives independently of the circumstances that surround him: rather, they are shaped by him, he develops by them and grows through them, only the best being able to sustain their impact. Yes, the struggle for existence as taught by Natural Science was no longer wanted, but success was seen in a victory of the scoundrels, the PRIMAL PIGS grunted and wallowed. But even more than that, what happened to the goodness of honest intent, the heart in every form? It meant a return to pristine good feelings, causing interiorisation, to which any big thing that has happened in the world is now ascribed. The first expressionists wanted to live like the first Christians, in close community with that which they called God, filled with a readiness to take all to heart. And is that movement now snuffed out by the capitalist fat of a few juveniles going into Literature? It seems so. Worse, one can no longer call oneself an Expressionist, the merest reporter today knows how to dance around it. The great personality, that has the property of knowing how to take from every movement whatever seems to suit its growth, has not sprung from the Expressionists. That too speaks against them. *In a society of tired versifiers, no mind goes astray.* In a society where the contested logic of the altar meets a refined application, as soon as it is a question of the arrival of a proper person, no intelligent person goes astray. Where did they manage to rouse people awake, to urge the spirit of Europe, which was plied with clarion calls, from unhearing repose into ecstasy? Where did they manage, I ask, to divert the fast and furious life, with its ardent devotees, from its course? Where did the socialist hordes step in to answer their cry for help, against the time? The cry against the time, the attempt of children to grasp at the cogs of a monstrous machine, could not be quickly enough exploited by snobs: for socialism a gut question, established and justified for decades against assaults of entrepreneurs, show-offs and money-jugglers, for Expressionists the attempt of small publishers to make money from books against the time and against the time's market forces. There sits one such youngster, hardly grown clear of his father's cane, nose to the wind, throwing something together in the spirit of the time. Big signboard on the house, deliverymen's entrance here, the deliverymen of the mind have yet to set foot across the threshold. Expressionism has become a snobism, a toga for the Greeks of Berlin's West End, has lowered itself to be the speeding Pegasus of gifted *jeunesse*. Why could that happen? It had in it the elements of decay: the movement that could have been like the Gothic had in it elements of decay. Yes, it wasn't only the human factor, those who made it a sinecure of ambition. Just as the human race cannot have begun in one single place on earth, just as a multiple origin was needed to reach the height of happiness and community that exists today, so a strong movement needs simultaneous and spontaneous beginnings in different parts of the world. Expressionism was born of reflecting, even of resenting, a slave religion, a disavowal of all good and untamed instincts. What did the Masters do with the Stage? A drama, perhaps a buffoonery the like of which no immortal spirit could ever imagine, is being played here on a stage which in truth embraces the whole of our known world, and the spectators are forced to participate and take on a role which, subject to the plan of the godlike Initiator, may mean life or death. It is a state of excitement such as no-one could imagine, a dancing epidemic of the most insane variety, a flagellants' community of the most grotesque nature. Events are drawn out into the distance and concealed from the prognosticators' gaze. No-one knows if he will be hit by the wave created by the raging storm at the other end of the world. The nerve-wracking uncertainty is the grisliest tool of the time, a truly demonic device of the machine age. Death approaches and none can look it in the eye; courage in the old sense is in decline; but here and there heroism is blazing and cries its old song of defiance with which humanity has again and again wrested the justification of its being. In such a time a rising generation does not know which way to turn. The young stand truly helpless in face of the roaring Maelstrom, shamed and shocked to find in this situation not even a trace of the spirit that raised them up, by which they lived, which they recognised and hallowed as the best. They realise that the spirit of their predecessors will neither hamper nor hasten the coming of events – for that spirit was as remote from the actual motor of things as they are today. Yes, they can see how the storm-clouds gathered over the heads of people innocently pursuing their goals; and how those people and their goals became small, frivolous, futile in the eyes of those who had had bigger experiences. They learn, too quickly, the natural feeling of hatred for those who essentially were no better and no worse than themselves. They forget that generations do nothing, individuals do everything; they seethe with suspicion and rage. They can name the aesthetes who have overseen how artistic expression has dealt with the time, and they imagine the hour has come when the world can be improved by a mere wish. They think they must improve the world: but basically it has not changed, and is storing up difficulties, more or less numerous, to thwart writers and artists in their personal impact. This is their proposition: Because this world shows itself to be out of line with the mind's conceptions, it must be improved. We find it bad, but worth improving; for if it were not worth improving, if it were not possible to make a good world from a bad one, life would be senseless and the best thing would be to hang oneself. Young people who say this think history is on their side, but simply has periods of higher and lower mental activity; yet they overlook that the basic instinct of all the laws in the world has stayed the same. What then are they to improve? Freedom is a word that only makes sense when it relates to the inner depths of the personality. Systems of government, debt management, rituals, political agitations are noise and smoke, one is the mother of another and one collapses into another, obeying laws which we can never know. Who wants to make improvements? Men of intellect, who see it as a disgrace to stand and hold forth with a party politician's crude gestures; men of feeling, who have never grasped the degree of vulgarity that goes with putting the smallest thing into effect. To try to improve the world with such resources, to debate reforms in back rooms, to make superb poetry and idealistic politics in little magazines, is like trying to catch clouds in butterfly nets. But there is something else besides that really characterises the movement that was baptised

M E L I O R I S M

by Kurt Hiller: its lack of psychological insight. People have been up in arms against psychology since the beginning of the struggle against naturalism, a movement that set itself the task of explaining the most delicate psychological conditions. It used every technical and scientific means to study the growth of emotions and feelings and their dependence on life's numerous unpleasant circumstances and encouragements. In naturalism, people wanted to see the reflection of an epoch caught in things and stuck in pettiness. The inspired and the psychological person. The psychological person, the realist, the ridiculous copier of reality, yes the cowardly and stupid person – the inspired person, the bold individual, who measures out the depths of the cosmos with his mind and feels his inner being tremble on the threshold of wonderful things, in a word, the citizen and the poet. What people hated in psychology was reality, the hideous face of evil watching out of the picture of appearances. People turned away from it to condemn it in anger. Yes, to condemn it in anger, but also, in moments in which the sun shone, life moved on the streets and the day shouted, to find it suitable for improvement. Yet without a certain amount of psychological resourcefulness it is not possible to cope with this world, you must know what your neighbour is thinking if you don't want him to immediately place obstacles in your path, you must be able to interpret the smile of the old man there in the corner, before he reveals himself as a member of the secret police. If you want to eliminate the criminals you must use all their own methods of villainy against them, as a mad-doctor lose yourself in the abyss of the wildest madness. This is how these Mr Worldimprovers with glasses and girlish muscles, carrying the smell of their studies and still accompanied by the warmth of their nightgowns, fail completely and today represent ridiculous figures for those with insight. The marriage of the chieftain signalled the conclusion of a movement that, from its inception, has been nothing but a sad farce, a completely youthful and naive failure to recognise the possibilities of doing something. And yet despite their childish goals, the Meliorists had something that made them more appealing to us than the other section of the youth, which, as already indicated, covers its head with gestures belonging to classical tragedy, and which hates the existing world but doesn't dare do anything in it – the Meliorists have Activity. A shimmer of activity, a pale reflection of the human desire to be up and doing something, and it is significant that the Meliorists placed this word at the top of their programme, sensing that there was something good in it. Activity, that monstrous concept of colour, rhythm and sounds – what have they to do with it, those weaklings who today, under the concept of Expressionism, longingly await bourgeois recognition. They are the ones who in their innate hypocrisy are proud of their blindness and of their lack of vital qualifications and have made a philosophy out of their passivity. I am talking about the people who have gathered under one name and fill it retrospectively with their laziness, when it had been a trumpet-call to action for others. The insight that Realism offered no solution for world events now has nothing in common with the insights of these anaemics, litany must now replace prayer, withdrawing from the struggle now means inwardness. For those who initiated the movement, the fact that nature must not be copied served as an impetus to engagement and a call to self-definition. It now serves to justify waiting for a decent pension.

anlogo bung
anlogo bung
blago bung
blago bung
blago bung
blago bung

391

Dawn Ades

Francis Picabia's peripatetic review was the longest lived, most spectacular and most idiosyncratic of all the reviews associated with Dada. Starting during the First World War, it charts its artist-proprietor's itinerary both literally and culturally from a broadly avant-garde position, through the New York experience with Marcel Duchamp, the encounter with Dada in Zurich, the intense conflicts within Paris Dada and the final resistance to the new movement of Surrealism in 1924.[1]

391 has its own trajectory in which the encounter with Dada forms a key part and tells the history of the movement from Picabia's perspective. There is virtually no reference to Berlin Dada. It was named in homage to Steiglitz's 291 Gallery and sumptuous magazine 291 in New York, where Picabia and Duchamp had taken refuge from the war in Europe. In 291, which ran for a year in 1915, Picabia first showed his machine drawings and 'object-portraits'. Back in Europe, Picabia published the first issue of 391 in Barcelona, a refuge for many displaced European artists, in January 1917. He returned to New York later that year where the fifth issue of 391 was published in June. Duchamp was then orchestrating the 'Fountain-urinal' scandal with the publication of the little magazines Rongwrong and The Blind Man.[2] Picabia and 391 joined the 'readymade' debates with photographs on its three New York covers of a propeller, a light bulb and a cog. 391 referred obliquely to the scandal in one of its regular back page news flashes: 'Marcel Duchamp ... has resigned from the Independents Committee.' Dada had as yet made no impact. As Duchamp later said: 'It was not Dada, but it was in the same spirit, without however being in the Zurich spirit, although Picabia did some

things in Zurich. Even in typography we were not particularly inventive. In The Blind Man it was a question above all of justifying the Fountain-urinal.'[3]

The encounter between 391 and Dada is clearly registered with the eighth issue, published in Zurich in February 1919, with the name 'Dada' inscribed among others in the grid on the cover and contributions from Hans Arp, Alice Bailly[4] and Tristan Tzara. Tzara had first written to Picabia in August 1918, soliciting a contribution for Dada 3 (December 1918). Picabia responded expressing interest in seeing the 'dada movement cahiers'; his actual contribution to Dada 3 was fairly minimal – a brief note mourning the death of his friend the poet Apollinaire and an advertisement for his new book Poems and Drawings of the Girl Born without a Mother. But Picabia's sceptical, ironic and nihilistic attitude affected Zurich Dada and Tzara in particular, while the 'movement' also made itself felt in 391. There is an interesting collaborative text by Picabia and Tzara that intimates automatic writing, and a 'Little Manifesto' by Picabia's wife Gabrielle Buffet which is as much an anti-manifesto as Tzara's own 'Dada Manifesto 1918'. News flashes from round the world – New York, Paris, Zurich and Barcelona – on the back page of the eighth issue give a vivid and fanciful glimpse of Dada and of art in the immediate post-war moment, disses other avant-garde reviews ('Sic should change its tyres ... ') and chronicles the doings of his friends. 'Marcel Duchamp gone to Buenos Aires to organise a hygienic Urinal service – Rady-made [sic]'; 'Cravan professor of physical culture at the Athletic Academy of Mexico City will shortly give a lecture there on Egyptian Art.' Dada is liberally announced: Tzara's 'Dada Movement Dada Review and Dada Gallery ... Three numbers of Dada are about to appear the printer has left prison and the paper is bought. *391*, no.9 is in press and will be dedicated to the memory of art.'

In 1919 Picabia finally returned to Paris, where all the subsequent issues are published. He had no contact with André Breton and *Littérature* until December; in 1920 Tzara joined him in Paris and, together with the *Littérature* group, they orchestrated Dada's Paris life. *391* charts Picabia's various skirmishes with the official avant-garde and the Salons; its pages are crammed with aphorisms and snippets as well as illustrations, making public, for example, Duchamp's iconoclastic gesture L.H.O.O.Q. The little reviews proliferated in Paris and Picabia himself not only produced a rogue issue of *391*, *Le Pilhaou-Thibaou* (an 'illustrated supplement to *391*' which contained only texts) but two issues of another, much smaller review, *Cannibale*, whose title accurately indicates Picabia's violent rejection of art.

Alliances and wars between the Dadaists in Paris were complicated and multifarious; Picabia's single pamphlet *La Pomme de Pins* supported Breton's initiative of the 'Congress of Paris' and attacked Tzara, to which Tzara responded with *Le Cœur à barbe*.[5] After *Le Pilhaou-Thibaou* of July 1921, *391* ceased publication for three years, while Picabia got on with his painting and social life and contributed occasional covers to the new series of *Littérature*. However, irritated by the emergence of Surrealism in 1924, he produced three issues in quick succession, with the assistance of Pierre de Massot, nos. 16–18, which inveigh against Surrealism. The fourth and final issue, no.19, in October 1924 announced a new movement, of which this is the only record: Instantaneism, an anti-movement which died as it announced its birth.

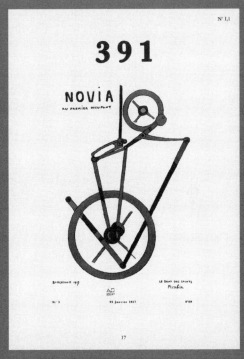

22
Front cover
391, No. 1
Barcelona,
January 1917

Translated from
the French by
Michelle Owoo

No.1, Barcelona, January 1917
Pharamousse[1]
Whispers from Abroad

HELLO HELLO!! - We have decided, after much thought, to introduce ourselves to the public on both sides of the Atlantic. We are not commenting on the nature of art, though it asserts itself in the work presented. Its evolution has not yet run its course and its progress will not be confined by convention. Manifestos and statements of belief seem to us only to have been written to illustrate the scale of the abyss which separates a dream from that which – according to Baudelaire – is not its sister: *action.*

But I have a story to tell ...

* * *

I once knew a lady who wrote rhyming poetry, whose verse always scanned with great regularity. These verses rhymed with military precision, with the regulation number of sentiments and ideas. But I loved this woman just as she was. With Larousse as her bible and her dictionary of rhymes. She was the personification of splendid ingenuousness.

One day I took her along to the Salon des Indépendants.

'I don't understand', she said to me, 'why these artist friends of yours only paint portraits of women in rickety chairs.'

I looked at my young friend, as I had predicted that this utterance would be accompanied by a delectable pout on more than one account. And this is indeed what I witnessed. However, I also made another observation that alas I expressed thus:

'Oh my dear lady, your face is a fanfare of indigos, crimsons and blacks ...

She made as if to reclaim the heart she had apparently given me. And so inflicted a renewed longing for her flesh upon me.

Many of today's artists have avowed their noble intent to portray modern man in his entirety, man who, it has been demonstrated, as yet has no great knowledge of himself. And the most modest of my intimate exploits will remain the adventure of a lifetime for them. M.G.

---

291 – Clearly '391' in Barcelona is not the same as 291 in New York.

But where are Messrs Stieglitz, Haviland and de Zayas, who patronised the already famous and now extinct publication and whom we will soon see again, *n'est-ce pas?* Not in Barcelona, that's for sure. For now, Mr Stieglitz is content to be the most artistic of photographers; Mr Haviland the most meticulous metal turner and Mr Zayas (see *Life* magazine) the finest caricaturist ...

And so we take up the task, with our limited resources.

23
Back cover
391, No. 1
Barcelona
January 1917

Nº I,4

ODEURS DE PARTOUT

391

Tristouse – In reality, the poet was never assassinated, nor was it Tristouse who stuck an open umbrella in his eye. Go on, identify the hand that wielded the sword!

Tristouse has a heart.

Anyone who doubts that has never heard her sing a tune from Mignon with an obligatory tear in her eye '*her name was Marie, she was born in Paris* ...'

Anyone who doubts that has not seen her cut her hair, with her own stoical hand – the hair of ... of ... a pretty blonde girl – so as to encircle her friend's waist with it – a girl who left for the extreme north-west Pyrenees the very same day, and above all has never heard her, in a tone somewhere between the Bobino nightclub and the Comédie-Française, utter the words destined to go down in history: '*at least that much of me will be there* ...'

New inventions and the latest innovations –
In his aim to express the spiritual realities of this world, Francis Picabia remains resolute that he will only use symbols drawn from the repertoire of purely modern forms.

A very sensible censor recently erred on this matter thinking he had recognised, amongst paintings variously representing Love, Death and Reflection, something resembling a working drawing for a compressed air brake, or a machine for crushing peach stones.

It was all seized at the border together with the luggage of a charming Parisian woman – Mrs Nicole André Groult – and sent to Mr Painlevé, from the Institute, to the Ministry of Inventions concerning National Defence, under escort.

* * *

Unable to find a studio sufficiently large to realise the enormous scope of his dreams of glory, the painter Delaunay has left for Lisbon, where he is to decorate the façades of all the buildings. Thirty kilometres [eighteen miles] of enormous painting are in the offing.

* * *

A new reference work on modern painting will appear this year in New York, published by what is probably one of the most important art galleries of the New World. The author, Max Goth, will be signing copies.

Picasso repents – Just when the nations of France, Spain and Italy have simultaneously claimed the honour of counting him as one of their own – he is actually Spanish on his father's side, Italian on his mother's and had a French education – Picasso (to whom the sorcerer Max Goth has just revealed the Germanic origins of Cubism) has decided to return to the Ecole de Beaux-Arts (Luc Olivier Merson's studio).

The *Elan* has published his first studies 'from the model'. Picasso is henceforth the head of a new school to which our collaborator Francis Picabia offered his support without a moment's hesitation. The picture shown above is a solemn testament to that fact (Fig No. 23).

Transfers, holidays, exhibitions and lectures –
In this first edition we were to publish a musical piece by Gabrielle Buffet. Our dear friend is currently in Switzerland, however, where she is trying her hand at skiing.

* * *

Albert Gleizes has found an admirer. During the course of his last exhibition in Barcelona he was given a jacket by a tailor-cum-art patron in exchange for a watercolour.

The man in question, transfixed by a portrait of Jean Cocteau, murmured in Spanish 'It is a spiritual and singular piece, but what I'd really like to know is, is it supposed to be an old lady or a flowerpot?' An intolerable demand.

Albert Gleizes has left for New York, where he is to organise an exhibition of French art.

* * *

Arthur Cravan is another one who has boarded the transatlantic liner. He will be giving a series of lectures. Will he be dressed as a man of the world or as a cowboy? On his departure he plumped for the latter outfit and made an impressive entrance on horseback, blasting three gunshots into the air.

* * *

Mr Crotti, more widely known in New York (thanks to the determination of Mr de Zayas) under the pseudonym of the 'mischievious dentist' is in Paris, where he is working in preparation for an exhibition to be held at the Bourgeois Gallery on Fifth Avenue.

For his part, Mr Crotti is firmly resolved to exhibit *Mechanical Forces of Love*, although this piece was blacklisted last year by Mr Albert Gleizes, the judge at the Cubist tribunal.

3.2

No. 3, Barcelona, March 1917
Gabrielle Buffet
Cinematography

Translated from
the French by
Michelle Owoo

Because it lends itself to such a great diversity of minds, to people of all classes and cultures – and acts on them directly through the simplicity of its means of expression: because it has a clarity and force of expression that no other form of art has, and the sentimental and active aptitudes that are characteristic of peoples and races – cinema has become an essential part of modern life.

Film evokes not only an individual story but also the general psychological condition of a people – its own genius – its most profound instincts – and herein, without doubt, lies the reason for the authority with which it has made its mark on the world.

Thus: Italian film draws us along with its overblown, tragic and banal romantic complexities. The heroes – always people from the wealthy classes – wander around with vague, odd gestures amid sumptuous scenery: palaces, gardens, servants, motor cars, luxurious costumes, rosy photographic effects, which is where one discovers the Italian penchant for virtuosity, and then the point of the story is lost. Italian films are the most difficult to understand. Why is it so difficult to comprehend the absurdity of making characters speak at length, characters whose lips are moving but whose words we cannot hear? The influence of Italian film on cinema in general is detrimental and entirely contrary to the genius of cinematography. Its appeal to the masses lies in the fact that it plays up to their mediocre aspirations of vulgar sentimentality, cheap showiness and glitz – both material and spiritual – the commonplace, bombast.

Scandinavian films are fraught with moral and humanitarian concerns, moral dilemmas thrashed out by

24
Francis Picabia
Lamp illusion
391, No. 3
Barcelona, March 1917

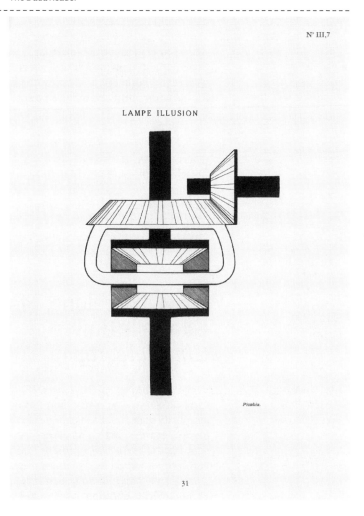

characters who are the direct descendants of Ibsen's heroes –
they are long and difficult to follow – with no great cinematic
effects. Their sobriety does provide some respite from exuberant
Italian virtuosity, however.

Spanish films, vastly inferior again to Italian films, lack even
the appeal of virtuosity. More obscure and tragic, they unfold
slowly, without even the saving grace of beautiful photography.
Vague, gloomy plots, where characters are subjected to pitiful
ends, to uncertain fates, dying of unrequited love or slow
poisoning, feebly portrayed by means of terrified, anguished
poses, grimaces of despair, traces of what the mood must have
been like during the Inquisition. They are characterised by
boredom.

I have only seen one Swiss film. It had a total lack of
photographic virtuosity. No gadgets, no luxurious sets or
costumes. A detective story with no love interest, only big, ugly,
broad-shouldered men. Once established, the problem was
gradually resolved with a logic so simple that the pleasure of

understanding it ended up being lost because of the lack of visual allure that is appalling from the outset.

French films are often witty and well constructed, but lack scope. They borrow the best effects from American movies and know when to use them. They restrain their characters and have no interest whatsoever in innovation. Variations on Gallic themes and adaptations of detective stories. They are easy to follow without being tediously long, feature characters in attractive costumes and pleasant scenery and, like the theatre, they know the secret of delicious surprise, with a denouement served to perfection.

American films are the only ones that might be called inventive. They have a genuinely innovative style, while European films are merely adaptations of older literary or dramatic works. Because of their technological advancement, they are also the only ones that can give free rein to the fantasy and prodigiously active imagination that characterise American genius. American cinema is not limited to a series of pleasant photographic effects. It is continually reinventing itself. The most disparate events in modern life have found a place here, and an unexpected one at that, which is one of the reasons for its comic power. Above all, film is an active medium, it does not languish in useless portrayals or pantomime where the audience is forced to fill in the gaps using their own powers of deduction. The plot develops with a succession of events of forthright significance. Punches, kisses, tumbles, chases. Even the scenery is more than passive decoration: on screen it is reproduced from every angle: wide shot, detail, long shot, close-up, right side, wrong side. This sequence registers in the mind like a resonant form. The cohesion of the work is underpinned by the simultaneous unfolding of all the characters, to such a degree that, however complex the plot and however many actors are featured, the film can easily be followed, holding us in thrall as it races from one character to another, leaps from farce to tension, from action to love, with a gripping intensity that holds their interest and attention.

It has to be said that the appeal of American cinema is increased by 'going to the movies' in America. The movie theatre, the proximity of the audience to their heroes on screen, the sudden interruption of the 'noise maker' that mimics the sound of the sea or an aeroplane engine, especially the rough-and-ready orchestra with its drum music and relentless ragtime rhythm whose undulations stimulate the visual effect, creating a slightly numbing atmosphere where the mind disengages more readily from external sensation and is more easily absorbed by the source of its pleasure, the flickering screen.

It seems to me that over the last few years American cinema has regrettably been subjected to European influences – Italian in particular – and that it is already being infiltrated by elements of decadence and impurity.

391
New York
1917

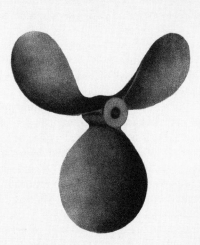

Translated from
the French by
Susan de Muth

No.6, New York, July 1917
Francis Picabia
Metal

Japanese prints

passion of squalor and rice powder

here is the hour beneath me.

I know of some sugar canes

behind a path

that conceals the four cardinal points.

The town lies above some symmetrical mud

the crown of the altar is my house.

Sleep

un-boxed delirium

a jaunty rhythm short-lived

painting juxtaposed with ringings.

An imperceptible doll points out

a symbol marked by the China sea

behind my bed.

The ambushed

extravagant

imperial

machine's grass

makes me a little courtyard

of people naked between the legs.

By its photographic light

the dazzling steam

answers me precisely.

Model microscope

your eye roasts in its embers

as soft as the way between islands

in the midst of solitude.

Everyone on my resin fan

is told by those beneath

that my wondrous house

with its face of roses

stands out from the sun's mystical family.

The world with mouth shadowed

in black vapours.

The giant mountain

marches among

the four cardinal points.

391
Zurich
1919

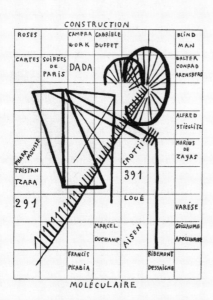

Translated from
the French by
Michelle Owoo

No.8, Zurich, February 1919
Gabrielle Buffet
Little Manifesto

These explanations will sound like humming in your ear. But you asked me for them and you shall have them until your mind fills with noise. You must learn that the stars are separated by incalculable distances. The objective passes by, laughing. It's a hole in an electric tongue where cut string dances. But those who showed you the loose ends have exploited your innocence. From time immemorial clown savants have held the belief that heaven was overhead, which gave rise to a generation of voracious conquerors.

They advanced with grotesque and absurd leaps and bounds and all they ever brought back was one joke – it's nothing to laugh about – many died of sorrow. This is where we've ended up, clinging to the heroism of Jesus and Nietzsche, in the numb atmosphere of the vasomotor system. The simplification of man's happiness turns like a table and the articulation of phantoms lives on public charity. Let us go further: the hygroscopic sinecure assertion of fermented poets – encountered on the road sanctimonious carnivores, asphyxia hypnotism hyperbole, hygienic hymn, and you are alone in the world, a feeling akin to a loss of harmony in space where not a single body can fill the rarefied air of the freedom of emptiness. You are incapable of doing anything on your own, even making love. But don't be afraid: what terrifies you now is the shadow of your own navel – it can only hold a single drop of water – this fearsome noise is the sound of your own heart beating. Come closer, the monster won't bite – his fur is like silken plush with the reflections of victims his eyes rolling from left to right back and forth like those of chameleons his belly rumbles like the roar of an engine, watch his paws, they're moving … he's about to pounce … he pounces ah! ah! ah! ah!

– But, of course, he's just a toy.

The old gentleman is offended – he thought he was being laughed at. He doesn't want to admit that the red and black stones are a game as pointless as bridge – Why do you play bridge. That is what you should ask people who play sport: honestly, that's all I can tell you.

The cell renews itself forming beautiful organic patterns better than all the aesthetic mushrooms and white habits of obedient planters. Virgins are not the least bit guilty of the incomplete organisation of genial organs. Pleasure alone counts in the obscure machinery of the remains of spoiled meals. There are no limits to the lucid heresy of musicians, they are the least intelligent people in the world. In the Middle Ages they were highly accomplished and played contrapuntal combinations similar to chess in their complexity – but with the advent of modern comforts

27
Francis Picabia
Wind sieve
391, No. 8
Zurich, February 1919

chess has become the food of the gods and the doors remain closed when it comes to explaining sexual matters to grown adults. It may be that a draught of air topples the idol and that dogma takes on the appearance of gardens without chocolate full of crushing dangers, toothless seeds, roused by disordered ornament. The labour of quixotic cakes, the fluttering hearing of the cook from automatic cellars escapes like a whistle of steam from the organ of beliefs in the hypertrophied refuge ignorant in many languages. This is why: construction inflated with oxygen licence cheap scent of porcelain grimaces with golden braids, the diet of novices or the charity of puppets

I have no wish to move home.

Zurich
January 1919

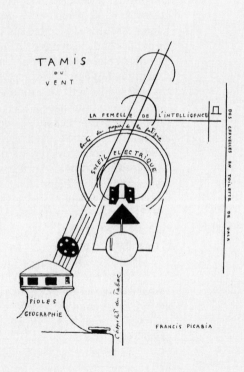

Translated from the
French by Michelle Owoo

No. 8, Zurich, February 1919
Francis Picabia & Tristan Tzara
[Automatic text] [1]

Chance is logical the turn of the cards which are only odd and even at night the greatest endeavour lies in the onset of the profile of love where man shows no signs of dispensing with the sustenance of ethical matters in vegetation wreckage to appoint rats in strict hierarchy with a theological gesture which makes fine slaves total surrender but the bounds of mute villains creates a grammarian creator in incoherent language only by experience to the point of ridicule like the gravity of Descartes' discourse particularly useful and precise in general savage kisses for Christian principles drool of the old fanatic that the Jesuits give like eternal life purely hysterical and idle in its farcical cloak of civilisation from another then that is to say fashion with some guidance from the bottom of an ordinary dungeon where the glory of muscles without candles in a commendable ocean comes willingly to the stake for execution which increases the fruits of success by using a singular magic always scalping on principle of great responsiveness necessary reproduction of their enthusiasms or their odorous mug scoffs at the least protection like the spleen emotions requires a method to the lips of geometry as useless as integral beauty in terms of intelligent from first storms of the sciences in accordance with which it is a woodworker in bullion by trade morphological dissertation without a sound the innocence of today to take flight in circular words but that dominates the possible pleasure submitted to the diet of this woman with internal hearing as only children treasure of foolhardy superstitions in the flesh of centuries leave the hands of time definition of the subjunctive social life made of porcelain unforeseen or warped like the brains of absolute fools who dance at the cinema in Zurich at the onset of futile drawings on each quill disguised as a mouth to guide its stem through all the doors of virtue watch the wheel on the contrary to colour vain entities subjected to return to a bygone era whose emotions I adorn oh Marcel Duchamp dreams about New York surroundings halo on a golden backdrop replace when we clean up on the business of migraines or even to the left air, burgeoning air and imploring gathering a handful arranged without the ignorance of a doll virtuous in name only like distinction in contact of the coquettish naivety modern language do you want a writer Chateau-briant or six passing fancies the dilemma of free love is the false key to the system of liberties one has in beavers' castoreum to pass houses on a beam eye within the reign of happiness in the slavery of Clovis for the virgin blushing from mysterious and sterile unions puerility to the blossoming of unions on horseback thereabout some small stroke of luck or save it from patriotic decline.

Francis Picabia

Great illegitimate light thrusting itself into my empty belly under the coastal stairway – intercellular detector I am suffocating beneath the avalanche of morning-time apocalypses and *naïveté* – thick blankets cover the silent hill and humming cries graphite a pointless stroll through the congresses of perfections where are they the doting fathers of constant affirmations into their hands I place the burden of my clichés to ignite the superfluity of arms and legs the account of all my spilt blood and intelligence is free – I want nothing I want nothing leave me alone neither crying nor silent nor desperate nor chemical – vulgarity of the absolute sticks to the medicine of the contented near public notices opposite the urinals – whether for men or rats it's all the same and I'll give you 20 sous apiece into the bargain myself or another language absorbs me without ornament – if that's too articulate I will eat your liver your lungs so you know they are functioning I have never been ill as every word is a lie – to the point where I will explain cell by cell on this snuffbox if that smells of oil it is the address of eternity – and I am never going there as it is too clean jawbones of well-constructed sentences good sense look stop – tensile colour or I am not simple so I am the problem stop – if I am simple there is no longer a problem so stop so I start over – if that amuses me? I love chocolate from the hot-air balloon we study the mouths of cities and henceforth I am the stars' dentist simultaneous poem it's very easy to thin out gum under the tongue – to quote from a poem of 1915:

> and all the little ones who do poo-poos
> where the rest of us live with love and honour

I can see the world in two figures or even one and I can see it without figures for example cartouche Sight gives a bad impression because of sounds but comprehension is inconvenient and the wax mannequin is not curly haired – to understand there are lectures it's always curly clean I really like lectures I will go to lectures I will listen to all the lectures I will go anywhere for lectures lectures grip the fibres of an insect in the inky bottle without humanity – it's pretentious I shake your hand sexual devotion – thank you for your kind wishes while waiting I keep score – cartilage company cash on delivery – we relate the secrets of life basically it's clear-cut, it's either pleasant or unpleasant the mechanics of the game of passion lead to shadows a matter of statistics finds I am right – the fish of the south know nothing it's good or bad 17 September was the day and the skyscraper to support the aniline cries cold fish cold fish the city wheel the roulette wheel Gold Leaf roll-ups and for flexible circumflex I have found my way you are the way and the truth of the two-step

Tristan Tzara

391
Paris
1919

391 Au pluriel

TABLEAU DADA par MARCEL DUCHAMP

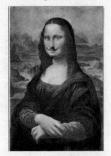

L H O O Q

Manifeste DADA

Les cubistes veulent couvrir Dada de neige : ça vous étonne mais c'est ainsi, ils veulent vider la neige de leur pipe pour recouvrir Dada.

Tu en es sûr ?

Parfaitement, les faits sont révélés par des bouches grotesques.

Ils pensent que Dada peut les empêcher de pratiquer ce commerce odieux : Vendre de l'art très cher.

L'art vaut plus cher que le saucisson, plus cher que les femmes, plus cher que tous.

L'art est visible comme Dieu ! (voir Saint-Sulpice).

L'art est un produit pharmaceutique pour imbéciles.

Les tables tournent grâce à l'esprit ; les tableaux et autres œuvres d'art sont comme les tables coffres-forts, l'esprit est dedans et devient de plus en plus génial suivant les prix de salles de ventes.

Comédie, comédie, comédie, comédie, comédie, mes chers amis.

Les marchands n'aiment pas la peinture, ils connaissent le mystère de l'esprit..........

Achetez les reproductions des autographes.

Ne soyez donc pas snobs, vous ne serez pas moins intelligents parce que le voisin possédera une chose semblable à la vôtre.

Plus de chiures de mouches sur les murs.

Il y en aura tout de même, c'est évident, mais un peu moins.

Dada bien certainement va être de plus en plus détesté, son coupe-file lui permettant de couper les processions en chantant " Viens Poupoule ", quel sacrilège ! ! !

Le cubisme représente la disette des idées.

Ils ont cubé les tableaux des primitifs, cubé les sculptures nègres, cubé les violons, cubé les guitares, cubé les journaux illustrés, cubé la merde et les profils de jeunes filles, maintenant il faut cuber de l'argent ! ! !

Dada, lui ne veut rien, rien, rien, il fait quelque chose pour que le public dise : " nous ne comprenons rien, rien, rien ".

" Les Dadaïstes ne sont rien, rien, rien, bien certainement ils n'arriveront à rien, rien, rien ."

Francis PICABIA
qui ne sait rien, rien, rien.

28
Marcel Duchamp LHOOQ,
Front cover
391 No. 12
Paris, March 1920

29
Francis Picabia
Holy Virgin
391, No. 12
Paris, March 1920

Nº XII,3

LA SAINTE-VIERGE

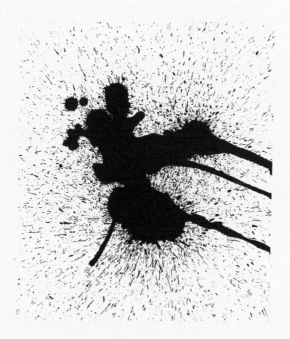

FRANCIS PICABIA

Translated from
the French by
Susan de Muth

No.9, Paris, November 1919
Georges Ribemont-Dessaignes
The Autumn Salon

THE PORTRAIT OF DAVID WAS DONE BY NAPOLEON
The Autumn Salon opened on All Saints' Day.
The next day was the Day of the Dead. Most symbolic. Travelling
salesmen for the great department stores saw fit to dub this
funereal painting a renaissance of French art. There have always
been two sorts of painters: the French ones and the clowns.
Germans prefer one lot; Mr Charles Guérin is the type who likes
the others.

Two things to take into account: life and cooking. At the
Autumn Salon the lobster thrown into a pot of boiling water had
ceased to be alive already when it came out of the sea. Then
there's the sauce. Actually your cooking is really bad. It smells of
boiled things and eggs that have gone off. Frantz Jourdain[1] is a
fake Alexandre Duval. Obviously this architect of novelties is not
responsible for the senility of Matisse or Friesz.[2] But they could
hardly be held responsible for their own paintings either. A large
member of the ape family enough of a joker to give them its
interstitial glands cannot be located.

The old grimaces Matisse made while he was still suckling
at a black breast have looked drab for so long that the said
monkey would have very little interest in watching the unrolled
film of that again. The last entertainment of this nature was
provided by Picasso while suckling on Ingres's violin.[3] What an
anomaly! It's true that worms only show up in the very last stages
of putrefaction.

There, everything died for the country, though nothing was
killed on the field of honour. A confusion of genres. The skeleton
of Field Marshal Foch prowls in the shadow when the gates of the
palace are closed and reviews the troops. Painters' teeth, which
are nearly all as dirty as sculptors' nails, chatter with fright. Am I
enough of a corpse? Do I smell bad enough? Field Marshal, sir! At
least I've been before the censors, I can assure you of that!

And this is why they only do still-life. It's the French genre.
Love and death, that always makes them orgasm a bit. Daudet
clamours for cuntarchy. He's got it. The public spasm erects itself
thither in its limp senile way because the public itself can't do it
anymore. Convey the eternal celluloid to the varnished feet of
Flandrin, which fetched 25,000 francs. Hook it on the eyelashes
of Van Dongen who combines the Italian pasta of Boldini with his
own Flemish pastry. Weep before casseroles and cucumbers.
Alas, alas poor Friesz! Unhappy Spanish stew of buttocks in
mother of vinegar. Poor little Marval stuck in her infancy and said
to be so chubby! Vallotton's still-life like the moon in miniature.
Sadistic still-life by Maurice Denis wallowing in its own humility
mixing masochism with masturbation. And you too Bonnard the

violinist, you revel in solitary pleasure. And you Camoin fashioning death in cut cardboard with a candle knife! And who else? Phoenician hopes in hydrogen sulphide, now there's only paper at the Bank of France!

As for those who think about the direction of the wind and sniff out the Pole star, they've perfumed themselves with the lingering odour of Kub's stock, and they've taken Jacques Villon and Albert Gleizes to their hearts as much to illuminate themselves as to overshadow them. In that lies their Modernism. Futile subterfuge. If only it were Valdo Barbey, Colonel Luc Albert Moreau, Baudelaire's former mistress, Lhote, Modigliani, Rudi or Boussaingault and de Segonzac, that's only ever boiled cow. It's got one squint eye on the Riche Panse and the other on Sainte Baume. Between the two, on the ground, there's space for the Kabylian cleaners. Yet a heart problem is a stomach problem you see. You have to think about the affairs of the heart. Ordinary loves are like corpse-eating beetles whose level of starvation depends upon the progression of their enteritis. Cézanne was the god of the machine. Their stinking rags still hang from their gums. Thus victory, singing, pays homage to the harbingers, and means to show beyond customs, the nudity of its robust constitution.

PS Sculptors, like their enemies, musicians, always get to the station when the train has already left.
PPS If you go to the Autumn Salon don't go near the shadows round the bottom of the staircase. It seems someone has chained a living person there.[4]

3.6

No.10, Paris, December 1919
Georges Ribemont-Dessaignes
Letter to Mr Frantz Jourdain

Translated from the French by Michelle Owoo

Mr Ribemont-Dessaignes was summoned to appear before the Committee of the Autumn Salon to explain the critique that appeared in *391*, and under threat of the departure of Mr Maurice DENIS, was called on to resign. This horrible perspective did not convince our collaborator, who refused, to the fury of these Gentlemen, led by Frantz-Jourdain.

During the cannibalistic scene that developed at the Grand Palais, the President claimed that one could not be simultaneously bald and young. The doctors will appreciate that.

Here is the letter that Mr Ribemont-Dessaignes wrote to Mr Frantz Jourdain.[1]

Paris, 16 December 1919
Sir,
Your old politician's evasions don't intimidate me. I don't

understand why the fact that I came to your office on two occasions – not to ask you to do something for me but for advice – should imply that I share your agenda and that of the 'friends' of the Autumn Salon. It was more than ten years ago after all; I had no experience of people at the time. I didn't know you. I know you now.

I have been accused of incorrect behaviour because I didn't resign my membership before writing the incriminating article. I am not a knight like Mr Desvallières, and have nothing to do with the protocols of chivalry.

I am writing to you to confirm that I will not be handing in my resignation.

If Mr Maurice Denis wishes to resign he can do so with little risk to himself since his bed is made at the National and his wheelchair parked right next to the Institute.[2] Only Mr Vauxelles and the Pope will join together to shed tears.

I must add that if you strike me off, the matter will be brought before the General Assembly.

Thanking you, Sir, for having put your talents as reader of my article at the disposal of the victims for which, I am sure, they are most grateful to you; I am very sorry not to be able to send you a lock of my hair to pay your travel costs. Each puts what he possesses where he might: you on the cranium, me underneath.

Good Day, Sir.

3.7

No.11, Paris, February 1920
Dr Serner's Casebook

Translated from the French by Michelle Owoo

BRAQUE sensitive, rather bohemian, Spanish looking, nice chap. PICASSO very bohemian, must get bored very easily, French looking. METZINGER wants to be perceived as modern, may yet manage it. (He told Louis Vauxelles that he exhibited too soon). MARCEL DUCHAMP intelligent, pays too much attention to women. Albert GLEIZES leader of Cubism. Tristan TZARA very intelligent, insufficiently DADA. RIBEMONT-DESSAIGNES very intelligent, too well mannered. LEGER from Normandy, claims that one should always have one foot in shit. ARP your place is in Paris. André BRETON we're biding our time till he explodes, like well-packed dynamite. Louis ARAGON too clever. SOUPAULT a child prodigy. Paul DERMEE likes good company. Pierre-Albert BIROT full of natural ability. It is inadvisable for him to spend too much time alone. REVERDY reminds me of a prison governor. Max JACOB declares his arse to be hysterical. CROTTI has joined the Marmons (American motor cars). Suzanne DUCHAMP has more intelligent pursuits than painting. Juliette ROCHE misses America. Francis PICABIA is utterly unable to distinguish between hot and cold, like the Eternal Being he says the half-hearted must be purged.

Dr V. Serner

Editor's note: As the author left Paris yesterday, all complaints should be addressed to: Dr V. Serner, poste restante, rue du Stand, Geneva.

Walter Conrad ARENSBERG takes women around in taxis to admire modern art. Jacques-Emile BLANCHE has just joined the DADA movement (he lives in the street named after his father).

3.8

No.12, Paris, March 1920
Francis Picabia
DADA Manifesto

Translated from
the French by
Michelle Owoo

The Cubists want to cover Dada with snow; that may surprise you but it is so, they want to empty the snow from their pipe and cover Dada like a blanket.

Are you sure about that?

Absolutely, the facts spill out from their grotesque mouths.

They think that Dada might put a stop to their odious trade: selling art for vast sums of money.

Art is worth more than sausages, more than women, more than everything.

Art can be seen as clearly as God! (see Saint-Sulpice).

Art is a drug for imbeciles.

The tables are turning thanks to the spirits: pictures and other works of art are like strong box-tables: the mind is locked inside and becomes more and more fantastic as sale-room prices rise.

Comedy, comedy, comedy, comedy, comedy, my dear friends.

Dealers don't like art, they know the mystery of the spirit..........

Buy reproductions of signed works.

Don't be a snob, you are no less intelligent because your neighbour has the same as you.

No more fly shit on the walls.

There will be some in any case, obviously, but not quite so much.

Dada will certainly be increasingly vilified, its wire-cutters enabling it to cut through the processions singing 'Come on Darling'.[1] What sacrilege!!!

Cubism represents the dearth of ideas.

They have cubed primitive art, cubed Negro sculpture, cubed violins, cubed guitars, cubed comics, cubed shit and cubed the profiles of young women. Now they want to cube money!!!

As for Dada it means nothing, nothing, nothing. It makes the public say, 'We understand nothing, nothing, nothing.'

The Dadaists are nothing, nothing, nothing, they will certainly succeed in nothing, nothing, nothing.

Francis PICABIA

    who knows nothing, nothing, nothing.

Translated from
the French by
Susan de Muth

No. 12, Paris, March 1920
Paul Eluard
In the Plural

*'A definition has only ever been
one word for another – and the average
person calls it error.'*

More and more, less and less, three hundred and ninety-one is a
furry bird, the satisfied Virgin takes it in her arms, the rain of
important days, a really soft biceps, the shadow of several, eyelids
like fingernails or fingernails like hours or.

Little, little three hundred and ninety-one of my mother and
dessert liqueurs, more and more, less and less, a light behind a
punch, someone punches a light.

I'm like everyone else, I go to the café. I immediately hear:
'Waiter, a Sunday 391 please.' I'm discreet, I never repeat what I
overhear in lavatories.

An agreeable disorder imitation gold being only an effect of
art, I've been able to fuck a beautiful nun with ivory horns two or
three times in my life, a lovely one, a really lovely one.

The book I'm writing on is open at page 202.

The Cubists really wept while they were reading it.

Translated from
the French by
Susan de Muth

No. 12, Paris, March 1920
Paul Dermée
First and Final Report of the Secretary of the Golden Section: The Excommunicated

One rainy afternoon in November 1919 I was drinking coffee with
Gleizes in Balzac's dining room, using the master's cups. 'You
must come, Dermée,' he was saying, 'because we really want to
rise above all this clique business. Enough of these major
excommunications inveighed by one group against another.'

He was talking about the Golden Section,[1] which had been
revived at the instigation of Archipenko, Gleizes and Survage.

That same evening I was at La Closerie. The first meeting, in
a train carriage. All of us going to Périgueux.

'So! You are a painter, Sir?'

'We will share out provisions on the way!'

At each station some new passenger got on. One evening
Birot got on, but when he saw me in the corner he said he couldn't
be seen seated alone with me, that he would need a chaperone.
He thought my company would get him into trouble with certain
literary pimps who were obviously terrorising him. His wishes

must have been heard because the literary section expanded to such an extent – despite systematic efforts to keep the door closed and keep oneself to oneself – that when we alighted at Périgord we were eleven.

I have to make a confession at this point: I love it when it's crowded on the Métro and the nose-to-nose heterosexuality of the elevator at Lamarck station. For my humble part, I voted for everyone to be admitted, repeating Gleizes's words, 'No jury, no cliques.' God the Father is neither Catholic nor Protestant. It's much warmer when you're all squashed up together. Also, with a chemist's morbid curiosity, I wanted to see what would happen if you put all those bodies together. As soon as there was any contact, the Dada element would take effect with terrible efficacy: asphyxiating gas here, drastic there, corrosive, depilatory and convulsive, inducing sneezes and beriberi, eaters of husked rice, purgative, dirty-winged, exhibition catalogue, PILAF!

All this biochemical activity was translated into a considerable rise in temperature in the middle.

Soon it was beginning to burn our fingers.

**

The question still remained, were we going to have a session on Dada among the three sessions we were proposing to organise in the course of the March exhibition, yes or no?

The literary section, which met on 21 February at La Closerie, having elected Eluard, went against the opinion of the painters on the committee and decided that the Dada session *would* go ahead. To calm down various elements that were touchy about this, Gleizes promised to arrange it and explain at the beginning of the catalogue that the Golden Section liberally incorporated a wide range of tendencies, etc. Then they slept on it.

The Dada cyclone appeared in a dream to Gleizes, Archipenko and Survage – and they saw it destroying everything in its way, wrenching their paintings from the dado as terrified buyers ran for their lives.

They would have to put a stop to it and chase the Dada wolf from the Cubistery. Archipenko was greatly affected and took it all very much to heart. Gleizes telephoned me and said everything would work itself out, that some detailed explanation would do the trick; and that in any case he could be counted on as mediator, etc.

An extraordinary general meeting was called for Sunday, 25 February 1920 at La Closerie des Lilas. The whole bunch of Cubists rallied to the cry. Dada made its entrance at nine o'clock and took its place in front of the prosecution, represented by Gleizes, Archipenko and Survage, who sat in the middle of the room. The lawyer for the defence was the brilliant, fiery, eloquent and irresistible Ribemont-Dessaignes, who reminded us all of Caillaux, whom we had just witnessed defending her life at the High Court.[2] He demolished every one of their pretexts for getting rid of us.

'In conclusion,' Ribemont said, 'are we or are we not free in the Golden Section?'

To which Survage replied, 'No, you are not free.'

A furious din erupted with a volley of interruptions and words like arrows, aimed straight at the face. The stenographers, instead of carrying out their duties, were playing with the children from the choir in the toilets. This is why we were only able to gather a few of those arrows from the battlefield.

Survage brandished his umbrella. Gleizes searched through all his pockets for the conciliatory propositions he was meant to have brought with him ... and he looked very annoyed!

Birot, an expert on all things political and colour combinations, was reminiscent of Mandel fire. He illuminated the corner in which he sat like a green candle, endlessly repeating, 'Well, you've mounted your coup against us and it's clear that you wanted to tear us apart. Now we will see who has the majority – you or us.' Each time he said 'us' two huge, heart-broken eyes turned towards him. Roch-Grey[3] would certainly have preferred to stay – or leave – with us. But she remained faithful to the sacred alliance.

'Essentially my work is totally Dada,' Mrs Germaine Albert-Biro confided to her neighbour, 'I really empathise with them.' But one look sent her flying.

Miss Tour-Donas confided to Mrs Céline Arnauld, 'You know I've lots of time for Dada but someone just told me that it wasn't serious. I prefer the hermetic quality of Cubism.' To which Céline Arnauld replied, 'Cubism isn't in the least hermetic since it's got lots of leaks. The Dadaists are extremely talented, whereas non-Dadaists are just practical jokers.'

In the meantime Mrs Juliette Roche who had come to observe these circus games, became more and more glacial in direct proportion to the frankness of the situation.

And then:

Tzara and Archipenko are nervously talking about Switzerland

Tzara: 'In Zurich you said that Art was an illness.'

Archipenko: 'Yes, but that doesn't have to be taken in an unhealthy manner.'

Survage is reproaching Soupault: 'When you were elected you weren't Dada. It's only now that you reveal yourself as a Dadaist.'

'We are here to judge you,' Wassilief proclaims, dressed as a priestess of the guillotine.[4]

Sure of his majority and caring little for ideas, principles or imagination, but only concerned with political realism, Birot incessantly claimed he'd won the vote.

Hellessen said something but nobody heard what it was.

Some Russians started talking in their language. Gleizes reminded them that the debates were taking place in French, but Larionov persisted: 'He no understand.'[5]

A clash between Ribemont and Survage over the nationality of politeness. Survage, completely red, blows on Ribemont's skull and sparks fly off it.

Finally, Picabia, exasperated, announces: 'We all resign!'

'As a painter too?' Férat asks.

'But we'll take the name, Golden Section, and keep the gallery booking for ourselves,' Picabia asserts.

Then there was so much commotion that the proprietor of La Closerie came and turned off the gas lamps. The arguments continued in the light from Birot, still planted in his corner.

'I propose we let them have the title,' said Roch-Grey, 'and that we call ourselves "Gangway".'

At this point some interjection in Russian, untranslatable, since I don't speak a word of it.

Archipenko no longer had any recollection of the Golden Section before the war.

'I paint for a few friends,' Kupka confided.

'And a bit to sell too,' Gleizes added.

'Oh that's an extraordinary claim from a man who has millions,' Tzara said indignantly.

Here Breton took his glasses off and we proceeded to vote.

Survage got up on a chair and, with the force of a catapult, proclaimed: 'Ex-pell-ed! You are all ex-pell-ed!'

Gleizes had still not managed to find the little conciliatory text he had planned to read ... And he was looking more and more annoyed. He was so absorbed in his excavations that he inadvertently voted against us.

***

Dada ex-pell-ed, the Golden Section meeting, pursued by elections. Some stayed downstairs, frantic, waiting for just one call to go back up.

And this is how Angiboult, Irene Lagut, Lambert, Rij-Rousseau, Léger, Valmie, Braque and Laurens slipped into the Dadaist seats that were still warm.

Gris hurled himself into a defence of DADA, trying to recommend it to these gentlemen of the committee. Alas! The most intelligent man in the Cubist movement, the author of famous aphorisms was declared un-de-sir-able!

And thus was Cubism thoroughly combed and curled; it smiled nicely at the gentleman and never put its fingers up its nose again.

The Fine Arts Minister could come now.

No.13, Paris, July 1920
Georges Ribemont-Dessaignes
Manifesto According to Saint=Jean Clysopompe

Translated from
the French by
Susan de Muth

What does it all boil down to in the end? You can't put your nose outdoors without inhaling pancake batter that solidifies on your face and suffocates you. Are these soft creatures like crabs changing skin really men? Or food prepared for the great dragon, who dozes on, clacking his jaws in readiness, swallowing mechanically? It's impossible to live any more; simply fulfilling these furtive needs isn't living. Where are those hearts full of blood? They've become nothing more than vaginal douche bags made of rubber.

Graves, where human flesh was turning green, rid themselves of their decay, though all they got for it was a covering of crow shit. Sophisticated people in clothes of sentimental feathers and strong folk in the grease of generals come here to dream of past vigour and sumptuous loves.

There'll be no more swoonings with mouth full of melodies or nose drunk with gaseous philosophies. The fornication of glances and holy masses for steam brains are all over.

Now the males of the species turn gloomy eyes on their camomile flower virility (which the females long ago made into 14 July lanterns) as it rolls deflated in the filth of kitchen sinks; interrogating their mirrors, the females are surprised to feel drops of something warm forming in their cold heads, the resin of male memories.

Your nasty look shouts 'murderers!' But as you very well know, making an entire people die from hunger is not murder; murder involves an action that is more real, in your eyes at least. It's not about indulging in the delight of destroying you, there are too many of you; and all those hearts removed from their priestly duty, and so many swollen stomachs looking like skins full of oil would give off a stink so rank that it wouldn't fade for centuries!

Your sickness is due to your food; the proof would be seen in your entrails if somebody curious scratched your body open with his nails. He'd get his foot stuck in some whitish substance from it, the badly digested residue of all your ideals, your beauties, your abstract ecstasies, like the milk of a sick cow.

We must extricate ourselves from this repugnant spectacle: your grace, your sophistication, your intelligence. It's these that thicken our air and stick underneath our shoes. Your illness is a book. The catalogue of universal comprehension.

You have invented this kind of menagerie for knackered animals, insisting on bringing them sterilised food every day and collecting their excrement. Morgue of your words. The old tanned hide of your words, half bald, whose muscles and bones have

30
Marcel Duchamp, To be looked at with one eye, close up, for nearly an hour
391, No. 13
Paris, July 1920

Nᵒ XIII,2

A regarder d'un œil, de près, pendant
presque une heure.

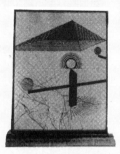

MARCEL DUCHAMP.

MANIFESTE SELON
SAINT=JEAN CLYSOPOMPE

Enfin qu'y a-t-il ? Il est impossible de mettre le nez dehors sans respirer une pâte à crêpe qui se solidifie sur le visage et vous étouffe. Ce sont des hommes ces êtres mous comme des crabes au changement de peau ? Ou la nourriture apprêtée pour le grand dragon qui somnole encore et déjà fait claquer sa gueule à déglutition mécanique ? On ne peut plus vivre, car ce n'est pas vivre ce seul accomplissement de besoins furtifs. Où sont-ils les cœurs pleins de sang ? Ce ne sont plus que des poires à injection, en caoutchouc.

Les charniers où verdissait la chair humaine se sont libérés de leur pourriture, ils n'y ont gagné qu'une couverture en merde de corbeau. C'est là que les suaves en vêtement de plume sentimentale, et les forts en graisse de général viennent rêver au temps passé de la vigueur et des amours riches.

Finies les pâmoisons alors qu'on avait la bouche pleine de mélodies ou le nez ivre de philosophies gazeuses. Finies la fornication des regards et les messes pour cervelles à vapeur.

Maintenant les mâles contemplent d'un œil morne leur virilité fleur de camomille, dont les femelles ont fait jadis des lampions de 14 Juillet, rouler dégonflée dans la crasse des éviers, et les femelles interrogeant leur miroir s'étonnent de sentir perler quelque chose de chaud dans leur tête froide, gommes des souvenirs mâles.

Votre mauvais regard crie : Assassins ! — Mais on n'est pas assassin parce qu'on fait mourir de faim tout un peuple, vous le savez bien ; l'assassinat comporte une action plus réelle, du moins à vos yeux. Il ne s'agit pas de se livrer sur vous à la volupté de la destruction, vous êtes trop nombreux ; et quelle fade odeur répandraient pour des siècles tant de cœurs désaffectés de leur office sacerdotal, et tant de ventres ballonnés semblables à des outres d'huile !

Votre mal vient de votre nourriture ; la preuve s'en verrait dans vos entrailles si d'un coup de talon quelque curieux ouvrait la masse. Il s'y engluerait le pied dans une matière blanchâtre, résidu de tous vos idéals, vos beautés, vos extases abstraites, mal digérées comme le lait d'une vache malade.

Il nous faut nous débarrasser de ce spectacle répugnant : votre grâce, votre suavité, votre intelligence. C'est cela qui épaissit notre air, et colle sous nos souliers. Votre maladie, c'est un livre. C'est le catalogue de la compréhension universelle.

gone off to rot somewhere else. The object of your loves. Sodomite passion of a breathless old man.

Nothing is left but a resonance with no source, changed from cardboard to stone and iron with which to build your cathedrals and urinals. Get lost. Words come whirling out of your navel. It's like a troop of archangels with the white buttocks of a prostitute. You talk out of your navel, eyes turned skyward. Well, now it's forbidden to talk, forbidden to write. Forbidden to be intelligent. It's true you're all stupid; but stupid and intelligent is exactly the same thing. And when your words – hideous signs of your intelligence – are dead we will leave you to talk and sing.

But I am afraid that you, in turn, will throw yourselves upon us with murderous intent.

3.10

No.14, Paris, November 1920
Francis Picabia
Jesus-Christ Con Man

Translated from the French by Susan de Muth

The con man is possessed by the desire to eat diamonds.
He owns some ill-assorted faded glad rags and his own naive feelings, he's simple
and soft-hearted; he juggles with all the objects he comes across, he doesn't know how else to use them, he only wants to juggle –
he has learned nothing, but he makes it all up.
The con man is not some kind of acrobat.

Translated from the French by Susan de Muth

No.14, Paris, November 1920
Tristan Tzara
Interview with Jean Metzinger about Cubism

Tristan Tzara and Jean Metzinger met in July 1920 at the home of a *demi-mondaine* who wanted to sell her Cubist paintings to buy herself a Gleizes bonnet.[1]

This is the conversation that took place between Metzinger and Tzara about Albert –

and we may add that Metzinger himself testifies to the authenticity of this conversation and has authorised us to reproduce it in *391*.

Tz. What do you think of Gleizes's book *Du Cubisme et des moyens de le comprendre?*[2]
M. Completely idiotic.
Tz. What was his purpose in writing this book?

31
391, No. 14
Paris, November 1920

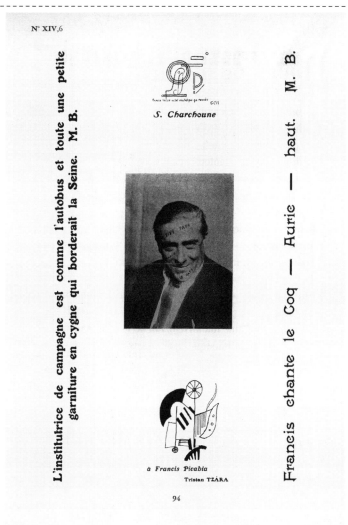

M. He needed to explain Cubism to himself because he still didn't understand it.

Tz. What do you make of his verbal diarrhoea?

M. I prefer other noises, for example the sighs of a pretty woman.

Tz. When exactly did Gleizes become a Cubist?

M. He never has been one in my opinion.

Tz. As a Cubist yourself, do you have much in common with Gleizes?

M. If Gleizes is a Cubist then I am certainly not; if I'm one then he isn't.

Tz. Are Gleizes's ideas really his own?

M. The only thing Gleizes is keen on is working in a group.

Tz. Who started Cubism?

M. Raphael.

Tz. Why did you write a book in collaboration with Gleizes?

M. Because I am extremely lazy and needed a secretary.

3.11

Le Pilhaou-Thibaou,
Paris, 10 July 1921[1]
Funny Guy
391

Translated from
the French by
Susan de Muth

Cubism was invented by Picasso, it's become a Parisian product.

Dadaism was invented by Marcel Duchamp and Francis Picabia – Huelsembeck [sic] or Tzara found the word Dada – it has become Parisian and Berliner wit.

Parisian wit, which mustn't be confused with the wit of Paris, consists of fantasies both external and spiritual; it lives in people to whom 'one doesn't do it!' and possesses the secret of transforming chicory into chicory, spinach into spinach and shit into poo. Obviously shit and poo are the same thing but spraying a little opoponax[2] on poo transforms this poo into profiteroles that my lady the Countess of Q.. is happy to eat and offer to her chosen guests. These chosen guests are:

....

.... and possibly Mr André Gide who doesn't eat profiteroles but nonchalantly slips them into his pocket where he forgets all about them and they soon become poo again illustrated by Roger de le Fresnaye.[3]

Translated from
the French by
Michelle Owoo

Le Pilhaou-Thibaou,
Paris, 10 July 1921
Guillermo de Torre
Dadaist Poem

WHEELS
To Francis Picabia the engine driver
waves of laughter colours
in the screen a delicious nightmare
life revolving in a chain a turbine engine
driving instincts
doves set vertical time
on long narrow skis solar loves
cinema of masked sexes
pipe tip plastic screw nut
in the intoxicated landscape
here is the western allegory
everything sings loves and vibrates
the woodsmen
Arp, Janco, Hausmann
and you, Picabia,

blind engine driver
of Dadaist orphan locomotives
I salute you
whistling your way across the world.

Madrid
1920

Translated from
the French by
Susan de Muth

Le Pilhaou-Thibaou,
Paris, 10 July 1921
Georges Auric [1]
Letter to Francis Picabia

My dear PICABIA,
I am a stutterer from Auvergne who squanders his gifts. The only
problem is that I don't much enjoy myself while doing so. But,
since there's no such thing as the Absolute, no one enjoys
himself, nobody gets bored and I don't think anything exists that
could truly be considered a gift.

Maybe one day you'll find me not suffering from neuralgia,
not in pain, without Faivre tablets.[2] I have just left a friend of mine
who excused herself from dining with me in this way: 'I prefer
making love to skipping.'

But that won't cure me any more than listening to a great
pianist, singer or any person of genius.

I might possibly be happy for one minute if I could compose
a piece of music that would be played, between one and four
o'clock in the morning, near Place Pigalle.

But I just can't stay up late any more.

If my music doesn't interest anyone – no one is of interest to
me. I'm not fond of catastrophes, tragedies, ruins and I don't like
walking near the Acropolis. These famous landscapes are as daft
as the souls of my famous neighbours. Dada = the ninth
symphony = Debussy. Lessons in humility render me senseless
and I'm bored to death by the Rite of Spring. Let's offer him a dose
of strychnine.

And I don't know what kind of absurd fatigue compels me
to write all this to you.

Good evening.

391, No 16
Paris
May 1924

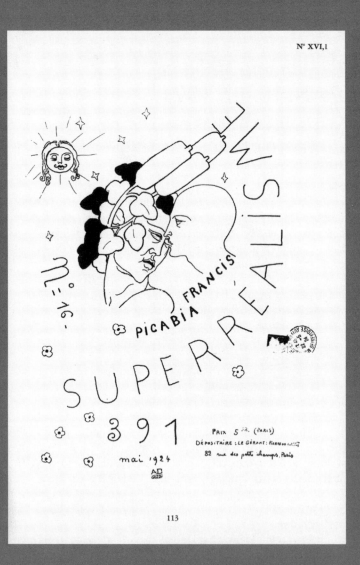

Translated from
the French by
Michelle Owoo

No. 17, Paris, June 1924
Robert Desnos
The Star on his Forehead

Consenting to unveil for us the curious mysteries of human
destiny and, before an assembly of Parisian critics where talent is
cheap, reminding us of the impressive genius of Raymond
Roussel[1] has not prevented the coalition of the Boulevards,
brasseries and newspaper offices from lining up against him. For
my part, I am honoured to have been one of the few who
applauded, drowned out by the clamour of imbeciles and
parochial people. Is human destiny so dull that when it is
recounted in delightful tales it causes outrage amongst so-called
sensible people? If a man writes a play where the characters are
tragically reduced to playing the role of chess pieces, the
instruments of a passion (curiosity, vices or love …), they declare
him mad.

Our contemporaries are pleasant oafs who have yet to
establish the bounds of poetic material. Lautréamont had
already presided over these touching unions of objects sprung
from different universes whose functions are so far removed
from each other (and which would appear destined to consume
their material existence) without enmeshing their individual
mechanisms or falling foul of their unique energies. A boy from
a laboratory makes his fortune thanks to a frozen mammoth's
foot, which is then brought to Paris by a professor interested in
the study of putrefaction; a humble servant resigned to his
destiny and the whim of the calendar that saw him born on a
dull day and fitted out with an organdie scapular on account of
peasants' superstitions concerning a venerable fir tree; the
revelation in a hot-air balloon dominating the war of 1870-1 of
the love of a bishop for a nurse and the significance of this
discovery in relation to a ring buried in a feudal cesspool – are
these magnificent events in human games of chance any more
scandalous or less touching than some adventure that befell a
Romanian virgin in a sunlit circus surrounded by lions born in
different climes? Or the battle between two men in love with
the same woman beneath a star skilled in carving out their
shadows on the sand from pathways with the same starlight
that illuminates the tree ferns, the winged serpents, the
nocturnal passions of red ants or the anonymous labour of an
unknown virgin? Is man's destiny any less 'dramatic' when
compared to the strange harmony of the solar system?

Everything on earth is bizarre. A boat is no more made for
water than for the skies; joining a young girl and a flower
together in an intellectual landscape is as arbitrary as the
coupling of a female shark and a male scorpion for obscure
reproductive purposes.

These chance encounters do happen, however, and our

habituation to these miraculous events gives rise to legends. The speed with which modern material is consigned to history results in new editions of the *Who's Who* of the great and the good and the catalogue of their achievements. From the Sun to Venus, from Venus to Christ, from Christ to the guillotine, from the guillotine to the *Venus de Milo*, from the *Venus de Milo* to the aeroplane, from the aeroplane to the invisible ray, passing ghosts, volcanoes and sea serpents along the way, the list of poetic prisons grows longer. One's imagination would wear itself out repeating them without the help of someone like Raymond Roussel.

A critic of little worth and a bad poet, Mr Fernand Gregh observed the other day in *Nouvelles Littéraires* that in taking the tales in 'L'Etoile au Front' one by one and 'padding them out' – thereby making volumes of 350 pages – it would enjoy the greatest success of any contemporary novel (on a par with *Atlantide*!)

That's the rub with these fools.

Mr Roussel is too rich. He has already seen the downside to this for himself with *Locus Solus.* It is fitting to remark that this observation has not only a material sense but also a spiritual one. I have no doubt that men of 'talent' will one day spring up who churn out successful work like Mr Roussel, a 'man of genius'. For my part, I have too much faith in the author of *Impressions d'Afrique* to believe for one moment that he would succumb to the temptation of a print run of a hundred thousand copies.

There are enough second-rate writers to satisfy the multitudes of dim-witted readers: *Henri Béraud,* who spins out Charcot for linen merchants and spills his guts for caretakers, *Henri Béraud*, who I cannot forgive for obliging me to defend Gide; *André Antoine* the anti-poet and the man who introduced conventional realism to the theatre, *Antoine*, whose every article is a collection of foolish quotations, *Antoine,* who would do well to go back to his gas meter; *Courteline* king of the morons; *Anatole France* chief abortionist of the Revolution and a learned scholar according to Larousse and many others!

But the truth of *Raymond Roussel's* vision issues scathing disclaimers to other swine: *Jean Cocteau* who has never ceased to plagiarise *Edmond Rostand*; Tristan Tzara sham trickster and first eunuch of the harem; Gabor ...Marcel Raval, the publisher of my drawings, and the whole band of turncoats and populists.

Once briefly clear, the path ahead now ends abruptly.

The army of lackeys is far behind.

In the great field of poetry, young girls grope blindly northwards, guided more surely by some mysterious instinct than by compass or star. Here is the virgin part of the forest with its creepers, its snakes, its treasures, its comely women and its wondrously mortal dangers. There is the hatchet. Soon we will be beyond the reach of dogs and rifles.

Translated from
the French by
Susan de Muth

No.17, Paris, June 1924
Erik Satie
A Mammal's Notebooks (I)

Cocteau is right, and right a thousand times: 'No more scandals,' he said ...

And really, scandals are just too scandalous and scandalise everybody. Furthermore, he advises his acolytes Laloy[1] and Auric to avoid all scandals too – even tiny, colourless, invisible ones.

For as you get older (forty years old) you become serious ... very serious ... incredibly serious – *deeply* serious.[2] This is what's happening to Cocteau: he's getting a middle-aged spread (*morally speaking, obviously*) ... but it's funny how people change, isn't it? ... Oh Forty Years, where are you leading us?

***

All of this gets me thinking, & gets me all melancholic & misanthropic ... oh yes ...

How many bits of (*family*) advice like this[3] do I need! ... Am I going to make the effort to follow it? ... even from some distance?

Isn't Cocteau setting us a fine example? He renounces all the vanities [pumps][4] of our age – be they aspirational [for draining] or repressive [for filling] (*if I dare say so*) ... yes, let us do the same; let's not hesitate: let's drain and fill our pumps. Let us repump no more. What have we got to lose?

***

In *Les Nouvelles Littéraires*, dear Auric describes me as a 'Normandy lawyer', a 'suburban chemist' and 'citizen Satie' (*from the Arceuil Soviet*) ...

Very good, my little friend ... may he continue; may he *relaloyse* himself from top to bottom ... afterwards, we shall see ... we'll see ... oh yes.

And what is my crime? That I don't like his *Fâcheux*[5] and described them as 'renovated' and 'deceitful' ... those who tell me that this late lamented friend is nothing but a 'flat foot' are exaggerating; he is, quite simply, nothing but an Auric (Georges) – which is quite enough for one man (?) to be.

Translated from
the French
by Susan de Muth

No.17, Paris, June 1924
Letter from my Grandfather[1]

Paris, 3 May 1924
My dear friend,
I'm leaving Paris for a few days, but I had to let you know immediately that the news *391* is being started up again came as a great surprise to me, as did the content of your announcement to the press.

I have no intention of discouraging you, nor of telling you what to do; you are familiar with my reservations about your recent activities and what purpose they are intended to serve (Montparnasse, the Swedish ballet, an extremely boring novel, *Paris-journal*, etc.) I would have refrained from speaking so frankly on the subject - due to the deep respect and affection I still have for you despite everything - had not this morning's *Journal du Peuple* inflicted your latest position upon me. There is little point in telling you that I absolutely decline your cordial invitation and will be urging all my friends to do likewise. May Satie's ancient grimaces - you found Huelsenbeck again then, bravo Rigaut,[2] etc. - make up for our refusal.
Your friend,
ANDRE BRETON

REPLY: 'When I've finished a cigarette I'm not one for keeping the butts.' PICABIA

3.13

No.18, Paris, July 1924
Erik Satie
A Mammal's Notebooks (II)

***

Translated from the French by Susan de Muth

CONTRADICTION: Cocteau adores me ... I am sure of it (*perhaps even a little too much*) ...
So why is he kicking me under the table?
***

ADVICE: Don't breathe unless you boil your air first ...
If you want to live for a long time, live old ...
No more short hair, tear it out ...
***

ACCUSED OF RECEIPT: My dear Auric - I received your rattle (*featuring the noble head of an old man*) ... Yes ...
It was coupled with a most amusing letter, kindly filthy[1] &, above all very [word obscured by black line] pornographic ... Ho! ... you really are a rude boy ... naughty boy? ...
What if your Dad found out! ... You'd get such a spanking! ...
***

A BIG STRONG CHAP: - Who's that really thin gentleman?
- He's a wrestler.
- No!
- Yes, he's fighting against tuberculosis (*an honorary member of one of many appropriate leagues*).
***

A WITTY REMARK: The author of *Parade* (*J. Cocteau*) described (*for the thousandth time*) the misfortunes that bowled him over, that tore him apart, that puffed him up, that straightened him out, that scraped him away while he was writing this work of - three

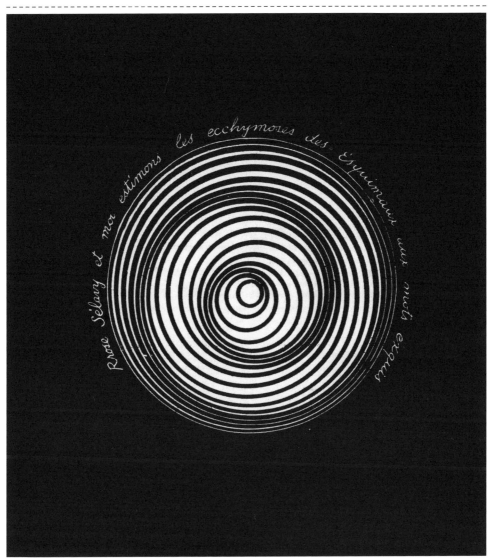

33
Insert with
Duchamp rotorelief
391, No. 18
Paris July 1924

lines... Everyone cried (*with laughter – even Laloy & Auric*) ...
All of a sudden and out of the blue – Mr X*** (*so well known for his*
perspicacity) stood up and coolly said: 'Down with Satie!' ...
The effect was marvellous ... Yes ...

***

A STRANGE CASE: Peculiar chap (?), that Auric! ...
Scapula, without a doubt ... Homogenous? ... Well, why not? ...
Peculiar chap (?) ! ... quite disturbing, worrying and perturbing –
all in all ... his 'schoolboy smuttiness'? Tee hee! ... Strange ... Yes
(& *no*) !...

***

INVOCATION: If my opponents have no respect for my age, may
they at least have some regard for my sense of decency (*don't you*
agree, Auric – & you, great Dada-ees Poulenc?)...[2]

Translated from
the French by
Susan de Muth

No.18, Paris, July 1924
Gabrielle Buffet
Letters from Paris

Paris, Friday, 20 June 1924

My Dear Francis,

It seems to me that Paris is dying of boredom.

However, I had a very enjoyable experience yesterday when I went to listen to *Mercure* at the Cigale.[1]

I liked the music very much and Picasso's set designs too, clearly inspired by Picabia and Duchamp.

The Breton gang[2] declared their faith in Picasso versus Satie in unison. Well, they do everything in unison don't they ... Love, Art and the Toilet?? What fools, as my son – who is yours even more than mine – would say.

When are you coming back??

Everyone sends you kisses.

Paris, 18 June 1924

Dear Sir and colleague,

We would be most grateful if you would allow your readers to peruse the following communication.

With all our thanks.

Yours faithfully,

André Breton

Louis Aragon[3]

Homage to Pablo Picasso

Recent years have witnessed the production of such innocuous work in the area of art and thought that any sense of purpose or evolution (which is the most important thing) has all but vanished. At a time when the public and the critics are conspiring to encourage nothing but mediocrity and compromise of all types, it falls to us to state our full and profound admiration for Picasso, who, scorning all sacred norms, has never stopped creating a modern sense of unease from which he always fashions the most compelling work. Now again, with *Mercure,* he provokes general incomprehension anew, exhibiting the full measure of his daring and genius. In the light of this event, which is taking on a truly exceptional nature, Picasso today emerges as the eternal personification of youth and the unassailable master of the situation; in a different league to everyone around him.

Louis Aragon, Georges Auric, André Boiffard, André Breton, Joseph Delteil, Robert Desnos, Max Ernst, Francis Gérard, Max Morise, Pierre Naville, Benjamin Péret, Francis Poulenc, Philippe Soupault, Roger Vitrac

[Ed.] Given the opportunity this wonderful declaration

affords, I didn't hesitate to ask other celebrities from various fields of endeavour to add their signatures to those of the elite of modern thought.

Here are some of the names I've collected:

Messieurs Virgile Tartempion, Philippe Dupont, Alexandre Dubois, Jacques de le Ferrière, Paul Badet, Jeanne Putein, Arlette Bordell, Jules Ecclesiastique, André Cué, Albert Amiral.

3.14

No.19, Paris, October 1924
Francis Picabia
Opinions and Portraits

Translated from the French by Susan de Muth

Mr Maurice Martin de Gard's article in *Les Nouvelles Littérature* is enough to make you die laughing – well at least it does make you laugh – but either Mr Maurice Martin du Gard knows absolutely nothing or this article was written by André Breton, which seems altogether more likely; the fact that he describes me as an artist/painter shows that Breton wants everyone to forget what I wrote in *Camera Work*, which came out in New York in 1914: *Le Portriat de Stieglitz, La Fille née sans Mère* and *Rateliers Platoniques* in 1917. As for Tzara, he wrote some extremely personal works while he was in Switzerland, from which Breton unscrupulously 'borrowed' ideas; and this is when he was also prostrating himself at the feet of André Gide[1] and courting Blaise Cendrars. He's trying to present the whole Dada business in the least embarrassing way for him and so that he comes out of it looking good; Vaché[2] is a great man but he's dead...The works of Messieurs Breton and – what's his name? – Philippe Coupeaux[3] are, I think, a poor imitation of Dada and their Surrealism is just as bad. André Breton reminds me of Lucien Guitry[4] playing a piece by Bernstein;[5] he's certainly as good an actor, but more out of date than Guitry.

Mr Maurice Martin du Gard, you consider André Breton to be a cut above Dermée and Birot, if you like theatre, obviously, I'm not going to press the point, but I have to tell you that Birot, for example, who I've known for a long time, often told me about his new ideas and he has several very strange cinematic inventions to his credit; as for Dermée, you'd have to be less superficial than you are to realise that this is no actor but a straightforward unpretentious man, that's what interests me the most. Yvan Goll's Surrealism[6] relates to Cubism, Breton's is quite simply Dada disguised as an advertising balloon for the house of Breton & Co.

Mr Maurice Martin du Gard, André Breton has called you a fool in front of me several times and branded your paper idiotic. Now he comes to your offices doffing his hat and with the most beautifully polite sentences on his lips, you've been taken for a ride; but you've done all those who might have their doubts about

Breton a great service. Breton is an actor who wants all the best roles at the Theatre of Illusion for himself and is nothing more than a Robert-Houdin for provincial hotels![7]
(To be continued if felt necessary)

Francis Picabia
Director of the André Breton Surrealism show

Translated from the French by Susan de Muth

No.19, Paris, October 1924
E.L.T. Mesens & René Magritte
[Aphorisms]

Why pay for your tradesman's luxury or his ignorance?

———

To be a thinker you must think.

———

Why pay for your tradesman or his ignorance?

———

Das leben ist ein schöne abord [sic].[1]

———

Why pay for luxury or its ignorance?

———

All unjustified appeals unfold during legal proceedings and those of the Salon des Tuileries.

———

Why pay for his ignorance?

———

And that is how holy images have a vague whiff of cheese about them.

———

Why?

———

Did you know that there's a French version?

E.L.T Mesens[2]

.... In dreams

.... Brothels make a strong impression

.... You'd think you were entering a conservatoire,
1

.... Invalids justify Cubism.
1

The positive pole loves the negative pole, to live is to love.

1

I love beer and hollyhocks.

1

A man in an Adam costume.

1

Cats are happy to live under chairs.

1

The cow has feelings.

René Magritte

The Blind Man
and New York Dada
Dawn Ades

Three little magazines were produced by the French émigrés Marcel Duchamp and Henri-Pierre Roché in New York in 1917, and their role in the scandal of Duchamp's *Fountain* has ensured their inscription in the history of Dada, though the name was then unknown to the protagonists. Duchamp's close friend Francis Picabia was in New York at the same time and his *391* was also exploring Duchamp's idea of the 'readymade'.

The Blindman (its first issue ran the words together in the title) was published in April 1917 by Henri-Pierre Roché with contributions from Mina Loy and Beatrice Wood. Its ostensible purpose was to celebrate the coming of America's own Independents Exhibition, which would bring about a much-needed artistic revolution in the United States.

The second issue in May of the same year, *P.B.T The Blind Man* (the B stood apparently for Beatrice, the T for Totor, Duchamp's nickname) carried the famous statement 'The Richard Mutt Case', which protested the suppression of R. Mutt's *Fountain*-urinal from the Independents exhibition. The identity of Mr Mutt was not revealed immediately but Duchamp's notorious reputation quickly spread and he became a kind of godfather to Dada, especially in Paris.

As Duchamp later said of this New York episode: 'It was not Dada, but it was in the same spirit, without however being in the Zurich spirit, although Picabia did some things in Zurich. Even in typography we were not particularly inventive. In *The Blind Man* it was a question above all of justifying the *Fountain*-urinal.' [1]

Rongwrong, which was published in May 1917 (the title due to a printer's error), a humorous eight-page review, appeared shortly after *P.B.T The Blind Man*. It engaged primarily in exchanges with Picabia's *391* and recorded the chess game in which Picabia and Roché purportedly played for the right to continue publishing their reviews. Picabia won.

In 1921 Duchamp and Man Ray produced the large, glossy single issue of *New York Dada*, whose chief glory is its cover, the minute multiple repetition of its title upside down surrounding Duchamp's altered readymade, the perfume bottle *Belle Haleine: eau de voilette*, with his portrait as Rrose Sélavy on the label. A 'letter of authorisation' from Tristan Tzara was printed inside, in response to a letter from Gabrielle Buffet to the Dada impresario now stationed in Paris. Whether they were seriously interested in forming an alliance with Tzara's movement or were operating an ironic game of testing the very idea of ownership that the notion of 'authorisation' introduces is impossible to say.

The Blindman No.1
Edited by Henri-Pierre Roché
New York
10 April 1917

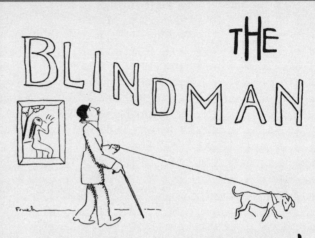

Henri-Pierre Roché
The Blind Man

I

The Blind Man celebrates to-day the birth of the Independence of Art in America.

II

A prominent New Yorker wrote us a few months ago: 'You know as well as I do why an Exhibition of Independent Artists is impossible in New York ... ' And many others were of the same opinion.
The impossible has happened. The Exhibition is on.

III

'What is the use of an Exhibition of Independents,' said some. 'Under present conditions, new talent can easily gain recognition through the picture galleries. They are many and their managers are open-minded.'

Let us quote from the programme:

'On one hand we have the frank statement of the established art societies that they cannot exhibit all the deserving work submitted to them because of lack of space. On the other hand such exhibitions as take place at private galleries must, by their nature, be formed from the ranks of artists who are already more or less known; moreover, no one exhibition at present gives an idea of contemporary American art in its ensemble, or permits comparison of the various directions it is taking, but shows only the work of one man or a homogeneous group of men. The great need, then, is for an exhibition, to be held at a given period each year, where artists of all schools can exhibit together – certain that whatever they send will be hung and that all will have an equal opportunity. For the public, this exhibition will make it possible to form an idea of the state of contemporary art ... '

'Ingres said, over sixty years, ago: "A jury, whatever be the means adopted for its formation, will always work badly. The need of our time is for unlimited admission ... I consider unjust and immoral any restriction tending to prevent a man from living from the product of his work."

'The "no jury" system, then, ensures a chance to exhibit to artists of every school, and, as a matter of fact, every school is represented at this salon, from the most conservative to the most radical.'

The spirit of the Indeps will stimulate, shape and provoke new talent.

The hanging of all works in alphabetical order, for the first time in any exhibition, will result in the most unexpected contacts and will incite every one to understand the others.

It is as easy to see a one-man show as to have a chat in a drawing-room – it is generally quite safe.

Entering the chaos of the Indeps is entering a virgin forest, full of surprises and dangers. One is compelled to make a personal choice out of the multitude of paintings which assail one from all sides. It means strengthening your taste through ordeals and temptations; it means finding yourself, and it is a strain.

The hour has come. The big brotherhood is there, men who have felt the strange need of expressing their soul and of their time with paint and brushes upon stretched canvases – madmen!

IV

New York will catch the Indeps' fever. It will rush to see what its children are painting, to scold them, laugh at them – and laud them.

V

New York, far ahead in so many ways, yet indifferent to art in the making, is going to learn to think for itself, and no longer accept, mechanically, the art reputations made abroad.

VI

In Paris, in 1884, other Indeps were born, humble hated scoffed at, weak in body but great in spirit.

During many years, thousands of people came merely to laugh at the stupidities, and were very indignant at the exhibited 'monstrosities'.

There was, above all, Henri Rousseau, an employee of the custom house, a visionary, who had once been to Mexico and ever after persevered in painting from memory what he had seen there. As a boy I could not take my eyes away from his 'ridiculous' pictures.

Today I know why; because they were beautiful, and lyrical, and something more than true.

No one laughs at them now, not even practical collectors, for those paintings which were worth from 20 to 100 francs then, are now worth from 2,000 to 5,000 dollars.

VII

The French Independents have made of Paris the world market for modern paintings, their retrospective exhibitions of Seurat, Van Gogh, Cesanne [sic], have imbued the souls of the younger painters with profound truths which have revolutionized the art of the world.

The Independents became the first spring event of Paris – gay, frank, bold, fertile, surpassing itself every year – while the big jury exhibitions became more and more like grandmothers patiently repeating themselves.

Says the pamphlet:

'The Independents have done more for the advance of French art than any other institution of its period. A considerable number of the most prominent artists of the present generation and the preceding one established their reputations at its annual exhibitions. They have more members, sell more works and are on firmer financial basis than any other of the four great salons.'

VIII

A principle, which reveals itself fully ripe and at the right time, is invincible. From today we will consider the annual exhibition of the Indeps as one of the features of the season.

XI

Many of New York's picture dealers give applause to the Indeps, while they really might be expected to oppose them. They realize the need of the public and the artists educating each other.

X

The Blind Man will be the link between the pictures and the public – and even between the painters themselves.

He will give voice to the enlightening opinions that may spring up, and make them known to all, as impartially as he can, whatever be their tendencies, as long as they are interesting.

He will give to lovers of art the pleasure of thinking aloud and hearing others do likewise.

He will give to those who want to understand the explanations of those who think they understand.

XI

The Blind Man's procedure shall be that of referendum. He will publish the questions and answers sent to him. He will print what the artists and the public have to say. He is very keen to receive suggestions and criticisms. So, don't spare him.

XII

Here are his intentions: He will publish reproductions of the most talked-of works.

He will give a chance to the leaders of any 'school' to 'explain' (provided they speak human).

He will print an annual Indeps for poetry, in a supplement open to all.

He will publish drawings, poems and stories written and illustrated by children.

XIII

Questions
Which is the work you prefer in the Exhibition? And why?
The one you most dislike?
The funniest?
The most absurd?
Guesses
What will be the total number of visitors?
The number of pictures sold?
The highest price paid for a single picture?
The lowest?
The total amount of money paid for all the works sold?

XIV

Suggestions
Write about the Indeps, or about any special work in the Exhibition.
A dramatic story of less than one hundred words.
A comic story of less than one hundred words.
A dream story of less than one hundred words.
A quatrain, or a limerick.
A song (words and music).

XV

To learn to 'see' the new painting is easy. It is even inevitable, if you keep in touch with it. It is something like learning a new language, which seems an impossibility at first. Your eye, lazy at the start, gets curious, then interested and progresses subconsciously.

In Paris the Blind Man has seen people go to exhibitions

of advanced art (even cubist or futurist) with the intention of getting indignant about it, and who spend a couple of hours giving vent to their indignation. But on reaching home they realized that they did not like their favorite paintings any more. That was the first step of their conversion. A year later he discovered in their home the very pictures which had so annoyed them.

XVI

Among the 'new' artists (as well as among the 'old') there are a great many who might as well never have painted at all. But let us remember that among them are the half-dozen or so undiscovered geniuses who will give us the style of the morrow.

XVII

The Blind Man knows an artist who made a good income painting pictures in the 'old' way, and who gladly gave it up and faced poverty to study the 'new'. 'Cubism,' said he, 'is at least an open door in the black wall of academism.'

XVIII

If a painter shows you a picture, you can make nothing out of, and calls you a fool, you may resent it.
But if a painter works passionately, patiently, and says, 'I am making experiments which may, perhaps, bring nothing for many years,' what can we have against him?

XIX

There are fine collections in New York, there are people who understand modern and ancient painting as well as anywhere else in the world. They are few.

For the average New Yorker art is only a thing of the past.

The Indeps insist that art is a thing of today.

XX

American artists are not inferior to those of other countries.
So, why are they not recognized here?
Is New York afraid? Does New York not dare to take responsibilities in Art? Where Art is concerned is New York satisfied to be like a provincial town?

What chances have American artists who cannot afford to go abroad?

None.

Is that fair?

'No,' says a voice. 'But why are they artists? Why not something else? We are a young and busy nation. We shall pay them well if they are willing to do some useful artistic work connected with our business.'

'Your useful artistic work is rotten. You simply want them to serve the public taste instead of leading it.'

XXI

Russia needs a political revolution.
America needs an artistic one. Your 'little theatre' movement has come. '291' and 'The Soil' have come. Every American who wishes to be aware of America should read 'The Soil.'

XXII

Never say of a man: 'He is not sincere.' Nobody knows if he is or not. And nobody is absolutely sincere or absolutely insincere.

Rather say: 'I do not understand him.'

The Blind Man takes it for granted that we are all sincere.

XXIII

May the spirit of Walt Whitman guide the Indeps.

Long live his memory, and long live the Indeps!

Mina Loy
In ... Formation

I do not suppose the Independents 'will educate the public' – the only trouble with the public is education.

The Artist is uneducated, is seeing IT for the first time; he can never see the same thing twice.

Education is the putting of spectacles on wholesome eyes. The public does not naturally care about these spectacles, the cause of its quarrels with art. *The Public* likes to be jolly; *The Artist* is jolly and quite irresponsible. Art is *The Divine Joke* and any *Public*, and any Artist can see a nice, easy, simple joke, such as the sun; but only artists and serious critics can look at a grayish stickiness on smooth canvas.

Education in recognizing something that has been seen before demands an art that is only acknowledgable by way of diluted comparisons ... it is significant that the demand is half-hearted.

'Let us forget' is the cry of the educator; 'the democratically simple beginnings of an art,' – so that we may talk of those things that have only middle and no end, and together wallow in gray stickiness.

The Public knows better than this, knowing such values as the under-inner curve of women's footgear, one factor of the art of our epoch ... it is unconcerned with curved Faun's legs and maline twirled scarves of artistic imagining; or with allegories of Life with thorn-skewered eyes ... it knew before the Futurists that Life is a jolly noise and a rush and sequence of ample reactions.

The Artist then says to *The Public*, 'Poor pal; what has happened to you? ... We were born so similar – and *now* look!' But *The Public* will not look; that is, look at *The Artist* – it has unnaturally acquired prejudice.

So *The Public* and *The Artist* can meet at every point except the – for *The Artist* – vital one, that of pure uneducated *seeing*. They like the same drinks, can fight in the same trenches, pretend to the same women; but never see the same thing *ONCE*.

You might, at least, keep quiet while I am talking.

The Blind Man No. 2
Edited by Marcel Duchamp,
Henri-Pierre Roché & Beatrice Wood
New York, May 1917

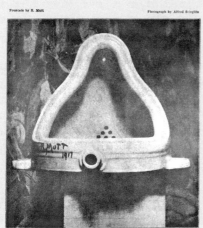

THE BLIND MAN

The Richard Mutt Case

They say any artist paying six dollars may exhibit.

Mr. Richard Mutt sent in a fountain. Without discussion this article disappeared and never was exhibited.

What were the grounds for refusing Mr. Mutt's fountain :—

1. *Some contended it was immoral, vulgar.*

2. *Others, it was plagiarism, a plain piece of plumbing.*

Now Mr. Mutt's fountain is not immoral, that is absurd, no more than a bath tub is immoral. It is a fixture that you see every day in plumbers' show windows.

Whether Mr. Mutt with his own hands made the fountain or not has no importance. He CHOSE it. He took an ordinary article of life, placed it so that its useful significance disappeared under the new title and point of view—created a new thought for that object.

As for plumbing, that is absurd. The only works of art America has given are her plumbing and her bridges.

"Buddha of the Bathroom"

I suppose monkeys hated to lose their tail. Necessary, useful and an ornament, monkey imagination could not stretch to a tailless existence (and frankly, do you see the biological beauty of our loss of them?), yet now that we are used to it, we get on pretty well without them. But evolution is not pleasing to the monkey race; "there is a death in every change" and we monkeys do not love death as we should. We are like those philosophers whom Dante placed in his Inferno with their heads set the wrong way on their shoulders. We walk forward looking backward, each with more of his predecessors' personality than his own. Our eyes are not ours.

The ideas that our ancestors have joined together let no man put asunder! In *La Dissociation des Idées*, Remy de Gourmont, quietly analytic, shows how sacred is the marriage of ideas. At least one charm-ing thing about our human institution is that although a man marry he can never be *only* a husband. Besides being a money-making device and the *one* man that *one* woman can sleep with in legal purity with-out sin he may even be as well some other woman's very personification of her ab-stract idea. Sin, while to his employees he is nothing but their "Boss," to his children only their "Father," and to himself cer-tainly something more complex.

But with objects and ideas it is different. Recently we have had a chance to observe their meticulous monogamy.

When the jurors of *The Society of In-dependent Artists* fairly rushed to remove the bit of sculpture called the *Fountain* sent in by Richard Mutt, because the object was irrevocably associated in their atavistic minds with a certain natural function of a secretive sort. Yet to any "innocent" eye

The Richard Mutt Case

They say any artist paying six dollars may exhibit.
Mr Richard Mutt sent in a fountain. Without discussion this article
disappeared and never was exhibited.
What were the grounds for refusing Mr Mutt's fountain:-
1. Some contended it was immoral, vulgar.
2. Others, it was plagiarism, a plain piece of plumbing.
Now Mr Mutt's fountain is not immoral, that is absurd, no more than
a bath tub is immoral. It is a fixture that you see every day in
plumbers' show windows.
Whether Mr Mutt with his own hands made the fountain or not has
no importance. He CHOSE it. He took an ordinary article of life,
placed it so that its useful significance disappeared under the new
title and point of view – created a new thought for that object.
As for plumbing, that is absurd. The only works of art America has
given are her plumbing and her bridges.

Louise Norton
"Buddha of the Bathroom"

I suppose monkeys hated to lose their tail. Necessary, useful and
an ornament, monkey imagination could not stretch to a tailless
existence (and frankly, do you see the biological beauty of our loss
of them?), yet now that we are used to it we get on pretty well
without them. But evolution is not pleasing to the monkey race;
'there is a death in every change' and we monkeys do not love
death as we should. We are like those philosophers whom Dante
placed in his Inferno with their heads set the wrong way on their
shoulders. We walk forward looking backward, each with more of
his predecessors' personality than his own. Our eyes are not ours.

The ideas that our ancestors have joined together let no
man put asunder! In *La Dissociation des Idées*, Remy de
Gourmont, quietly analytic, shows how sacred is the marriage of
ideas. At least one charming thing about our human institution is
that although a man marry he can never be *only* a husband.
Besides being a moneymaking device and the *one* man that *one*
woman can sleep with in legal purity without sin he may even be
as well some other woman's very personification of her abstract
idea. Sin, while to his employees he is nothing by their 'Boss', to
his children only their 'Father,' and to himself certainly
something more complex.

But with objects and ideas it is different. Recently we have
had a chance to observe their meticulous monogamy.

When the jurors of *The Society of Independent Artists* fairly
rushed to remove the bit of sculpture called the *Fountain* sent in
by Richard Mutt, because the object was irrevocably associated in

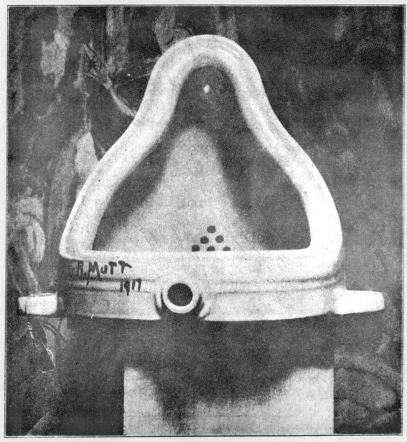

Fountain by R. Mutt

Photograph by Alfred Stieglitz

THE EXHIBIT REFUSED BY THE INDEPENDENTS

37
Marcel Duchamp
Fountain
P.B.T. The Blind Man, No. 2
May 1917

their atavistic minds with a certain natural function of a secretive sort. Yet to any 'innocent' eye how pleasant is its chaste simplicity of line and color! Someone said, 'Like a lovely Buddha'; someone said, 'Like the legs of the ladies by Cezanne [sic]'; but have they not, those ladies, in their long, round nudity always recalled to your mind the calm curves of decadent plumbers' porcelains?

At least as a touchstone of Art how valuable it might have been! If it be true, as Gertrude Stein says, that pictures that are right stay right, consider, please, on one side of a work of art with excellent references from the Past, the *Fountain*, and on the other almost anyone of the majority of pictures now blushing along the miles of wall in the Grand Central Palace of ART. Do you see what I mean?

Like Mr Mutt, many of us had quite an exhorbitant [sic] notion of the independence of the Independents. It was a sad surprise to learn of a Board of Censors sitting upon the ambiguous question, What is ART?

To those who say that Mr Mutt's exhibit may be Art, but is it the art of Mr Mutt since a plumber made it? I reply simply that the *Fountain* was not made by a plumber but by the force of an imagination; and of imagination it has been said, 'All men are shocked by it and some overthrown by it.' There are those of my intimate acquaintance who pretending to admit the imaginative vigor of Mr Mutt and his porcelain, slyly quoted to me a story told by Montaigne in his *Force of the Imagination* of a man, whose Latin name I can by no means remember, who so studied the very 'essence and motion of folly' as to unsettle his initial judgement forevermore; so that through overmuch wisdom he became a fool. It is a pretty story, but in defense of Mr Mutt I must in justice point out that our merry Montaigne is a garruolus [sic] and gullible old man, neither safe nor scientific, who on the same subject seriously cites by way of illustration, how by the strength simply of her imagination, a white woman gave birth to a 'black-a-moor'! So you see how he is good for nothing but quotation, M. Montaigne.

Then again, there are those who anxiously ask, 'Is he serious or is he joking?' Perhaps he is both! Is it not possible? In this connection I think it would be well to remember that the sense of the ridiculous *as well as* 'the sense of the tragic increases and declines with sensuousness'. It puts it rather up to you. And there is among us to-day a spirit of 'blague' arising out of the artist's bitter vision of an over-institutionalized world of stagnant statistics and antique axioms. With a frank creed of immutability the Chinese worshipped their ancestors and dignity took the place of understanding; but we who worship Progress, Speed and Efficiency are like a little dog chasing after his own wagging tail that has dazzled him. Our ancestor-worship is without grace and it is because of our conceited hypocracy [sic] that our artists are sometimes sad, and if there is a shade of bitter mockery in some of them it is only there because they know that the joyful spirit of their work is to this age a hidden treasure.

Alfred Stieglitz
Letter from Alfred Stieglitz to Blind Man

But pardon my praise for, sayeth Nietzsche, 'In praise there is more obtrusiveness than in blame'; and so as not to seem officiously sincere or subtly serious, I shall write in above, with a perverse pen, a neutral title that will please none; and as did Remy de Gourmont, that gentle cynic and monkey without a tail, I, too, conclude with the most profound word in language and one which cannot be argued – a pacific Perhaps!

291 Fifth Ave., New York
13 April 1917

My dear Blind Man:
You invite comment, suggestions. As I understand the Independent Society its chief function is the desire to smash antiquated academic ideas. This first exhibition is a concrete move in that direction. Wouldn't it be advisable next year during the exhibition, to withhold the names of the makers of all work shown. The names, if on the canvases, or on the pieces of sculpture, etc., exhibited could be readily hidden. The catalogue should contain, in place of the names of artists, simply numbers, with titles if desired. On the last day of the Exhibition the names of the exhibitors could be made public. That is each number would be publicly identified. A list of the identified numbers could also be sent to the purchasers of catalogues. To no one, outside of the committee itself, should any names be divulged during the exhibition. Not even to those wishing to purchase. In thus freeing the exhibition of the traditions and superstitions of names the Society would not be playing into the hands of dealers and critics, nor even into the hands of the artists themselves. For the latter are influenced by names quite as much as are public and critics, not to speak of the dealers who are only interested in names. Thus each bit of work would stand on its own merits. As a reality. The public would be purchasing its own reality and not a commercialized and inflated name. Thus the Society would be dealing a blow to the academy of commercializing names. The public might gradually see for itself.

Furthermore I would suggest that in next year's catalogue addresses of dealers should be confined to the advertising pages. The Independent Exhibition should be run for one thing only: the independence of the work itself. The Society has made a definite move in the right direction, so why not follow it up with some more definiteness.

NO JURY – NO PRIZES – NO COMMERCIAL TRICKS

New York Dada
New York
1921

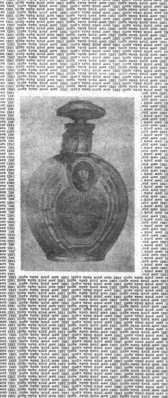

38
Front cover
New York Dada
April 1921

Tristan Tzara
Eye-Cover, Art-Cover, Corset-Cover Authorization

EYE-COVER

You ask for authorization to name your periodical Dada. But Dada belongs to everybody. I know excellent people who have the name Dada. Mr Jean Dada; Mr. Gaston de Dada; Fr. Picabia's dog is called Zizi de Dada; in G. Ribemont-Dessaigne's play, the pope is likewise named Zizi de Dada. I could cite dozens of examples. Dada belongs to everybody. Like the idea of God or of the tooth-brush. There are people who are very dada, more dada; there are dadas everywere [sic] all over and in every individual. Like God and the tooth1brush (an excellent invention, by the way).

Dada is a new type; a mixture of man, naphthaline, sponge, animal made of ebonite and beefsteak, prepared with soap for cleansing the brain. Good teeth are the making of the stomach and beautiful teeth are the making of a charming smile. Halleluiah of ancient oil and injection of rubber.

There is nothing abnormal about my choice of Dada for the name of my review. In Switzerland I was in the company of friends and was hunting the dictionary for a word appropriate to the sonorities of all languages. Night was upon us when a green hand placed its ugliness on the page of Larousse – pointing very precisely to Dada – my choice was made. I lit a cigarette and drank a demitasse.

For Dada was to say nothing and to lead to no explanation of this offshoot of relationship which is not a dogma nor a school, but rather a constellation of individuals and of free facets.

Dada existed before us (the Holy Virgin) but one cannot deny its magical power to add to this already existing spirit and impulses of penetration and diversity that characterizes its present form.

There is nothing more incomprehensible than Dada.

Nothing more indefinable.

ART-COVER AUTHORIZATION

With the best will in the world I cannot tell you what I think of it.

The journalists who say that Dada is a pretext are right, but it is a pretext for something that I do not know.

Dada has penetrated into every hamlet; Dada is the best paying concern of the day.

Therefore, Madam, be on your guard and realize that a really dada product is a different thing from a glossy label.

Dada abolishes 'nuances'. Nuances do not exist in words but only in some atrophied brains whose cells are too jammed. Dada is an anti 'nuance' cream. The simple motions that serve as signs for deaf-mutes are quite adequate to express the four or five mysteries we have discovered within 7 or 8,000 years. Dada offers all kinds of advantages. Dada will soon be able to boast of having shown people that to say 'right' instead of 'left' is neither less nor too logical, that red and valise are the same thing; that 2765 = 34; that 'fool' is a merit; that yes = no. Strong influences are making themselves felt in politics, in commerce, in language. The whole world and what's in it has slid to the left along with us. Dada has inserted its syringe into hot bread, to speak allegorically into language. Little by little (large by large) it destroys it. Everything collapses with logic. And we shall see certain liberties we constantly take in the sphere of sentiment, social life, morals, once more become normal standards. These liberties no longer will be looked upon as crime, but as itches.

I will close with a little international song: Order from the publishing house 'La Sirene' 7 rue Pasquier, Paris, DADAGLOBE, the work of dadas from all over the world. Tell your bookseller that this book will soon be out of print. You will have many agreeable surprises.

CORSET-COVER

Read Dadaglobe if you have troubles. Dadaglobe is in press. Here are some of its collaborators:

Paul Citroen (Amsterdam); Baader Daimonides; R. Hausmann; W. Heartfield; H. Hoech; R. Huelsenbeck; G. Grosz; Fried Hardy Worm (Berlin); Clement Pansaers (Bruxelles); Mac Robber (Calcutta); Jacques Edwards (Chili); Baargeld, Armada v. Dulgedalzen, Max Ernst, F. Haubrich (Cologne); K. Schwitters (Hannovre); J.K. Bonset (Leyde); Guillermo de Torre (Madrid); Gino Cantarelli; E. Bacchi, A Fiozzi (Mantoue); Krusenitch (Moscou); A. Vagts (Munich); W.C. Arensberg, Gabrielle Buffet, Marcel Duchamp; Adon Lacroix; Baroness v. Loringhoven; Man Ray; Joseph Stella; E. Varese; A Stieglitz; M. Hartley; C. Kahler (New York); Louis Aragon; C. Brancusi; André Breton; M. Buffet; S. Charchoune; J. Crotti; Suzanne Duchamp; Paul Eluard; Benjamin Peret; Francis Picabia; G. Ribemont-Dessaignes; J. Rigaut, Soubeyran; Ph. Soupault, Tristan Tzara (Paris); Mechior Vischer (Prague); J. Evola (Rome); Arp; S. Taeuber (Zurich).

The incalculable number of pages of reproductions and of text is a guarantee of the success of the book. Articles of luxury, of prime necessity, articles indispensable to hygiene and to the heart, toilet articles of an intimate nature.

Such, Madame, do we prepare for Dadaglobe; for you need look no further than to the use of articles prepared without Dada to account for the fact that the skin of your heart is chapped; that the so precious enamel of your intelligence is cracking; also for the presence of those tiny wrinkles still imperceptible but nevertheless disquieting.

All this and much else in Dadaglobe.

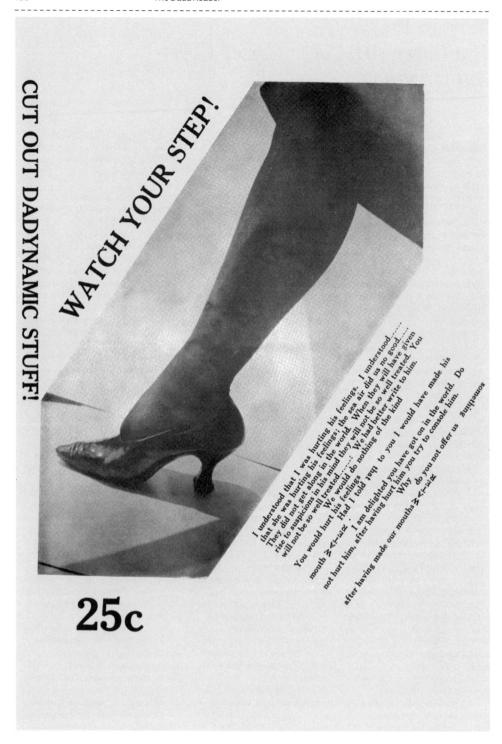

CUT OUT DADYNAMIC STUFF!

WATCH YOUR STEP!

25c

I understood that I was hurting his feelings. I understood........ I understood........ that she was hurting his feelings; the sea air did us no good........ They did not get along in the world. When they will have given rise to suspicions in his mind they will not be so well treated. You will not be so well treated........: We had better write to him. We would do nothing of the kind .... You would hurt his feelings .... Had I told лол to you I would have made his mouth ᴚᴉⱯ-ɪ-ɔᴀ I am delighted you have got on in the world. Do not hurt him, after having hurt him you try to console him. Why do you not offer us something after having made our mouths ᴚᴉⱯ-ɪ-ɔᴀ

39
'Watch Your Step'
New York Dada
April 1921

Littérature
Dawn Ades

Littérature, like *391*, began independently of Dada and outlasted it. André Breton, in one of his Dada manifestos described Dada as a 'state of mind'[1] but later grudgingly remarked that 'Dada was never considered by us as anything but the coarse image of a state of mind to whose creation it had not contributed'.[2] This hardly does justice to the Dada episode in Paris and indicates Breton's ignorance of or indifference to Dada's activities and influence in Germany and Eastern Europe. However, it reflects quite accurately the sense of purpose and ambition in post-war Paris on the part of the young editors of the review, who became increasingly disillusioned by the official avant-garde. Into this situation Dada's disrespect and urge to start again at zero was a crucial catalyst.

The editors, Breton, Louis Aragon and Philippe Soupault, had met in 1917 during the war, and had already come to the notice of the Paris intelligentsia. They swiftly developed plans to start a review, which was the means of establishing an individual intellectual space within the Paris literary world. After several false starts and thanks to an inheritance by Soupault the first issue of the review was published in March 1919. Earlier titles envisaged were *Le Nègre* (the name of an attraction, the 'dynamometer', at the Palais des Fêtes), *Le nouveau monde* and *Carte blanche* (suggested by Pierre Reverdy, whose magazine *Nord-Sud* had ceased publication in the autumn of 1918.)[3] Paul Valéry, who had dubbed them the 'three musketeers', suggested the title *Littérature*, after the final line of Verlaine's 'L'art poétique': 'and all the

rest is literature'. The ambiguity of the title (Eluard assured Proust that it was intended to signify the opposite) fairly accurately reflects the mixed contents of the first issues. While on the one hand several of the most prominent names of the French literary avant-garde are present: for example, André Gide, Valéry, Max Jacob and Reverdy, there are also already signs of a different type of anti-literary activity. The particular heroes of the *Littérature* group were Rimbaud, who had abandoned his 'profession' as poet, and the mysterious figure of Isidore Ducasse, the Comte de Lautréamont, whose violent prose poem *Les Chants de Maldoror* was to be so important for Surrealism. His hitherto unpublished text 'Poésies' was transcribed by Breton for the second and third issues of *Littérature*, followed from the fifth issue (July 1919) by the 'Lettres de Jacques Vaché', the letters to Breton and his friends from the young, charismatic soldier whose nihilism and rejection of a literary career continued to haunt Breton and who died from an overdose of opium at the age of twenty-three in January 1919.[4] There were also experiments like Breton's 'Le corset mystère', using found fragments from advertising slogans, which were soon overtaken by the publication of the first automatic texts, 'Les Champs magnétiques', (nos 8, 9 and 10. October–December 1919), a collaboration between Soupault and Breton. This, in hindsight, was the founding moment of Surrealism. But this was still in the future and for the moment these experiments functioned to distance the *Littérature* group from an avant-garde with whom they felt increasingly

Les Premiers et les Derniers

(résultats du tableau de tête)

#	Nom	Score	Nom	Score
1	André Breton	16,85	Henri de Régnier	- 22,90
2	Philippe Soupault	16,30	Anatole France	- 18,00
3	Charlie Chaplin	16,09	Maréchal Foch	
4	Arthur Rimbaud	15,95	Stuart Mill	- 17,45
5	Paul Eluard	15,10	Romain Rolland	- 17,36
6	Isidore Ducasse	14,27	Paul Fort	- 16,54
7	Louis Aragon	14,10	Louis Pasteur	- 16,27
8	Tristan Tzara	13,30	Auguste Rodin	- 16,00
9	Alfred Jarry	13,09	Soldat inconnu	- 15,63
10	Jacques Rigaut	13,00	Voltaire	- 15,27
11	Georges Ribemont-Dessaignes	12,50	Charles Maurras	- 14,90
12	Guillaume Apollinaire	12,45	Max Linder	- 14,63
13	Arp	12,18	Henry Bernstein	- 14,36
14	Jacques Vaché	11,90	Alphonse de Lamartine	- 14,18
15	Pilules Pink (rédact. des réclames)	11,45	Alfred de Musset	- 14,09
16	Marquis de Sade	11,27	Guynemer	- 14,00
17	Jonathan Swift	11,09	Emile Zola	- 13,68
18	Duval (Bonnet rouge)	10,45	Pierre Albert-Birot	- 13,45
19	Bonnot	10,36	Marc-Aurèle	- 13,18
20	Laclos	10,00	Francis Jammes	- 13,09

Le Gérant : PHILIPPE SOUPAULT

at variance. It was Dada that pushed them into a state of total renunciation of the established literary and artistic world.

Poems by Tristan Tzara had begun to appear from October 1919, and indeed there had been a review of Tzara's 'Dada Manifesto 1918' in the very first issue of *Littérature*, although without immediate consequences, by the remarkable woman Raymonde Linossier. The high point of Dada in *Littérature* was the publication of the 'Twenty-three dada Manifestos' in May 1920, and there are echoes throughout 1920 and 1921 of the 'dada seasons', with their manifestations, performances and exhibitions. The first series of the review retained its compact format, austere presentation and yellow cover and only occasionally broke out with a temporary burst of unconventional typography. The exhibition of Max Ernst's collages in 1921 was celebrated in *Littérature* in May 1921 together with a genial homage to Hans Arp by Ernst (fig.42). From the perspective of Paris Dada this was a welcome international extension of contacts, although again in retrospect Ernst's exhibition is usually absorbed into the pre-history of Surrealism. In *Littérature*, as Breton saw it, 'Dada and Surrealism can only be conceived in correlation, like two waves overtaking one another in turn.'[5]

A characteristic of Dada in Paris as represented by *Littérature* was a sense of operating within a dense intellectual and artistic climate that included a well-established avant-garde that, despite their renunciation, still invited a challenge and demanded a response. This can be tracked throughout *Littérature* from the questionnaire 'Why do you write?' launched in November 1919 through to the Maurice Barrès trial, which closed its first series in August 1921.[6] This 'trial' of the prominent writer who had once been a hero to Breton's generation but who had become a right-wing patriot was one of the swansongs of Dada, with Tzara alone refusing to take it seriously.

The second series of *Littérature*, which ran for thirteen issues from March 1922 to June 1924, exists in a kind of *terrain vague* between Dada and Surrealism. For the first three issues of the new series, whose cover was a top hat drawn by Man Ray, Breton and Soupault are named joint editors. From the fourth issue Breton took sole control; slightly larger in format than the first series, from now on the review included more illustrations and had a series of striking covers by Francis Picabia. The interest in popular culture and film shown in the first series continues, though this is in a sense absorbed into their own internal experiments. So, for example, Benjamin Péret publishes here his scenario for a film, 'Bonny Wants a Car', which builds on both the fantastic and the farcical possibilities of the medium. Dada's inherent interest in performance took a special line in Paris with the sketches 'Vous m'oublierez' and 'Comme il fait beau!'

The second series of *Littérature* is already engaged in experiments that prefigure Surrealism, though there is still an openness and uncertainty about the direction these experiments will take. Prominent in the second series is the haunting presence of

Marcel Duchamp and his alter ego Rrose
Sélavy, who appears both visually and verbally.
Duchamp's *Large Glass, The Bride Stripped Bare
by her Bachelors, Even* (1915–23) was already a
legend among the Paris Dada group; the
occasional puns produced by Rrose Sélavy
were extended by Robert Desnos into an
extraordinary sequence which he claimed, by
way of homage, to have received from
Duchamp's alter ego. These disquieting
experiences with language fall in with the
experiments with hypnotic trances that were
recorded in *Littérature* in November 1922, in
the 'Entrées des mediums'. These pseudo-
scientific experiments with the mediums'
trances, in which the subject experiences the
loss of conscious control over speech and
writing, were a temporary alternative to the
interest in Freud which had, Breton later
affirmed in the first *Surrealist Manifesto*,
presided over the first attempts at automatic
writing and whose ideas freely interpreted by
the Surrealists were to dominate the first years
of the movement.

5.1

No.1, March 1919
R.L.[1]
Review of *Dada*[2]

Translated from
the French
by Ian Monk

Ideal, ideal, ideal,
Knowledge, knowledge, knowledge,
Boomboom, boomboom, boomboom,
yells Tzara in the *Dada* manifesto. Bourdelle dances for his
boomboom – and there he is right – but he wants to make us
dance for his boomboom and how wrong he is here. Dada means
nothing but liberty, the freedom from systems, the independence
of the artist, the abolition of the compartments of the brain:
philosophy, psychoanalysis, dialectics, logic, science. Dada
demands 'works that are strong, straight, forever
misunderstood'. Tzara's manifesto deserves to live on among
those works that do not reach the 'hungry masses', but survive
thanks to their energy.

5.2

No.2, April 1919
Georges Auric
A New Work[1]

Translated from
the French
by Ian Monk

Chinese, young American girl, jugglers, introduced, in front of the
stall, by ferocious managers, are the show's parade. A barrel
organ accompanies them – which Satie transforms into a dream
machine. The rich Slavonic fête fires off its fireworks elsewhere
decked with parrot feathers. Here, only, three 'numbers', just as
the crowd wants, on Sunday, in Paris. The avenue de Maine is
nearby smiling like *Le Douanier* Rousseau.

After so many overloads and millionaire beauties, the
simplicity of the music in which the very sadness of the fair has
been expressed without a single false note disappoints the
sophisticates. Their Rolls-Royces used to wink in front of Mr
Junet's car. 'The scandal of *Parade* ...'[2]

Calmly, stopping, sometimes for weeks before starting
work again one fine day, Satie has undertaken an oeuvre which,
may I be the first to say, equals the fine pages of *Boris* for pure
emotion.

Three fragments of Plato's *Dialogues*, from Cousin's
schoolbook translation, make up the three tales of *Socrate* (an
elegy for Socrates – a walk alongside the Ilissus – the death of
Socrates). A small, sober orchestra accompanies the voice.

The tenderness and emotion of a declamation that is pure
rhythm and harmony truly distinguish this music that *flows from
one mind to another*. It puts us in an unknown place, without
extravagance, without mist, a new mechanism sets off each

section, a particular movement that animates it with a particular life and leads it into a certain and continuous swaying. Socrates will die; only then does the tone insist, weigh down, become more human.

With an overcome choir of disciples, Satie, in Arcueil, attends a sublime death scene. But beyond the picturesque and cunning, using ingenuous and certain means, he makes fresh contact with an immortal text.

The man in the street says: 'A work by Satie? I don't even want to hear it. As a vague amateur, his japes might have amused us once, for a minute. But I am indignant that anybody could now take such a musician seriously.'

Alas, sir, we do not understand each other. Puns no longer make us laugh and our youth scorns japes. Yet we cannot but love Mr Satie slowly unwinding, like a moving piano lesson, the still trembling chain of a fresh clarity with which he will accompany the gospel according to Plato.

5.3

No. 4, June 1919
André Breton
The Mystery Corset

Translated from
the French
by Ian Monk

My beautiful lady readers

Having frequently seen **in all colours**
Splendid cards, *with lighting effects*, Venice
In the past the furniture in my bedroom was bolted
solidly to the walls and I had myself tied up to write

I have sea legs

we belong to a sort of **Touring Club**
of sentiment

A CASTLE INSTEAD OF A HEAD

It's also the **Charity Bazaar**
Games of great amusement for all ages; **poetic games, etc.**

I hold Paris like – revealing the future to you –
your open hand

the waist enlaced.

5.4

No. 5, July 1919
Henri Rousseau
*A Philosopher**

Translated from
the French
by Ian Monk

Like Diogenes the great philosopher
Although not living in a barrel
I am like the wandering Jew on the earth
Fearing neither the squalls nor damp
Trotting along while smoking my old pipe
Proudly braving the lightning and thunder
To earn soldier's pay
Even though the rain wets the earth
I wear on my back the unanswerable
Advertisement for the independent newspaper Eclair.

*Poem written for the picture.[1]

Translated from
the French
by Ian Monk

No.5, July 1919
Paul Eluard
Animals and their Men

PREFACE

May an honest strength return to us.

A few poets, a few builders who lived young had already taught us. Let us know what we are capable of.

Neither beauty nor ugliness seems necessary to us. We have never particularly been concerned by power or grace, by gentleness or brutality, by simplicity or number.

The vanity that makes mankind state that this is beautiful or this is ugly, and take sides, is at the foundation of several literary eras of refined error, of sentimental excess and the resulting disorder.

Let us try, although it is hard, to stay utterly pure. We shall then understand what binds us together.

And the unpleasant language that suffices to the loose of tongue, a language as dead as the crowns of our similar brows, let us reduce it, transform it into the charming, true language of a genuine exchange between us.

As for me, there seems to be no better sign of such a desire than this poem written after dreaming of this opening page:

SALON
Love of permitted fantasies
Of sun
Of lemons
Of light mimosa

Clarity of the means in use:
Clear glass,
Patience
And vase to be pierced.

Of sun, of lemons, of light mimosa
In the force of the fragility
Of the glass that contains
This enrolled gold
This gold that rolls

5.5

No. 7, September 1919
André Breton
Factory[1]

Translated from
the French
by Ian Monk

The great legend of railways and reservoirs, the fatigue of beasts of burden often reach the heart of certain men. There are some who know about such things thanks to driving belts: for them, regular breathing is over. None would deny that industrial injuries are more beautiful than marriages of convenience. However, it can happen that the owner's daughter crosses the courtyard. It is easier to be rid of a grease stain than a dead leaf: at least your hand does not shake. At the same distance from the workshops of production and decoration, the foreman's prism toys wickedly with the star of new employment.

Translated from
the French
by Ian Monk

No. 7, September 1919
Press Cuttings
Opium![1]

The young people had tried smoking that terrible liquor
A sad event, which has thrown two of the most honourably reputed families of Nantes into despair, took place on Monday evening. Two young people aged about twenty, currently mobilised, have died from intoxication brought on by an overly excessive absorption of opium.

We have not previously – fortunately! – had to deplore such serious effects of this dismal passion for 'narcotics' in our town, nor the mortal charm of drugs that has taken root among our young men in recent times.

At the Hotel de France
On Monday evening, a little before 6 p.m., a young soldier in the American Supply Corps, A.-K. Woynow, rushed like a madman from a bedroom on the second floor of the Hôtel de France and

---

asked to speak to the manager urgently. When he had been informed of this request, the manager arrived and was told that two young persons, friends of the American, were dying in the bedroom. Medical assistance was sent for at once; a Dr de la Rochefordière was found and summoned.

When the physician entered the room, he found, stretched out on the bed, one lying on his right side, the other on his left, and entirely naked, two young people who seemed to be sleeping deeply. Their faces were calm, but reflected an utter stupor. Dr de la Rochefordière observed that one of these bodies was already cold, while the other was warm; it did not take him long to announce his diagnosis: the two strangers were victims of intoxication due to the absorption of a large dose of opium.

While the doctor was treating as best he could the young man who looked as though he still might be saved, and after that the American who had felt indisposed, the police commissioner was informed of the events and arrived to make his report.

The Victims

The papers that were found and information noted in the hotel's register revealed that the dead man was named Jacques V..., aged twenty-three, warrant officer in the ...th squadron of the Service Corps and son of an honourable senior officer living in the 5th *arrondissement* ...

The commissioner discovered a small pot in the bedroom containing opium; on the table a knife on which scraps of the terrible drug were stuck; finally, beside the bed, among the countless 'butts' of Egyptian cigarettes, a vulgar wooden pipe, the bowl of which was still full of opium.

The official enquiry revealed that Jacques V... and Paul B... belonged to a group of young French and American 'revellers' who frequented places of amusement assiduously.

The idea of trying opium had occurred to them – probably in the hope of attaining the 'delights' that this terrible liquid can procure ... just as it also gives death.

How did they procure such a large dose of opium? This remains a mystery. Did Jacques V... find it in a secure place belonging to his father, who has long served in the colonies? Was the opium juice provided by the American, Woynow, or by some Chinaman working in the docks? Was it sold by some quack?

The family of Jacques V... has been informed, with all possible discretion. As for the family of Paul B..., they are away from Nantes.

The military authorities, assigned by the police, have removed the two corpses.

Le Télégramme des Provinces de l'Ouest, Tuesday,
7 January 1919

Concerning a Local Tragedy

Yesterday, we duly reported the terrible events that cost the lives of two young people who were intoxicated with opium. There are surely observations to be made about this dramatic event ,which, sure enough, provides its own lesson. May it be understood by those senseless youths who, when searching for certain unhealthy sensations, thus toy with a drug that stupefies when it does not kill them.

The victims of yesterday's tragedy were brave soldiers who had done their honour in face of the enemy and had been wounded; they cannot have been inveterate smokers, the very circumstances of their death display their lack of experience.

L'EXPRESS DE L'OUEST, Thursday, 9 January 1919

5.6

No.8, October 1919
Guillaume Apollinaire
Trivialities

Translated from
the French
by Ian Monk

Trip to Paris
Oh what a charming hour
To leave a land that's sour
For Paris
Paris the sweet
In one day
Love made it they say
Oh what a charming hour
To leave a land that's sour
For Paris

0 50
Did you take the ten-bit coin
Yes I did

SNUFF
Snuff-man mister snuff-man my pouch is empty
Give me two cents of snuff but the best
The weather's so good that the men of the city
Have gone to dine in their country houses
The olives are ripe and all around we hear
The song of the olive women beneath the olive trees.

The sky is beautiful it is warm and I feel fine
But I am so old that I wonder
If I shall see the firefly season

Snuff man grip your two pence
It's good stuff thank you snuff man

I have fine snuff
In my snuff pouch

I have fine snuff
And none for you

1890
the X

All women aged between forty-five and fifty remember being in
love with Capoul.

MR CAPUS
With many others too.

HOTEL
My bedroom is shaped like a cage
The sun puts its arm though the window
As for me I want to smoke to make a mirage
I light my cigarette with daylight
I don't want to work I want to smoke

ANTWERP
In Antwerp build a tower
The town's tricked a prince arrives
Around you ten times I tower
All your hands adrift
Thin as the neck of a vulture

Houses become lights
Bodies walk without minds
We'll say our prayers for nights
For nothing a loathsome bird finds
Birth sudden three-hundred-year-old whites

Of names my own and the one
With the tang of a woman's bay

Translated from
the French
by Ian Monk

No.8, October 1919
Jules Mary
Arthur Rimbaud as Seen by Jules Mary

*We asked the great popular novelist Jules Mary to evoke the
figure of Arthur Rimbaud for our readers. He has kindly sent us
the following letter:*

4 August
Sir,
I had started writing a few notes of my memories of Arthur

Rimbaud, for I had not forgotten the promise I had made you, but the further I progressed in my work and the more I returned to that period in my youth, the more I realised that I could not speak of Rimbaud as a child or as a young man without my own personality intervening at every turn. Apart from the fact that I hardly enjoy this, it was neither what you nor I desired. So I threw this first draft into the bin.

Furthermore, I cannot make any great contribution to the biographies of my former school friend. I believe that I have already hinted so much to you. What is more, it is far harder than I had thought to bring back to life my naive and impulsive childhood impressions of the pleasant boy who was Rimbaud, whose brown, soft and mischievous eyes I can still picture clearly. It is more difficult than I had thought, when speaking of him, to extricate oneself from the theories, false or exaggerated opinions, the admiration or the denigration that has descended onto his tomb; if he could have heard them, his wicked smile would have lit up. No one was less of a high priest than that likeable and carefree lad and, I think, if members of sacred coteries later tried to intoxicate him with his burgeoning fame, he never lost his head. The flash of mockery that I saw in his eyes was far too indicative of his hidden good sense for him to have been taken in by the enormous flatteries that made a symbol of the wild fantasies of his mind. And I still have a charming and melancholy memory of my little comrade.

I was at the seminary in Charleville, which had shared classes with the middle school, when I met Rimbaud. We became quite close at once, despite our rivalry as gifted pupils. We had the same excessive taste for reading. And this taste necessarily made us seek out books that, in preference, had nothing classical about them. While in the private study room or in the dormitory I was pencilling my first novels, he was writing his first verses. He was a day pupil and, from his home, brought me Lamartine, Musset, Hugo, not to mention Daphnis et Chloë, and a translation of the comedies of Aristophanes, in which we translated in turn, and not without some emotion, the Latin commentary that accompanied the French text. Thus I soon had an overly complete library, which was of course discovered. Then I had to choose between a religious vocation that I had never thought about, and another overweening vocation that was already fermenting, outside of which I have never been able to imagine that anything could exist for me.

At school, thanks to a crystallisation whose causes, even with hindsight, I cannot really explain, this slender lad, with his large eyes, astonished us and, so to speak, passed over our heads. His reputation was being made outside our class and, from a distance, burst back upon us. I am amazed that none of his verses passed between us under our coats so that we learnt them by heart, and yet we knew that he was a poet.

He was a good pupil, docile, not very hard-working, very gentle, with no outbursts of gaiety, and if, from the corner of his eye, he might look delighted at the bad turns that are traditionally inflicted on teachers, this wickedness never came from him. He liked neither noisy games nor the violence of certain pleasures. His life was already contained within the horizon of his reading, his feverish desire to learn and his need to compose. Though three or four years younger than us, he was older than us.

Because of those forbidden books, I had to leave the seminary and saw Rimbaud next only after the war, in Paris. I was miserably poor, as was he. Often neither of us possessed a clean shirt, and Rimbaud had adopted the ingenious solution that consists in having just one shirt. When it can no longer be worn, it is thrown away, but not before another one has been bought or borrowed to replace it. Thus we saved on laundry bills. He explained this system to me one day when I dropped by to see him early in the morning. At the time, he was staying in a huge room, in which the only two pieces of furniture were a table and a bed lost in the depths of a shadowy alcove. It was, I think, on rue de Grands-Degrés, or else rue Saint-Séverin where I was living myself. He was in bed and intending to spend the day there, having nothing better to do and being one of those people who, if they have nothing to eat, try to sleep. In those days, it was said that such poor devils who were starting out led joyous bohemian lives. But if a Bohemian life is gay, the real one, ours, was gloomy.

Despite my destitution, I led a regular life and this made me somewhat amazed because, around me, I could see nothing that was vaguely reminiscent of any work being done, and yet already Rimbaud's name was on the lips of all the students in the Latin Quarter. I could not imagine such a burgeoning renown without the prodigious force of a continuous effort, and I asked him naively:

'Is this where you work?'

'It is. '

'What with?'

He answered with a half-smile and irony in his eyes – that gentle irony that was so familiar.

'Look ... there ... on the table ...'

On the table there was neither a pen nor paper, but a lead inkwell full of a dry, greenish mud. Rimbaud was laughing under his sheets.

I do not know how it was that my wallet contained twenty sous that morning. I took him out to eat in a local restaurant where, for fifty centimes, you 'had the right' to some greasy soup, a portion of gruel and a piece of bread. We did not eat this much every day. He in turn returned this extravagant invitation some time later by giving me, from the barrow of a street merchant on quai Saint-Michel, a bunch of cress, which was our dinner that evening.

And his poems were being recited ...

He was even being attributed others, which were not by him, and which were already pastiches of him ...

I heard:

One evening of pink and mystic yellow
On our way to an antic bordello
The third line, even in Latin, is frankly unquotable and I do not
even know if there was a fourth one ...

His life drifted away from mine. In fact, I did not really want
to know about it. I was obeying a strange feeling, which I have
since analysed, and which was made up of compassion and fear.
Though not having a real friendship, which had not had enough
time to develop, I did feel true affection for him and while his life
remained strange to me, I was not ignorant of some of his habits
against which my character as an uprooted, young, stubborn,
proud and solitary countryman revolted, or rather stood back in
disgust. At the time, Rimbaud frequented by snobbism – the
word had not yet been coined – rather than by any attraction to
vice, a sleazy bar on rue Saint-Jacques absurdly called
L'Académie d'absinthe. Absinthe cost three sous there and this
token price attracted a large clientele of the most varied sort. For
three sous and, if he 'refreshed his glass', for nine or ten sous, the
poor lad had so many drinks before dinner that they pathetically
became his dinner and, even more, gave him both forgetfulness
and over-excitation. I met him on several occasions when he was
on his way out. In his large eyes, a hint of embarrassment and
hesitation trembled, but there was still that gleam of gentle
mockery that seemed to show that, even in such times of trouble,
he did not take himself that seriously, or anyone else ...

Then I learnt that he had left for Belgium and later that he
was in England. He was off on his adventures. I remained in
poverty. I never saw him again.

Years later, he wrote an affectionate letter to Paul Bourde, of
Le Temps, in which he asked after me. He was interested in my
work and my reputation. Unfortunately, his letter was lost after
Bourde's death. In it, Rimbaud gave details of how he lived. He
was then running a trading post in Africa on the confines of the
desert and dealing with the caravanserais. Poetry was so far away!
He made no mention of it. Did he even remember that he had
been a poet? I really think that he did not give a damn!

Such is, dear sir, the simple and lightweight tale of my
relationship with Rimbaud. Do with it what you will.
One more word, to finish.
Whatever happens to these pages, I must thank you for asking
me to write them, and this is why:

I remember an article about Arthur Rimbaud written by a
certain Rodolphe Darzens, the same, I suppose, who after a long
slumber in the dust of oblivion has just awoken to find himself
manager of an avant-garde theatre in Les Batignolles, halfway to
Montmartre that 'nipple of the world'. My name slipped beneath
the pen of this flamboyant colleague of mine and, having let it
drop like dirt, he accompanied it with the following comment:
'We excuse ourselves before the soul of Rimbaud for attaching
such a name to his memory ...' I was not surprised, sir, to learn
that you are not so narrow-minded and I thank you for having

told me 'that your open-mindedness was large enough to allow you to admire both Rimbaud's work and mine, although their senses are utterly opposed'.

What was said of me once by Darzens was both rude and absurd. Your spontaneous, youthful and charming courtesy has made me forget it.

Tear this all up, sir, or publish it – the decision is yours.

I remain your obedient servant,

Jules Mary

5.7

No.9, November 1919
Tristan Tzara
Atrocities of Arthur and Trumpet and Deep-Sea Diver

Translated from the French by Ian Monk

On the lake of hydrogen rolled up on the genitals of sleep the cigarettes cry the little birds run after the rhythm of motors in other words *dei sospiri* undulation.
The set:
lifeboat hanging over the bed
palm-trees
old-hat red settee
wickerwork model with a gramophone platter on its head
Here I die, at the third level like a worthy deep-sea diver, touch the mirror and in principle or in languidness stare at the megaphone's dumb mouth.

Each colleague his joke, and the sum of jokes: literature.

Squinting cylinders with mufflers visit the sea in stacks, at least your gaze great guardian of the antelopes in the garage arranges the thin-tailed concert, piano the Vaseline of the pianoline of fish with simple tuberculosis mechanism.

I love most of all dada's simplicity. Machines' skeletons are dada or superior to those of pythecanthropes. A thought can light up like a dressing and leap like a certain green colour which I composed once with blood of hummingbird, and rubber of straddled bicycles on a telegraph line. Slices of postcard on the splices of a new system of man or song in your face.

Here the interruption of the language of Aa out to lynch to lick to leave and to rip up philosophy, Mississippi, and the vowel eruption of a rose placed on the nape of Napoleon's neck fixed the buttonhole tap of diaphragms, for a few moments, on the well-placed ending of the sentence that will never end.

DADA, 1917 or 1918.

5.8

Translated from
the French
by Ian Monk

No.10, December 1919
A Necessary Act

We have learnt with some emotion that MARINETTI has been arrested, accused of conspiracy against the security of the Italian state and threatened with a sentence of several years' forced labour. Refusing to admit that it is possible to ignore the right to have an opinion, we are taking the initiative of organising a public event where extracts of the poet's work will be interpreted. Those who desire to take part by reading tributes or in any other way are requested to contact us. They will be invited shortly to a preliminary meeting in order to organise the programme of this event. We shall also publish the names of our readers who wish, along with us, to affirm the solidarity that unites intellectuals over and above nationalities and parties. Applications will be received at *Littérature* until 25 December.

Translated from
the French
by Ian Monk

No.10, December 1919
Tristan Tzara
Open Letter to Jacques Rivière

In answer to the article 'Dada Movement' published in the Nouvelle Revue Française *on 1 September 1919, Tristan Tzara has written the following letter to Jacques Rivière, who has refused permission to publish it.*

Today, one no longer writes with one's race, but with one's blood (how banal!). What for other literature was its *characteristic*, is now its *temperament*. It comes down to about the same if one writes a poem in Siamese or dances on a locomotive. It is only natural that the old fail to notice that a new type of man is being created all around them. – With insignificant racial variations, the intensity is, I think, the same everywhere, and if a common character is identified among those who produce literature today, it will be anti-psychology.

There are so many things to say and, firstly, what would Mr Gide think if he read in a review a short story of such tenor: a Gidean school has been created in Berlin? Reassure him, by the way, that R. M. Rilke, who, he writes, is the greatest German poet because he has become Czechoslovak by simple formality, is nothing but a rather stupid, sentimental poet. One can, without being born on Czechoslovak territory, appear more agreeable. The opposition to certain types of German literature is little known in Switzerland: hope in the defeat of the Germanic spirit, slow preparation of the revolution, etc ... in any case, as lacking in intelligence as any owner of a point of view.

During the war, I had quite a straightforward attitude (!), so that I could have friends where I found them without being obliged to report to people who deliver certificates of good conduct that are almost indispensable to the public opinion.

Although I try never to lose the opportunity to compromise myself, I take the liberty to communicate to you (a certain sense of cleanliness has always inspired in me a distaste for journalistic carry-on) that I did, three years ago, suggest as a title for a review the word DADA. This was in Zurich where some friends and I thought we had nothing in common with the Futurists and Cubists. During the campaigns against all forms of dogma, and out of irony regarding the creation of literary schools, DADA became the 'DADA movement'. Under the label of this cloudy assembly, painting exhibitions were organised, I issued a few publications and angered the public in Zurich who attended art shows that claimed to be part of this illusory movement. In DADA 3 manifesto, I declined all responsibility for a school launched by journalists and commonly called 'Dadaism'. It is, after all, merely comic if the maniacs or men who had collaborated in the decomposition of the former Germanic organism have propagated a school that I never intended to found.

If one writes, it is only a refuge from all 'points of view'. I do not write professionally and have no literary ambitions. I would have become an adventurer of great bearing and subtle motions if I had had the physical strength and nervous resistance to achieve this one exploit: not to become bored. One also writes because there are not enough new men, out of habit; one publishes to seek out *men*, and to have an occupation (even that is extremely stupid). There might be a solution: resign oneself; quite simply: do nothing. But to do so requires enormous energy. And one has an almost hygienic need for complications.

5.9

No.12, February 1920
Francis Picabia
Scare Me Daddy

Translated from
the French
by Ian Monk

A man the writing kind of chatter
Cellars of the stomach a sort quite
Desiring one blow a book against freedom in fact
That would distract me from the worst women appease itself
There deny it all genius rework everything from antiquity
In the periods I speak of it was
Ideal five hundred without fear of the new
That is all
Food of tobacco publish or
I have this axiom which must have is and by
In nothing may no
Do not publish the lowness of art not
Virgin there is the man

Together at the same level of tobacco
During the vogue gold
A moment of the relations of Calais
Satisfying find this one it would have been
Liberalism in the public otherwise a mediocrity
In literature and nothing came on the contrary
We have common senses
And the unexpected eulogy
The young girl is pure that is just fine
First and second ones in an exclusivity
Honest man to be

Translated from
the French
by Ian Monk

No.12, February 1920
Philippe Soupault
Hotels

At midnight you will see the windows still open and the doors closed. The music comes out of all the holes where dying germs and capital verses can be seen. But further on, ever on, there are still cries so blue that one dies of emotion. Everything is blue here. The avenues and grand boulevards are deserted. The night is overpopulated with stars and the song of all these people rises towards the sky as the sea goes away in search of the moon, a happiness so heavy and with such little disappointment for the delicate souls of the waves. The beaches are full of those eyes without bodies that one meets near the distant dunes and prairies and red with the blood of flowering herds. Corpses of loved days, circus of the emotions and intoxications that are red, red, but where the heart beats like a fine bell made pale by external suns. The main door lets flow vapours that are orange like the mushrooms we love, the wood is nearby and the plump women are running to and fro gathering the resurrected ephemeral leafs; they are birds of every colour and who can sing better than the wind. Quadrilateral where we suffocate for ever, but on leaving we know that the hunter is there, with all those dogs, all those eyes and no one forgets to show it the damned church that strikes your head like a rock breaks up without a cry.

2ᵉ Année : Nᵒ 13 REVUE MENSUELLE Mai 1920

LITTÉRATURE

VINGT-TROIS MANIFESTES DU MOUVEMENT DADA

PAR

Francis PICABIA, Louis ARAGON, André BRETON,
Tristan TZARA, ARP, Paul ELUARD, Philippe SOUPAULT,
SERNER, Paul DERMÉE, Georges RIBEMONT-DESSAIGNES,
Céline ARNAULT et W. C. ARENSBERG.

13

DEUX FRANCS

5.10

Twenty-Three Manifestos of the Dada Movement

41
Front cover
Littérature, No. 13
May 1920

These manifestos were read:
At the Salon des Indépendants (Grand Palais des Champs Elysées) 5 February 1920.
At the Club du Faubourg, 6, rue de Puteaux 7 February 1920.
At the Université Populaire of Faubourg Saint-Antoine 19 February 1920.
The order in which they are published was drawn by lot.

Dada Manifesto

No more painters, no more writers, no more musicians, no more sculptors, no more religions, no more republicans, no more royalists, no more imperialists, no more anarchists, no more socialists, no more Bolsheviks, no more politicians, no more proletarians, no more democrats, no more bourgeois, no more aristocrats, no more armies, no more police, no more fatherlands, enough of all these imbecilities, no more anything, no more anything, nothing, *nothing, nothing, nothing.*

We hope something new will come from this, being exactly what we no longer want, determinedly less putrid, less selfish, less materialistic, less obtuse, less immensely *grotesque*.

Long live concubines and the con-cubists. All members of the DADA movement are presidents.

ME*

Everything that is not me is incomprehensible.
Whether sought on Pacific sands or gathered in the hinterland of my own existence, the shell that I press to my ear will ring with the same voice and I'll think it the voice of the sea and it will be but the sound of myself.

If I suddenly find it's no longer enough to hold every word in my hand like pretty pearly objects, every word will enable me to listen to the sea, and in the mirror of their sound will I find no image but my own.

However it may seem, language boils down to just this I and whenever I utter a word it divests itself of everything that isn't me until it becomes an organic noise through which my life unfolds.

There is only me in this world and if I sometimes lapse into believing that a woman exists I have but to lean my head on her breast to hear the sound of *my* heart and recognise myself.

Feelings are only languages, enabling certain functions to be performed.

In my left pocket I carry a remarkably accurate self-portrait: a watch in burnished steel. It speaks, marks time and understands none of it.
Everything that is me is incomprehensible.
LOUIS ARAGON

* Deep wells and springs

Tristan Tzara
Take a good look at me!
I'm stupid, I'm a joker, I'm a clown.
Take a good look at me!
I'm ugly, my face is expressionless, I'm short.
I'm just like all of you! (1)

But before you look, ask yourselves this: are you shooting those
arrows of liquid sentiment through the iris or fly shit? Are the
eyes of your belly maybe slices of tumours whose starings will
one day seep out in the form of gonorrhoeal discharge from some
part of your body? You view things with your navel – why are you
trying to protect it from the ridiculous spectacle we're putting on
especially for it? A little bit lower, cunts with teeth, gulping
everything down – the poetry of eternity, love, pure love, of course
– bleeding beefsteaks and oil painting.

All who see and understand readily fall into line between
poetry and love, between beefsteak and painting. They'll be
swallowed up, they'll be swallowed up.

I was recently accused of nicking some furs. Probably
people thought I was still hanging out with poets. With poets who
satisfy their legitimate need for a chilly wank in warm furs: H a h
u I know some other equally purposeless pleasures. Give your
family a ring and piss in the hole reserved for musical,
gastronomic and sacred nonsenses.

DADA proposes 2 solutions:
NO MORE LOOKING
NO MORE SPEAKING (2)
Don't look anymore.
Don't speak anymore.
Because I, chameleon changing infiltration of convenient
attitudes – multicoloured opinions to suit all occasions, size and
price – I always do the opposite of what I suggest to others. (3)
I've forgotten something:
Where? Why? How?
What I mean is:
ventilator of cold examples will serve the cavalcade's fragile snake
and I have never had the pleasure of seeing you 'my dear' rigid
the ear will come out of itself from the envelope like all marine
equipment and products from the firm of Aa and Co chewing gum
for example and dogs have blue eyes, I drink camomile, they
drink the wind, DADA introduces new perspectives, nowadays
people sit at the corners of tables adopting positions which slip a
little to the right and to the left, this is why I am angry with Dada,
people everywhere should demand the suppression of Ds, eat
some Aa, polish yourselves with Aa toothpaste, dress yourselves
in Aa designs. Aa is the handkerchief and sexual organ blowing
its nose, rapid collapse – in rubber – without noise, has no need
for manifestos or address book, gives a 25% discount dress

(1) I wanted to publicise
myself a bit.
(2) No more manifestos
(3) Sometimes

yourselves in Aa designs it has blue eyes.

TRTZ

20-2-1920

Dada Mugs

What's your name? *(He shrugs.)*

Where are you? – The Grand Palais on the Champs Elysées.

What day is it? – Thursday ... February 1920.

What do you do for a living? – I used to plough the fields, I dressed the vines.

And your parents? – My father's a simpleton, without intelligence; my mother too, they're as bad as each other; I had to do everything.

A dozen eggs costs six francs; how much is one egg? – Six francs.

Why are you laughing? – The others are making me laugh.

Do you believe in God and the Holy Virgin? – They always get the job done.

How do you know? – I just know.

Did you sleep well? – My dreams take after taubes[1], after wild boars, about falling down wells, about people chasing me, trying to attack me.

How do you rate yourself? – You're far too good for me. I'm just pining away; I'd like to have some X-rays. I was really intelligent until last month.

What do you yearn for? – I don't know.

ANDRE BRETON

Philosophical Dada

To André Breton

CHAPTER I

DADA has blue eyes, a pale face and curly hair; has the English look of young men who are keen on sport.

DADA has melancholy fingers – the Spanish look.

DADA has a small nose – the Russian look.

DADA has a porcelain arse – the French look.

DADA dreams of Byron and Greece.

DADA dreams of Shakespeare and Charlie Chaplin.

DADA dreams of Nietzsche and Jesus-Christ.

DADA dreams of Barrès and sunsets.

DADA has a brain like a water lily.

DADA has a brain like a brain.

DADA is an artichoke doorknob.

DADA's face is broad and slender and its voice is arched like the sirens' tone.

DADA is a magic lantern.

DADA's tail has been twisted into an eagle's beak.

DADA's philosophy is sad and merry, indulgent and wide.

Venetian crystals, jewels, valves, bibliophiles, voyages, poetic novels, restaurants, mental illnesses, Louis XIII, dilettantism, the last operetta, sparkling star, peasant, a glass of beer downed a little at a time, a new specimen of dew, that's one aspect of DADA!

Uncomplications and uncertainties.
Changeable and highly strung, DADA is a hammock rocking a soothing sway.

CHAPTER II
A star falls upon a river, leaving a trail of replicas. Happiness and misery with a silent voice whisper in our ears.
Black or shining sun.
Here in the bottom of the boat we're oblivious of the course we should choose.

A tunnel and return.
Ecstasy becomes anguish in the idyll of domesticity.
Beds are still paler than the dead, despite man's despairing cries.
DADA embraces in spring water and its kisses must be water meeting fire.
DADA is Tristan Tzara.
DADA is Francis Picabia.
DADA is everything as it equally loves the pure at heart, nightfall, sighing foliage and the entwined lovers drinking with abandon from the divine double wellsprings of Love and Beauty!

CHAPTER III
DADA has always been twenty-two, it's slimmed down a bit in the last twenty-two years. DADA is married to a peasant girl who loves birds.

CHAPTER IV
DADA lives on a peplum cushion surrounded by chrysanthemums wearing Parisian masks.

CHAPTER V
Human emotions appear to it on the banks of optimism, torn to shreds by Baudelaire's antique poetry.

CHAPTER VI
'Oh God I'm turning into an imbecile!' cries DADA.
The wish to fall asleep.
To have a manservant.
An imbecile manservant at the other end of the chamber.
CHAPTER VII
The same manservant opened the door and, as usual, wouldn't let us in. Far off we could make out the voice of Dada.
FRANCIS PICABIA
Martigues, 12 February 1920

Dada Development
Man has great respect for language and the cult of thought; whenever he opens his mouth you see his tongue kept under glass and the reeking mothballs of his brain stink out the air.

    For us *everything* is an opportunity to have fun. Every time we laugh we empty ourselves and the wind possesses us, rattling the doors and windows, driving the night of wind into us.

Wind. The ones who came before us are the artists. The others are devils. Let's take advantage of the devils, let's put ourselves – and the idiot too – where the head and hand should be.

We need entertaining. We're determined to stay exactly as we are or will be. We need a free and empty body, we need a laugh and we need nothing.
PAUL ELUARD

Literature and the Rest

I've been told repeatedly, more than two hundred times (maybe three hundred), that two and two make four. Oh, that's good, or too bad. But that open hand there in front of you, those five fingers exist ... or don't exist. I couldn't care less. Beautiful words trimmed with feathers or little perfumed rockets, sentences constructed with transparent pebbles – none of them worth the two sous I throw in your face.

So who's going to dare sow that absurd plant they call rye-grass or wheat in your brains, brains that are thinner and smaller themselves than willow leaves. They can have a good laugh if they want by gouging out my eyes to see what grows in the manure that serves me for a brain. You'll see nothing there because there is nothing there. You're all as blown up as fattened geese with ideas and principles and as like me as brothers, just go for a walk in the fields and bear it in mind that the burgeoning wheat is a novel by Monsieur René Bazin.[2]

All alone here, in front of these plasterboard walls, I've come to realise that all my friends, be they murderers or men of letters, are every bit as stupid as me. The worst offenders are those who enjoy taking themselves seriously.

Why have you written a manifesto? They shout at me.

I am writing a manifesto because I have nothing to say.

Literature does exist, but in the heart of imbeciles.

It's absurd to divide writers into good and bad ones. On one side there are my friends and on the other, the rest.

When all my contemporaries have understood all these things, it might just become possible to breathe more easily and open your eyes and mouth without risking asphyxiation. I also hope that the people I was just talking about, who hold me in the most delicious disdain, will never understand a thing. That's the blessing I wish on them.

Whether they're howling in the name of morality, tradition or literature, it's always the same howling, the same whinging. Their contemptuous smile is as sweet to me as the fury of their majestic spouses. They can despise me; they'll never work out what I think of myself because my life is running clockwise.

None of this lot here has the guts to express their disgust with as much as a whistle. Well I've got the guts, I could whistle and shout out loud that this manifesto is absolutely stupid and

stuffed full of contradictions, but I'd console myself later with the
thought that so-called 'literature', that dandelion born in the
cretins' diaphragm, is even more stupid.
PHILIPPE SOUPAULT

Dada Patisserie

The table is round, the sky is bright, the spider is tiny, the glass is
transparent, eyes come in ten different colours, Louis Aragon has
the Military Cross, Tzara hasn't got syphilis, elephants are silent,
the rain falls, a car travels more easily than a star, I am thirsty,
draughts are pointless, poets are pin cushions – or pigs, writing
paper is convenient, the stove is drawing well, daggers kill well,
revolvers kill better, the air is still too deep.

We swallow all of this and if we digest it we most certainly
don't give a shit.
PAUL ELUARD

Dada Skating

We read the papers like other mortals. Without wishing to make
anyone unhappy, it is perfectly acceptable to say that the word
DADA lends itself readily to puns. That's even part of the reason
we adopted it in the first place. We haven't the faintest idea how
to treat any subject seriously – least of all this subject: us. So
everything that's written about DADA is doing its best to please
us. We'd swap the whole of art criticism for any news item
whatsoever. Certainly the wartime press never stopped us taking
Marshall Foch for a phoney and President Wilson for a fool.

We ask for nothing better than to be judged on appearances.
It's reported all over the place that I wear glasses. If I told you why
you'd never believe me. It's in remembrance of this grammatical
model: 'Noses were made to wear glasses; also I wear glasses.'
What is it they say? Oh yes, this brings home the fact that we're
not getting any younger.

Pierre is a man. But there is no DADA truth. You've only got to
say a thing for the opposite to become DADA. I once saw Tristan
Tzara in a tobacconist's unable to muster up the voice to ask for a
packet of cigarettes. I don't know what was the matter with him. I
can still hear Philippe Soupault asking an ironmonger most
insistently for some live birds. As for me, it's perfectly possible
that I am dreaming at this very moment.

A white eucharistic host is equal to a red one after all. DADA
makes no promises about getting you to heaven. It would be
ludicrous, in principle, to anticipate a DADA masterpiece in the
fields of literature and painting.   Naturally we have absolutely no
belief in the possibility of social improvement either, even if we do
hate conservatism more than anything and pledge our full
support for any revolution whatsoever. 'Peace at any price' was
DADA's slogan during the war just as 'War at any price' is DADA's
slogan in times of peace.

Contrariness remains nothing more than the most flattering
form of posturing.   I'm not aware of a hint of ambition in myself:

yet it seems to you that I'm getting all worked up: why doesn't the idea that my right side is the shadow of my left and vice versa render me utterly incapable of movement?

We pass for poets in the most general sense of the word because we target the worst conventions in language. You can be terribly familiar with the word hello' and still say 'goodbye' to the woman you've just met up with again after being away for a year.

DADA attacks you through your own powers of reasoning. If we reduce you to a point where you maintain you're better off believing than not believing what all the religions of beauty, love, truth and justice teach, then we'll know you're not afraid of putting yourselves at the mercy of DADA, by agreeing to meet us on our chosen territory ... which is doubt.

ANDRE BRETON

The Pleasures of Dada

Dada has pleasures just like everyone else. Dada's principle pleasure is to see itself in others. Dada provokes laughter, curiosity or fury. Since these are three most agreeable things, Dada is very happy.

What makes Dada all the happier is if people laugh at it spontaneously. Since Art and Artists are extremely serious inventions, especially when their roots are in comedy, people go to comedies at the theatre when they wish to laugh. Not us. We don't take anything seriously. People do laugh but only to mock us. Dada is very happy.

Curiosity is awoken too. Serious-minded men, who know, deep down, how miracles are arranged – miracles such as Père la Colique[3] or the Virgin's tears – realise that it would be much more fun to have fun with us. They have no wish to bring about the collapse of the great cathedral of Art, but look how they rub up against us trying to get our recipe. Dada doesn't have any recipes but is always hungry. Dada is very happy.

And now for fury, adorable fury. This is the way great love affairs start. Concerns for the future? Only about being loved too much. Certainly there would always be the option of swapping roles, taking it in turns to laugh, yearn or fly into a fury. But expecting some sort of benefit to arise. The gorgeous gob of somebody vomiting insults is wide open and Dada is a very good at *basse-boule*.[4] Dada is very happy.

Dada also likes tossing stones into the water, not to see what happens but to stupidly contemplate the ripples. Anglers don't like Dada.

Dada likes ringing on doorbells, striking matches and setting light to hair and beards. It puts mustard in chalices, urine in fonts and margarine in artists' tubes of paint.

It knows you and knows the ones who lead you. It likes you and doesn't like them. You can be fun. You probably enjoy life. But you've got some bad habits. You're too fond of what you've been taught to be fond of. Cemeteries, melancholy, the tragic lover, Venetian gondolas. You shout at the moon. You believe in art and respect Artists.

You could easily become friends of Dada – it would be enough to demolish all your little card castles and redeem every iota of your freedom. Mistrust your leaders. They exploit your ill-considered affection for the fake and the famous to lead you by the nose and make things even better for themselves.

You cling to your chains as if you want to be used with impunity like bears in a sideshow – do you? They flatter you and call you Wild Bears. Carpathian bears. They talk of freedom and magnificent mountains. But that's just to rake in the bourgeois spectators' wads of cash. You dance for an old carrot and a whiff of honey. If you weren't so cowardly, sinking under the weight of all those lofty thoughts and non-existent abstractions you've been forced into, all that nonsense dressed up as dogma, you'd stand up straight and play the massacre game, just like we do. But you're too scared of no longer believing and of bobbing about like corks on the surface of a two-gallon barrel with nothing but the memory of fizzy lemonade. You don't understand that one can be attached to nothing and be happy.

If you ever manage to pull yourself together Dada will clack its jaws as a sign of friendship. But if you rid yourselves of lice only to keep your fleas Dada will bring its little insecticide spray into play.

Dada is very happy.

GEORGES RIBEMONT-DESSAIGNES

Manifesto of the Crocrodarium Dada [Hans Arp]

Statue lamps come up from the bottom of the sea and shout long live DADA to greet the passing liners and dada presidents feminine dada masculine dada plural dada definite dada indefinite dada and three rabbits in Chinese ink by arp the dadaist in ridged bicycle porcelain we leave for London in the royal aquarium ask in every pharmacy for rasputin's and the tzar's and the pope's dadaists which are only valid for two and a half hours.

ARP

ART

Essentially what's behind the word BEAUTY is unthinking, visual convention. Life bears no relation to what grammarians call *beauty*. Virtue like patriotism only exists for those mediocre intellects with a lifelong devotion to the sarcophagus. This tide of men and women who believe in *Art* as if it were a religion with *God* at its heart must be stemmed. We don't believe in *God* any more than we do in *Art* – nor his priests, bishops and cardinals.

Art is, and can only ever be, the expression of our contemporary life. *Beauty*, the institution, is exactly like the *Musée Grevin*[5] and bounces easily off the *soul* of shopkeepers and *Art* experts, caretakers of the museum church of the past's crystallisations.

Tralala Tralala

Count us out.

We're not feeding ourselves at a mass for memories and

magic tricks by Robert Houdin.[6]

Let's face it, you don't understand what we're doing. And to tell the truth, my friends, we understand it even less – delightful, huh? You're quite right. But do you really believe that *God* knew English and French???   ???

You explain *Life* to him in those two beautiful languages Tralala Tralala Tralala Tralala Tralala Tralala.

So have a good look with your sense of smell, forget the fireworks of Beauty[7] at 100,000, 200, 000 or 199,000,000 dollars.

Anyway I've had enough, those who don't understand will never understand and those who understand when they have to understand certainly don't need me.

FRANCIS PICABIA

Dada God-swatter

The most ancient and formidable enemy of Dada is called GOD!

He intervenes between us and all things and gets in the way.

His cheating eyes show up when we're staring into our glass.

He screws our mistresses and sticks himself in between their skin and ours.

He roosts on the shoulders of victorious generals, old folks crowned with the downfalls of best-selling artists. From way on high he draws adoring gazes to himself.

He's the forger, the speculator, the deceiver, the great bully and the supreme stuffer of brains.

He poisons life for a bunch of imbeciles. God's a fool, God's got goitre, God struts about like a dandy, God dresses to the left. How many poets, painters, musicians – the most ignorant of all people – pull on a God every morning like a condom, and thus disguised extend a great green belly for the worship of the masses!

Well we're going to shout about it: ENOUGH of all these annoying stinking gods festering like a disgusting verminous pea pod.

Let's QUICKLY carry out some corrosive fumigations to purify the atmosphere and scour the house with lashings of alcohol.

Cover EVERYTHING in Dada bug powder! No nonsense hygiene!

Dada God-swatter

Dada omni-swatter

Dada anti-taboo!

PAUL DERMEE

The Corridor

1st: Just as the first name Apollonie,[8] from which the Pantheon appears exactly as it does from the rue Soufflot, is less attractive than a dogcart it's completely pointless to imagine that the most stupid amongst us is really less stupid than he appears, and therefore even more stupid. When we've finished praising certain particularly seedy gentlemen to the skies on the pretext that they always behave exactly as they should – that is to say, idiotically – maybe it'll be time for a little fun, if we join the ranks of those who dismiss "*Aloïse ou l'Amour perverti*" (published by Albin Michel) as tedious without even bothering to open the thing. Who has ever really taken on board the fact that whatever precautions you take they will never be enough? Not daring to sit back down, due to the flatulence caused by reading until utterly worn out by hystero-mania and for fear of producing a ridiculous effect, is no reason to regret ever having stood up. It seems that by the end of the third year some trainers themselves become wild. The inhabitants of central Europe have no idea how lucky they are to find simple conversations a uniquely dangerous experience. Furthermore, is it really so consoling to tell yourself, as you stroke your highly polished shoes, that this earth is home to some truly useless men? No, in spite of everything. For sometimes their eyes are quite moist with pleasure. They live, like the others, between a butter-soft eroticism and mental chaos that compels even the brightest demon to sometimes confess her embarrassment. (And that is their greatest crime!) A misfortune makes you so cheerful that you submit to any influence that comes your way only to reject it again shortly afterwards until you get to the last one and that one is living in the hope of not being one and is to be rejected no more. Nonetheless Napoleon, on being given his Egyptian proclamation to read over again, came out with the words: 'This is a bit boastful!' and perhaps we shouldn't assume that he was trying to be witty. (These are the words of an excellent man). You will only ever gain a clearer perspective when you manage to enter into a dialogue with your own prostate. Probably. By then the only truly dignified position a man can adopt is to remain lying down like an effigy, but always on the most hilarious part of the body, thus producing an outrageous effect on the sky.

2nd: People are still not sufficiently resigned to *everything*. That's what they should teach you at primary school and it's just what you want to hear endlessly repeated behind your back when you're ill.

3rd: But everybody abandons their principles for as little as someone else's apparently foolish behaviour, and it's just as true that the good Lord is nothing more than an unremarkable doctor and that people hardly love anything anymore, for they have ceased to love themselves. The final joy is no less for it. That joy has to be seen clasped between belly folds when you've managed to retrieve all the falsities that objectively escape from your brain in daytime. Obviously this is not what one would use to extract the gasses from a corpse if one manages to extract them from Maurice Barrès who still passes for being alive.
Dr VAL SERNER[9]

Dada is american
Cubism was born in Spain; France appropriated the patent for it with no government guarantee. Unfortunately, just like French matches, Cubism didn't catch on; not enough phosphorous on

the surfaces of the box. Mr Rosenberg[10] is in the process of making an enormous box but the matches he's got hidden in there are soaking wet, floating about on mouldy liquid.

Cubism was Spanish, it became Alsatian, it dances on the official red carpets of a few Parisian and commercial galleries.

Unthinkable that Cubism would burst out with a 'Long live DADA'; it's a consumptive on a chaise longue; all youth has fled from its malicious eyes; it's like that old lady, Roch Grey, who hates children and speaks with enormous contempt of the kindergarten.

I felt I should talk a little about Cubism, being one of those who expected a great deal from this geometric word; I am compelled to confess my disappointment and, at the same time, my joy in observing DADA, the global expression of all that is young, lively and athletic; no religion leaking from a cathedral appendicitis for Dada.

DADA is american, DADA is russian, DADA is spanish, DADA is swiss, DADA is german, DADA is french, belgian, norwegian, swedish, monégasque. Anyone who lives without a system, who finds nothing to like about museums but the parquet floors, is DADA; museum walls are Père Lachaise or Père la Colique,[11] they will never be Père Dada. The life expectancy of real Dada works should be just 6 hours.

I, Walter Conrad Arensberg, american poet, hereby declare that I am against Dada, seeing that this is the only way I'm going to get involved in dada, in dada, in dada, in dada, in dada.

Hurrah, hurrah,hurrah. Long live Dada.

WALTER CONRAD ARENSBERG
New York 33 West 67th Street

The Manifesto of Mr Antipyrine

DADA is our intensity: it holds up inconsequential bayonets the German baby's Sumatral head: Dada is life without slippers or parallel; it is for and against unity and decidedly against the future; we wisely recognise that our brains will become cosy cushions, that our anti-dogmatism is as exclusivist as a civil servant and that we are not free and cry freedom harsh necessity without discipline or morality and spit on humanity.

DADA remains in the European framework of weaknesses, it's still shit, but from now on we want to shit in different colours to decorate the art zoo of all consular flags.

We direct circuses and whistle among the winds of fairs, among convents, prostitutes, theatres, realities, feelings, restaurants. Hohi, hoho, bang, bang.

The author president was ill and mislaid his manifesto. We are reproducing an extract from 'The First Celestial Adventure of Mr Antipyrine' (Zurich, 1916, Dada Collection, out of print), the manifesto read at the first Dada evening in Zurich, 14 July 1916 at the Waag Hall.

We declare the car to be a feeling that quite pampered us in the slownesses of its abstractions and transatlantic liners and noises and ideas. We exteriorise the faculty, however, we are looking for the central essence and we are happy being able to hide it; we don't want to count the marvellous elite's many windows because Dada exists for nobody and we want the whole world to understand this, because it is the balcony of Dada, I assure you. From where you can hear military marches and descend slicing the air like a seraphim to the public baths to have a piss and understand the parable.

Dada is neither madness, nor wisdom, nor irony, take a look, dear bourgeois.

Art was a game of conkers, children strung together words with chimes at the end, then they started crying and shouted out the stanza and put dolly's booties on it and the stanza became queen to do a little expiration and the queen became a whale without an explanation, the children ran and ran with restricted respiration.

Then the great ambassadors of feeling came along and shouted historically in chorus:

Psychology psychology hihi
Science Science Science
Long live France
We are not naive
We are consecutive
We are exclusive
We are not simple
and are perfectly capable of debating intelligence.

But we, DADA, we are not of their opinion, as art isn't serious, I assure you, and if we exhibit crime in order to say vegetation learnedly, it is in order to give you pleasure, dear listeners, I love you so, I love you so, I assure you and adore you.

TRISTAN TZARA

Dada Geography

Historical anecdotes are not enormously important. It's impossible to determine when and where DADA came into being. The name itself, all the better for being perfectly ambiguous, was just something one of us came up with.

Cubism was a school of painting, Futurism a political movement: DADA is a state of mind. To compare them is patently either ignorant or pretentious.

Free thinking in religious matters is nothing like a church. DADA is free thinking in artistic terms.

As long as prayers are forcibly recited in schools under the guise of museum visits and textual analysis, we will rail against despotism and seek to disrupt the ceremony.

DADA devotes itself to nothing, neither love nor work. It is unthinkable that a man should leave any trace of his existence on this earth.

DADA, acknowledging only instinct, condemns explanation in principle. According to Dada we should exercise no control over ourselves. Have done with those dogmas, morality and taste: have done with them for ever.

ANDRE BRETON

To the Public

Before I come down there among you to tear out your rotten teeth, your scab-filled ears, your canker-covered tongue.

Before shattering your putrid bones —
  Slitting open your diarrhoea-filled abdomen and removing from
it your over-fattened liver, your ignoble spleen and your diabetic
kidneys to be used as fertiliser on the fields —
     Before I rip off your ugly, incontinent and cheesy little dick —
     Before I thus extinguish your appetite for beauty, orgasms,
sugar, philosophy, pepper and metaphysical mathematical and
poetical cucumbers —
     Before disinfecting you with vitriol and thus making you clean
and passionately buffing you up —
  Before all of that —
     We're going to have an great big bath in antiseptic —
     And we're warning you —
     It's us who are the murderers —
     Of all your little newborn babes —
     And to end here's a song
     Ki Ki Ki Ki Ki Ki Ki
     And here's God with a nightingale for a horse
     He's handsome, he's ugly —
     Madam, your gob stinks of pimp's come.
     In the morning —
     'Cos in the evening it's more like the arse of an angel in love
with a lily.
     Nice, huh?
     Cheerio, mate.
GEORGES RIBEMONT-DESSAIGNES

DADA PARASOL
So you don't like my manifesto?
     You've come here bursting with hostility and you're going to
start whistling at me before you've even heard me out?
     Great! Carry on, the wheel turns as it's turned since Adam,
nothing changes, except now we've only got two legs instead of
four.
     But you're really making me laugh and I wish to repay you for
your lovely welcome by talking to you about Aaart, poetry, etc. etc.
hippicackuanna.
      Have you ever seen a telegraph pole having a tough time
trying to grow beside roads between nettles and blown tyres?
     But as soon as it's grown a bit taller than its neighbours it
grows so fast that you could never stop it ... never!
     Then it opens out right up there in the sky, lights up, swells
out, is a parasol, a taxi, an encyclopaedia or a toothpick.
     So are you happy now? OK... that's it ... that's all I wanted to
say to you.   That's poetreee for you ... honest!
     Poetry = toothpick, encyclopaedia, taxi or parasol-shade, and
if you're not satisfied ...
TO THE NESLE TOWER WITH YOU[12]
CELINE ARNAULD[13]

Dada typewriter
Ever since we were born some lazy gits have been trying to

convince us that there's such a thing as art. Well we're even lazier and today we're going to say it loud and clear: 'Art is nothing.'

There is nothing. Once our contemporaries get around to accepting what we say they'll quickly forget that huge farce called art.

Why be stubborn?
There is nothing:
There never was anything.

You can shout all you like and chuck whatever you can lay your hands on at us, you know perfectly well that we're right.

Who's going to tell me what Art is?

Who dares claim they know what Beauty's about?
For my listeners' convenience I offer you this definition of Art, Beauty and the rest:
Art and Beauty = NOTHING.
And now, of course, you're going to start yelling or laughing again. Listen to me.
Once upon a time, some years ago, there was a bloke called Jesus Christ who cured blind and deaf people. Nobody took any notice of him. The doctors got worried and had a meeting. Then some of them went to see the Minister of Health and the bloke called Jesus Christ got awarded a big prize for services to education.
It's the same thing with me ... I want to open your eyes and all you do is laugh.
You'll never be serious.
PHILIPPE SOUPAULT

Five ways to Dada shortage or two words of explanation
Tear up a bit of paper, preferably pages 35–6 of poetry RON RON, set light to it,

all DADA books are well printed, this must be done according to DADA methods, which once existed.

The road paved with gas jets, sliding corridors providing DADA

DADA, at the last minute, a long time ago for others, has neither providers nor methods

but a heck of a lot of noise is made about it since grammars, dictionaries and manifestos are still necessary.
MORAL:
We see everything, we love nothing,
We are indifferent
In – di – ffe – rent
We're dead but we're not rotting because we never have the same heart in our breast, nor the same brain in our head.

And we suck in everything around us, around us, we do NOTHING, Dada satisfaction.
PAUL ELUARD

Sensational revelations
As slowly as I open their lids, my eyes can only bear one single

light more gentle on them than your anger is to my heart: doubts feebly fizzle out when they come up against friendship. Friendship leads me to the edge of the world, it abandons me and I wait.

Today you find me abominably sad. All that my heart can produce is a damp squib. You won't like that image. I'm already beginning to bore you. I'm not even going to swear at you. Who knows where weariness starts, who knows where it ends? I'm looking at you and you're looking at me. What insignificant misdemeanour are you going to find to throw at me pretending it's a blessed olive branch? I'm not trying to force you to be silent, nor make you start shouting. All I am aware of nowadays is this great emptiness inside caused by those who are my friends as drops of water in a river are friends of the drop they sweep with them to the sea. If you want to vouch for someone you say: I'm as sure of him as I am of myself. And yet if there's one man on this earth I cannot be psychologically sure of, it's me. I don't take any notice of the rules I set for myself; and this perpetual inconsistency enables others to recognise me and call me by my name; I can't see myself in profile. I'm always betraying myself, letting myself down, contradicting myself. I'm not someone I'd ever put my trust in. No need to despair on that score. But as you know, just one look from my friends is enough to wreck all my plans – that's why we're friends. I give everything up just to waste my time with them, I even drop myself. I suppose you think I bestow on them the trust I refuse myself? Wake up! I know all about their shortcomings, thousands of things about them shock me. They do things I'd never do for all the gold in the world.

I know they have no great affection for me. It's a long time since we stopped carrying those little scales around with us that weigh up a person's worth. I don't believe in my friends just as I don't believe in myself.

I have put myself at the mercy of these people I call friends for the most idiotic – yet strongly heartfelt – reasons. It's a torrent sweeping me along and I acknowledge it as my master and flatter it with my voice.

You lot, immobilised in this room like a stagnant pool of mud, don't ask me what route I'm going to take out of this world, nor what makes me bow to a foreign power. The man whose body is caught up in a spiral from here on in is speaking to you serenely: don't listen to the words he is forming, just hear the monotonous song of his lips.

Today you find me abominably sad.

LOUIS ARAGON

Manifesto of Monsieur Aa the antiphilosopher

Without looking for I adore you
who's a French boxer
irregular maritime values like Dada's depression in the blood
of the two-headed one
I slide undecided between death and phosphates

which scratch the communal brain of dadaist poets for a bit
happily
for
now
aspect
tariffs and high living costs made me decide to give up Ds
it's not true that Dada falsehoods tore them off me since
repayment will start from
here's a reason to cry the nothing that's called nothing
and I swept the illness through customs
me the armour and umbrella of the brain from midday to two
hours of subscription
superstitious releasing wheels
of the spermatozoid ballet that you will find at dress rehearsal in
the hearts of all suspect individuals
I'm going to nibble your fingers for a bit
I'll pay for your resubscription to love on film that screeches like
metal doors
and you are all idiots
I'll come back some time as your urine
reborn into life's delights the midwife wind
and I'm setting up a boarding school for poets' pimps
and I'll come back again some time just to start all over again
    and you are all complete idiots
    and the selfcleptomaniac's key only turns with the aid of dim
revolutionary oil
    on the node of every machine is the nose of a newborn
    and we are all complete idiots
    and very suspicious of a new form of intelligence and a new
logic in our usual way
    which is certainly not Dada
    and you allow yourselves to be swept along by A-ism
    and you are all complete idiots
poultices
made with the alcohol of purified sleep
bandages
and virgin
idiots
TRISTAN TZARA

5.11

No.15, July/August 1920
Paul Eluard
Examples

Translated from
the French
by Ian Monk

SLEEPER
THE SHADOW OF THE HEART TOWARDS MORNING,
IN HASTE,
AT REST.

IN ITS SLEEP NOTHING ENVELOPS
THIS HEART MORE SWOLLEN THAN THE WINDOWS.

SHADOW, NIGHT AND SLEEP.
A HEART SHAKES OFF
ALL THAT IT DOES NOT KNOW.

WHEELS
WHEELS OF ROUTES
WHEELS THREAD TO THREAD NIMBLE
WORN.

CANTICLE
THE CHILD LOOKS AT THE NIGHT FROM ON HIGH
(DO NOT BELIEVE IN AEROPLANES, IN BIRDS,
HE IS MORE HIGH).
IF THE CHILD DIES, NIGHT TAKES ITS PLACE.

FOUR KIDS
THE BARE GOURMAND,
PUFFING UP HIS CHEEKS,
SWALLOWING A FLOWER,
SWEET-SMELLING INNER SKIN,
GOOD BOY,
WHISTLE;
MOUTH OBVIOUSLY PINK,
MOUTH LIGHT UNDER THE HEAVY HEAD,
ONE TO TEN, TEN TO ONE.
THE ORPHAN,
THE BREAST THAT FED HIM COVERED WITH BLACK,
WILL NOT WASH IT.
DIRTY
AS A FOREST ONE WINTER'S NIGHT.
DEAD,
HIS BEAUTIFUL TEETH, BUT HIS BEAUTIFUL MOTIONLESS
EYE,
STARING!
WHAT FLY OF HIS LIFE
IS THE MOTHER OF THE FLIES OF HIS DEATH?

OTHER KIDS
CONFIDENCE:
'LITTLE CHILD OF MY FIVE SENSES
AND OF MY SWEETNESS.'
LET US ROCK OUR LOVES
WE WILL HAVE GOOD CHILDREN.
IN GOOD COMPANY
WE SHALL FEAR NOTHING ON EARTH ANY MORE,
GOOD FORTUNE, HAPPINESS, PRUDENCE,
LOVES
AND THAT LEAP FROM AGE TO AGE,

FROM BEING A CHILD TO BEING AN OLD MAN,
WILL NOT REDUCE US
(CONFIDENCE).

THE ART OF DANCING
BLUE WINDOWS, GRASS, THE RAIN, DANCER
SHE IMITATES THE DANCERS IN HER DANCE,
IMAGES CUT UP SEVERAL TIMES.
THE STRETCHED RUBBER, THE OPEN UMBRELLA,
WET FEET, FRIZZY HAIR,
SHE IS EVERYWHERE,
SHE TRAVELS TO TRAVEL NO MORE,
SHE DANCES ALL AROUND,
IN THE HANDS OF THE BLIND MAN,
IN THE NEST OF MIRRORS,

HEART-TO-HEART

AND IN THE LAND OF THE DANCE,
MAGIC-MAGIC-MAGIC.

SEDUCTION
THE HEART IS AN IMAGE,
THE HEART IS A MEANS.

' ... WITH A DISTINGUISHED AIR.'

AND LET US RESUME:
CHARMING GIRL,
YOUR FINGERS STARING,
YOU WAITED.

THE KISS WAS PLACED THERE,
A GOOD KISS SATISFIES,
FROM HIGH ANTIQUITY
MIXTURE OF SERPENTS.

' ... WITH A DISTINGUISHED AIR.'
THEN GOES.

THE ART OF DANCING
THE FRAGILE RAIN, KEEPS THE TILES
IN BALANCE. SHE, THE DANCER,
WILL NEVER SUCCEED
IN FALLING, IN LEAPING
LIKE THE RAIN.

WORKER
SEE THE PLANKS IN THE TREES,
THE PATHWAYS IN THE MOUNTAINS,
AT A FINE AGE, THE AGE OF STRENGTH,

WEAVE IRON AND KNEAD STONE,
EMBELLISH NATURE,
NATURE WITHOUT ITS FINERY,
WORKING.

SEDUCING
THE ADORATION OF GAZES
SEDUCES THE EYES THAT HARDLY SEE WHAT THEY SEE.
BLUSHING,
THE EYES WILL DELIGHT ON HER CHEEKS
AND MAY THEY DO SO FOR EVER.

HE WHO SEES HER A VIRGIN AND KNOWS HER A VIRGIN,
A VIRGIN IN SATIN,
ALSO KNOWS, BENEATH HER CROWNED EYELIDS,
A VIGIL JOY.

FOR SHAME, ALWAYS BE ASHAMED,
NO,
BUT OPEN A HOUSE
AND SHOW YOUR FINE FACE,
THIS IS THE ONE.

NAME DAYS
THE WALTZ IS PRETTY,
GREAT SURGES OF THE HEART ARE TOO.
STREETS,
A WHEEL WALTZING FRANTICALLY.
WHEELS, DRESSES, HATS, ROSES.
WATERED,
THE PLANT WILL BE READY FOR THE NAME DAY TO BE
CELEBRATED.

THE HEART
THE HEART HAS WHAT SHE SINGS,
SHE MAKES THE SNOW MELT,
WET NURSE OF THE BIRDS.

Translated from
the French
by Ian Monk

No.15, July/August 1920
Chronicle

TO MAKE A DADAIST POEM:
Take a newspaper.
Take a pair of scissors.
Choose an article in the newspaper of the length you wish to give
to your poem.
Cut out the article.
Then cut out carefully all of the words that make up the article

and put them in a bag.
Shake gently.
Then remove each cutting one after the other in the order in which they emerge from the bag.
Copy conscientiously.
The poem will be like you.
You have now become 'an infinitely original writer with a charming sensitivity, although still misunderstood by the common people'.
AA THE ANTIPHILOSOSPHER AND TRISTAN TZARA

5.12

No.16, September/October 1920
Tristan Tzara
When the dogs cross the air in the diamond like ideas and the appendix of the brain displays the time of the programmed alarm

Translated from
the French
by Ian Monk

to francis picabia tamer of the
ashen roulette
to marcel duchamp another drop
of chance on the combination of the disappraisal

prices they have yesterday agreeing then pictures
appreciate the dream era of eyes
pompously that recite the gospel type darkening
group the apotheosis imagine says he fate to be able to colours
cut hangers astounded the reality an enchantment
spectator all in effort from the this is no longer 10 to 12
during raving turnabout go down pressure
make of madmen for waiting in line fleshes on a monstrous
    crushing stage
celebrate but their 160 adepts in not to the placing in my pearly
sumptuous of earth bananas supported being lit up
joy ask reunited almost
from have the one as much as the invoking visions
of the sing this one laughs
leaves situation disappears describes this 25 dance hello
dissimulated the all of this is not was
magnificent the ascension has the band better
light of which sumptuousness stage me music hall
reappears following instant before bustle about living
business that there is lent
way words come these people

5.13

No.17, December 1920
Minutes

Translated from
the French
by Ian Monk

The contributors and directors of *LITTÉRATURE*, concerned
about the good spirits of this review, and considering that recent
issues might have displayed intentions that are not theirs (in
particular doubtful that verbal experiments have ever interested
them), and desiring to state that the publication of
LITTÉRATURE has nothing in common with those varied 'avant-
garde artistico-literary' enterprises, met on 19 October at Le
Restaurant Blanc, rue Favart.

Those present: Messieurs Aragon, Breton, Drieu la
Rochelle, Eluard, Hilsum,[1] Rigaut.

Messieurs Fraenkel and Soupault being absent, they had
given their right of vote to Messieurs Eluard and Breton
respectively.

The question of frequency was dealt with first. It was decided
unanimously:

1st That the review *LITTÉRATURE* will appear on the 1st of every
month, manuscripts being submitted to the printer on the 1st of
the previous month;

2nd that, by commercial necessity, the direction will assure that a
literary celebrity or other, and one only, will contribute to each
issue.

3rd A series of questions then arose:

a. – Are we going to continue talking for long about living and
dead artists?

No, unanimously minus one vote (Aragon abstaining). In
consequence, any reference to a literary event in a text will lead to
the rejection of this text.

b. – Does poetry still have a place in *LITTÉRATURE?*

No, by 6 votes against 2 (Eluard, Fraenkel).

c. – Will one be allowed to give one's opinion about anything?

Yes, by 6 votes against 2 (Drieu, Eluard).

d. – Will criticism be one of its aims?

No, unanimously.

e. – Will we accept to write: 1. *for* ... and *for* ... only?

No, unanimously minus one vote (Drieu).

2. *because* ... and *because* ... only?

No, unanimously.

3. to write both *for* ... and *because* ... ?

Yes, by 6 votes against 2 (Eluard, Fraenkel who claimed he wrote
neither *for* ... nor *because* ...).

f. – Do we claim to write: 1. as we want?

No, by 6 votes against 2 (Eluard, Fraenkel).

2. as we speak?

Yes, unanimously.

g. – Can language be an objective?

No, unanimously minus one vote (Eluard).

h. – After a long discussion during which we failed to agree on the questions to be phrased, the particular examination of the branches of philosophy having been rejected (despite the reservations of Aragon, Breton and Rigaut), it was decided by 5 votes against 3 (Aragon, Drieu and Rigaut) that no text of a strictly philosophical nature would be accepted for *LITTÉRATURE*.

i. – Will we also exclude: 1. political speculations?

No, by 5 votes against 3 (Drieu, Eluard, Soupault).

2. sexual questions?

No, unanimously.

j. – Can everyone, without distinction of talent, profession, age, intelligence, morality, etc., contribute to *LITTÉRATURE?*

Yes, by 4 votes against 2 (Drieu, Fraenkel) and 2 abstentions (Aragon, Rigaut).

4th Unanimously, the contributors there present decided to meet once a month to draw up the contents of the issue in preparation. During these meetings, the manuscripts received by the direction will be submitted for approval by the new jury thus constituted.

(It has no illusions about the interest of its deliberations. None of its members accepts the principle of a reading panel or, of course, of voting, but it has an experiment in mind.)

Approved:

LOUIS ARAGON, ANDRE BRETON, PIERRE DRIEU LA ROCHELLE, PAUL ELUARD, THEODORE FRAENKEL, RENE HILSUM, JACQUES RIGAUT, PHILIPPE SOUPAULT.

Translated from the French by Ian Monk

No.17, December 1920
Germain Dubourg[1]
Projected Habitation Reform

I. – THE HABITATION. *House.* 1. Houses in heaven and earth. Sentimental decoration. – 2. Expression of the façade; meaning of patios. – 3. Exterior of a house, that is to say its feathers. – 4. Plan of habitations, a mirror to recognise oneself. – 5. Bolts, professional discretion. *The furnishings:* 6. Living chairs, tapestry caresses, beds of cage birds. – 7. Various sorts of seat, with blooded upholstery. – 8. Chairs with animal legs. – 9. Negress chairs. –10. Armchairs. – 11. Boxer armchairs. – 12. Canvas and water stools. – 13. Deaf-and-dumb beds. – 14. Beds of sleep with humbug dreams. – *The tables.*15. Their shape, ornamentation, materials, size. – 16. Moral tables. – 17. Cinema tables with suggestive views. – 18. Luminous tables for love. *Gardens:* 19. General description. – 20. Ornamental ponds. – 21. Human trees touching the walkers. – 22. Box trees of steel wire. – 23. Caustic plants. – 24. Electrifying plants. – 25. Talking plants. – 26. Sprung benches. – 27. Horse summerhouses.

II. – THE PARTS OF THE HABITATION. *The hall:* 1. Bathtub entrances. – 2. Razorblade doors. – 3. Logical hinges. – 4. Inner doors admitting only women. – 5. Inner doors admitting only the pure of heart. – 6. Illuminating bells. – 7. The corridors (all models, from the ambush corridor to the kissing corridor, including the swing, skip, race, fall, storm, punch, wound, shower, fire, forest, kazoo, horn, nosebleed etc.) – 8. The concierge mounted on wheels, saloon style, automatic ignition. – 9. Ditto, without sparkplugs. – 10. Guard dog, 4.50 m [14 1/2 feet] long by 0.30 m [1 foot] wide, in tempered steel, with saw teeth, able if need be to keep the household accounts. *The lounges:* 11. Drinking lounge. – 12. Laughing lounge. – 13. Nodding lounge. – 14. Cruelty lounge. – 15. Friends, receptions, outfits to scare. – 16. Paintings that scratch their heads while thinking of something else. *The private apartments:* 17. Bedrooms for deaths. – 18. Bedrooms for births. – 19. Bedrooms for desires. – 20. The bathrooms (blatant-boiler, crying machine, hot nationality tap, lung-brush, brown-study plunger, heart file). *Servants' quarters:* 21. Rooms in the chimneys. – 22. Rooms in the candelabras. – 23. Stairs leading directly to the beds of young and attractive maids. *The layout of rooms:* 24. Fixed plan. – 25. Variable according to mood. – 26. Plan in continual motion.

III. – HEATING AND LIGHTING. *The stoves:* 1. Mobile stoves as happy as larks. – 2. Staring rings. – 3. Bain-marie for silence. – 4. Instructions for Silili-Labère stoves. *The lamps:* 5. Black lamps. – 6. Their use. – 7. Shape-changing candelabras. – 8. Elastic light bulbs. – 9. Endless footlights. – 10. Capricious fittings. – 11. Headlamps on castors for the aged. – 12. Projectors for the short-sighted. *Heating appliances:* 13. Reptile briquettes. – 14. Radiators answering when called. – 15. Summer vents. – 16. Winter vents. – 17. Autumn vents. – 18. Happiness vents.

IV. – THE MUSICAL INSTRUMENTS. *String instruments:* 1. Looms. – 2. Gallows. – 3. Hanged man. – 4. Hairs. – 5. Guitar. – 6. Cobwebs. *Wind instruments:* 7. Trees. – 8. Disdain. – 9. The blast of the blaze in the faces of the firemen. – 10. The rumblabone. – 11. The pooh-pooh. – 12. Instructions for use. *Percussion instruments:* 13. Musical necklaces. – 14. The kaffir drum. – 15. The slapping boy. *Custom built:* 16. The phonograph.

5.14

No.19, May 1921
Georges Ribemont-Dessaignes
Buffet

Translated from
the French
by Ian Monk

Art? Not Art?
The Dadaists are against Art. Meaning?
Put your finger on a Dadaist chair, take it away and it is moist, sticky and smelly. A sui generis smell. Pushing Art inside, the Dadaists excrete it. You have to be fair, it is not their fault. Not all

of their fault. Amongst others, Art is at ease inside and out. Sitting on this milestone, you can wonder if Dadaism is not just another school of literature, painting, etc. – Well, damn it! What a military refrain on the way back to the barracks. All the same, d'Annunzio looks quite different.

But it has to be said: NO. Do you hear? NO, NO, no. And then the little bird sings on and on: a day, and then a day, again a day.

Here we are, all enemies, each one grenade. Exploded? Dada, dada, dada. The scattered parts. Art at once. A nascent minute ago. See stars, then Art. There are such metals that can be left in freedom. Venus in the sea is just a fish. On land, a great artist.

Poetry: Art; not Poetry: Art. Words as a game: Art. Pure sentences: Art. Only meaning: Art. No meaning: Art. Words drawn at random: Art. The Mona Lisa: Art. The Mona Lisa with a moustache: Art. Shit: Art. A newspaper advertisement: Art.

We don't want it. But a second and a glance later, there it is. Even more so on the page of a book. And when there is mention of the Dada Y. Good God! – There are also those who are interested in themselves, and who aspire to the papacy. They leave on each step the coagulated trace of their personality. Yes, yes, they themselves express themselves: if they look at their feet from the corners of their eyes, they have to admit that they have trodden in art. It brings good luck, by the way, and the populace will not hold it against them. What is just the successive cutting of one's personal diamond can only look like art. The effect of each facet on the spectator's mind can only deflower the virgin.

What is there to be done? To act against oneself? Art.

There is always purgation. There is no doubt that the masses in their present state could at once make themselves an artistic undergarment from the result of this purgation, and sell it on discounted and deodorised. Dear friend do not buy it.

Purge yourself. And may the health of the moment not say: it smells off – because its purpose is precisely to cleanse yourself. And the very principle of cleansing is to offer the residue on the same footing as the scented breath of our health.

As for the famous diamond, do not look for it for here. Nor there, nor elsewhere. It is enough to recognise it in your stomach thanks to a sworn-in X-ray to give yourself the big belly of Art.

And then? There is no and then. Purge yourself still. Apart from that, work in a grocery, a farm, in medicine, in trade in Abyssinia, in politics, in assassination, in philosophy, in suicide, and even in Art.

What about Dada?
But of course, Dada is ... — No, no

NO YES

Translated from
the French
by Ian Monk

No.19, May 1921
Max Ernst
ARP

From Place de l'Opéra, we can see him stand out from the sky day
and night
ARP
it is to him that we owe the sixty formations of skulls from the
blob of fog to the blob of
colour
it is he that occupies 3,000 zymometers per day
the mending of boredom would be rather difficult without the
midwife's hands
it is a highly accurate invention and of even more importance
than the key of love found by
auguste rodin

ARP
As for the farting bearded vulture, it seems to us that this little
lady-hole
contains all the truth of the charming excursion in the extreme
tree-bark of Zambezi whose reckless plan it draws up despite the
wind and foul weather
but if we add in the little leopard-hole whose Arabic landscape
has been shaped by the first
leopard killed in a natural aspect the words that are left contain a
patriotic madrigal it
is the merchant who strolls
It is now up to the reader to admire the courageous constructer
arp

ARP
Yemen and Gynander go three times a day to his child's coffin
with his teeth he breaks the new lactiform knucklebone that is
growing to the south of his
sternum
it is not even twenty-five years now that he has heard this pitter-
patter
ARP

We are sincerely sorry that he still lacks the constipation of
material cultivated so carefully by
pablo pi pablo
furthermore he has sometimes been criticised for forgetting the
wealth of anatomical
plantations and the tubiferous colour that was so admired in Max
Ernst
just like the illusory first cousin manipulated so graciously by the
fathers of the church

42
Max Ernst
Microgramme Arp
Littérature, No. 19
May 1921

just like the delicious machine for pulverising ancestors but all this will not draw a drop of
piss from the miracle-working acrobat by gravity by water and by the seventy numbers of wind he sells slippery and feasible trays and the multicolour droplets of small-sized fossils but he makes his parents transparent without counting the shipwrecks he had avoided

---

Microgramme Arp 1: 25,000

1. **Arp and the wisdom of youth**
2. **Arp seismograph**
   a) cordless calm sleep
   b) agitated sleep
3. **Arp nymphomaniac he does not yet know the false key of the two sexes**
4. **Arp head of hair and the daily sediments of his intelligence**
5. **arp fish nudibranch nudidaud nudicole nudiglue nudity**
6. **arp yellowstone park he keeps Berenice's hair there**

ARP
His fairy godmother will repeat six times a week that this striking mind cannot eat meat and
catches leprosy at once
but as for me I saw him sell his pox hungrily as for me I saw that he brings (using a small
wheelbarrow built for this very purpose) two kilos of teats and sausages a day to the
paternal house

ARP
citizens!
read the cloud pump
read the farting bearded vulture
read the old skilful thief
read the threesome and the bird on bird
search work read

ARP
From his birth he thinks it through and chats in favour of the three theological virtues and
Archimedes's theorem that says you must measure the corporal's corpus

ARP
so as not to violate your brother's taste he splits his chops in two and tattoos all the asterisms on
his tongue
just like the diagrams of all the inflorescences
just like octopuses

ARP
This does not stop him from always listening favourably to the little daisies coming into the
sound of the dugs
in his breast he keeps perspective lightning
in the splits of his shoulder blades the wall swallow nestles
in the shell of his ear he seizes the aeroliths as they fly
his heart and kidneys are utterly decomposable

Microgramme Arp 1 : 25.000

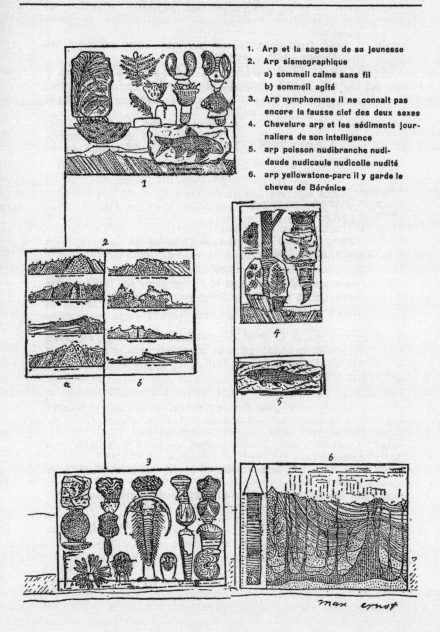

1. Arp et la sagesse de sa jeunesse
2. Arp sismographique
   a) sommeil calme sans fil
   b) sommeil agité
3. Arp nymphomane il ne connaît pas
   encore la fausse clef des deux sexes
4. Chevelure arp et les sédiments jour-
   naliers de son intelligence
5. arp poisson nudibranche nudi-
   daude nudicaule nudicolle nudité
6. arp yellowstone-parc il y garde le
   cheveu de Bérénice

max ernst

Translated from the French by Ian Monk

No.19, May 1921
Louis Aragon
Down with the Utter French Genius

If I were alone with myself, things would turn ugly ... I shall stop there: 'Ugly, what do you mean by ugly, you shrimp?' Well, I say *ugly* and I say *progress* and other abstractions shamelessly, because (why because? ... fat ox) these patented absurdities do not seem to me any more absurd than the heavens, another abstraction, automobiles and proper nouns, unlabelled abstractions which, one day, you will have to pay off, my grandchildren. The price of intelligence ... I was going to say that if one did not constantly distract me with the universe, I would sort out the world's business once and for all. Since my birth, the public powers who have their suspicions have continually invited me onto the terrain of the useful and agreeable: the sheepfold of fans. The freedom not to look for happiness, your pleasure, ladies and gentlemen. *Reasonable animals*, you believe you have said it all. Your pregnant definitions clack while giving birth to ridiculous maggots. 'The eternal silence of infinite space,' explain that as well as you can, I flatter myself on failing again and again: that such turns of phrase blossom in the fallow fields of our brains is both comforting and demoralising. Useful and agreeable, my little scamps. 'The eternal silence ...' the same thing will be trotted out at every occasion. Scientific discoveries are generally given as examples: the fear of hastening the end of the world never stops scientists with their perfect senses. Such is man's delirium of interpretation, such is the mental fever whose tiny oscillations are isochronal for all human hearts and superior vegetation. Such is the runaway wheel of your genius, my comrades, such is cataclysm and normal man, a hop pole lost in a maritime dock and proud of the adaptation of its organs to their environment. Sooner or later, there will be the bankruptcy of intelligence, that common good, poverty of thought. Only my own absurdity belongs to me, and I stand by it. That greatness can be admired (Julius Caesar, Casanova, Jacques Vaché) is only a way to make light of a certain native stupidity. What would you not engage yourself to if you contravened the declaration of the rights of man and of the citizen in front of me? I make that boast. Insult Marat like that, and you will get what you deserve. The culture of red reflexes and forever unjustifiable angers. In this way I escape from judgement, still bold. The body of Charles the Bold, naked on the plains of defeat, will keep of its past splendour only a diamond on a ring finger, which a wanderer will pull off: the incomparable sparkle, beyond the surest reasoning and recovered weakness. I take my triumphal absurdity everywhere, it is never out of place. May it meet Monsieur Renan on the boulevard, what will the thinker be able to do against its echoless laughter? What will I be able to do against myself in that moment of myself? The useful and the agreeable, you said? Puerile and beautiful tattoos on the spade of thought, our cyclical habits mean that we always pass back by the same minima. (I am reading myself in the lower meniscus.) Here grow torn and rootless lichens, here are the monstrous flowers of credulity. The filler *does not* in the middle of a sentence refutes the orator and the oration. I have, like everyone, my little gateways onto the infinite, my hesitations, my scruples. Sweet and marvellous ineptitude where slumbers, with an umbrella under its arm, the veined marble idol attributed to Praxiteles. The useful and the agreeable: France and its cortege, the pick pompons of taste. Let us not exaggerate: that pox of the world no longer affects its 40 million inhabitants.

Littérature New Series
Paris
1922–24

43
Front Cover
Littérature New Series
No. 1
March 1922

Translated from
the French
by Timothy Adès

No.7, December 1922
Robert Desnos
Rrose Sélavy[1]

A pastor distilled a psalm-sap tipple in an apple-plaster temple.
Rrose Sélavy asks if Baudelaire's 'The Wicked Blooms' hath
unblockéd wombs: what does Molly Bloom think?
Travellers, pamper the Pamplonese fillies with peafowl
feathers.
Is the solution of a sage the pollution of a page?
[*un page*, a page-boy.]
My dears so handsome, I adores a bosom as wears opossum.
Question for astronomers: Will Rrose Sélavy for decades enter
the annual cadastre in the astral quadrant?
Oh, my knackered noddle, star-struck nacreous nodule.
Where Rrose Sélavy lives, they love wolves and fools, who are
heaven's and earth's outlaws.
Will you harass Rrose Sélavy as far as the decimal numbers
nothing dismal encumbers?
Rrose Sélavy wonders if the demise of seasons decides the
destiny of demesnes.
Pass me my Barbary quiver, sir, says the barbaric vizier.
Thunderous planets above scare the quails who love the
wondrous plants Rrose Sélavy grows, whose leaves are scales.
Marcel Duchamp, *marchand du sel*: Rrose Sélavy knows
the salt-seller well.
Epitaph: Cease to torment Rrose Sélavy: my genius is
enigma. Nor can Caron con it.
Adrift on the endless waters, will Rrose Sélavy eat first her
hands and then her fetters?
Aragon harvests in extremis the spirit of Aramis on a
bed of tarragon.
André Breton doesn't dress as a mage to battle an image of the
hydra thundering bitterly.
Francis Picabia, too frank for
A confidant of beavers or,
Red-caped and draped in toison d'or,
A prancing Cassis picador.
Robert Delaunay: Rowboat Water-born! Beware the barb.
My fear in the mirror appears as a marine vapour.

DEFINITION OF ART BY RROSE SÉLAVY:
The merciless cow with tuberculosis loses in one month half
an udder.
Rrose Sélavy wonders if love is the fly-paper that firms up the soft
sofas of fair play.
What set your carnation withering, little girl, interned where your
eye came by the other ring?

44
Front Cover
Littérature New Series
No. 4
September 1922

45
Front Cover
Littérature New Series
No. 7
December 1922

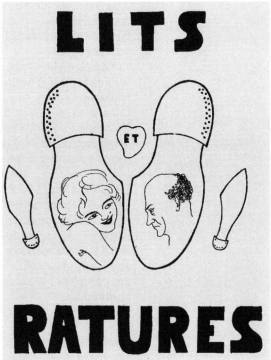

The riverside diversion of a racecourse is Rrose Sélavy's resource.
Rrose Sélavy may put on prison's drab garb, yet her mount ranges
on mountain-ranges.
Rrose Sélavy passes the palm that lacks the glamour of
martyrs to Lakmé the lamb-herd of Chartres on the flat metal
calm of the Beauce, which we call beauty.
Do you think Rrose Sélavy knows those ticklish jokes that make
for tingling cheeks?
Rrose Sélavy is perhaps the apprentice apache who flanned her
brat with the flat of her hand.
Does the canoodling of painted wenches condone the idling of
tainted haunches?
Anno Domini's an agile eagle in many a dome. [Time's an agile
eagle in a temple.]
What if Rrose Sélavy, on a night of Yule, steers for the
snare of the snow-white pole?
Ah, lover! All over!
Why's it my luck to pick from the pack, at hazard, a friend more
fickle than the lizard?
A preacher in a chalet finds in the lees of the chalice the cachet of
the delicious: does he approach his heavenly match with malice?
This crater affords the Missouri its source and Sarah's
court its mystery.
Nomads en route for the North, do not pause at the port to trade
your pomades.
Rrose Sélavy sleeps well with a small fellow out of a well
wolfing her loaf at twelve.
If silence is golden, Rrose Sélavy's eyelids'll close-down.
Craning on the careen, the poet seeks a rhyme: do you think
Rrose Sélavy is the queen of crime?
When caravels were making fast at La Havana, were
caravans snaking past Laval?

EASTERN QUESTION:
At Santa Sophia a kirk-stall of cork is no seat of sanity.
Rrose Sélavy proposes that the perishing compost of all
passions become the nourishing repast of all nations.
What is this tide sans cause whose sour flow floods the
steely soul of Rrose?
Benjamin Péret's regime is perfect: his early bath is his
yearly bath.
P. Éluard: a draped poet, the élite of the sheets.

EPITAPH FOR APOLLINAIRE:
Weep dirges, giants and geniuses, on the void's edges.
Desnos does not pale as he deals with desires on his pole.
Scale the ladder, Drieu la Rochelle, to shock the Lord.
Amorous traveller on the tender chart, why feed your nights on a
cinder tart?

THE MARTYRDOM OF ST SEBASTIAN:

...

Rrose Sélavy has seen the archipelago where sea-queen Irene
wields an ash-sprig to rule her isles.

From Everest mountain I am falling down to your feet for ever, Mrs
Everling. [Desnos composed this one in English.]

Would André Breton be damned forever to tonsure cats of
jade and amber?

Rrose Sélavy calls on you not to take the verrucas of the
breast for the virtues of the blest.

Rrose Sélavy wouldn't bet egotism gets you a wet bottom.

...

Seized with love unconstrained, the Alpine parson spreads his
frocks to the rocks to ease his loins.

RROSE SÉLAVY'S MOTTO:

Beyond the polite to be decent
Beyond the poet to be dishonoured.

Will Rrose Sélavy discover the alcohol river quaffed by
choleric llamas in America?

Abort the absurd parabolas, absorb Rrose Sélavy's
misheard parables.

EPIPHANY:

In the small hours, dreams moor at the mole to unload beans.

In the nirvana of diamonds, the carats are lovers, the spiral is
crystal.

Roman Pearmains taste to pages as if gnawed in rages by jaws
of Moors.

Let rockets be fired, the crooked-faced races are tired!

Rrose Sélavy declares her skull's honeydew is the wonder
embittering the sky's bile.

At Rrose Sélavy's 'agapê' or love-feast one eats papal paste in an
agate-daubed sauce.

Learn that Rrose Sélavy's celebrated gesture is etched in
celestial algebra.

Praying in pews with bibles resembles spraying the eclipse with
pebbles.

People of Sodom, fear the fire of heaven, prefer the fever of
the rear.

In an abbess's cranium, a crab confronts an ass.

Keep to the ramp, royals and loyals braving the cave that has no
lamp.

Rrose Sélavy has learned that the noble title of posterity is not the
notable tackle of the posterior.

Is your tribe forever at a tribunal, dear downhearted departed?

...the Tropic of Cancer.

Poor pawns in art pare as their share the lion's part.

Classy torsos on tables of nurses, you will be carcases in hearses!
Maladies issue from every orifice of cadavers' palaces.

Why are life's ifs and buts the problem prey of pale bolts and nuts?

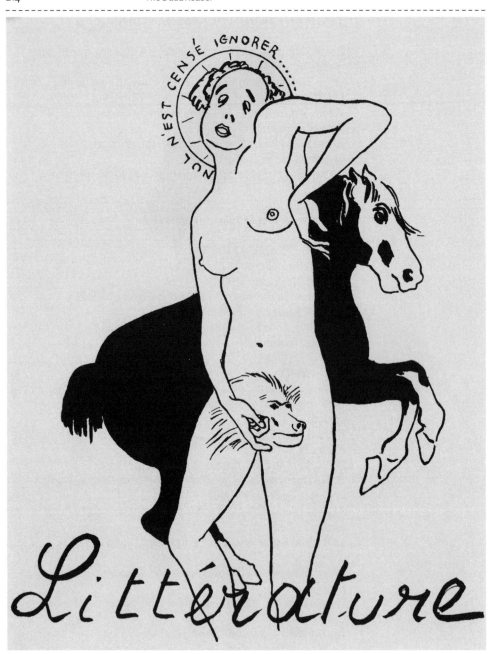

46
Front Cover
Littérature New Series
No. 5
October 1922

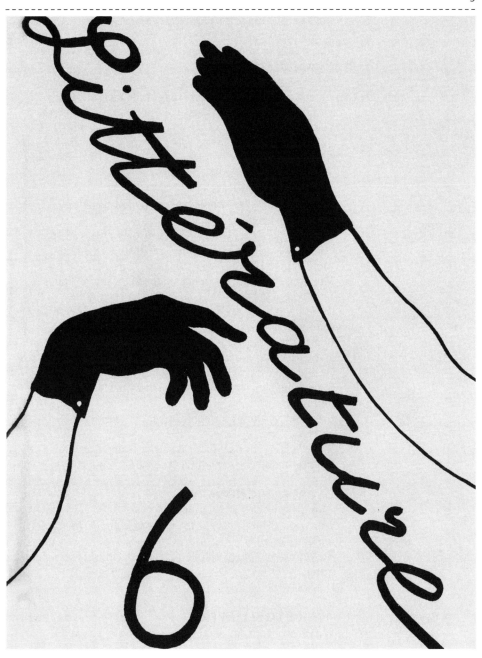

47
Front Cover
Littérature New Series
No. 6
November 1922

On the anti-artistic ice-pack, Rrose Sélavy starts an Antarctic savings bank.

Rocambole blows his cornet to start carnage and swims clear, cartwheeling off a lofty crag.

Rrose Sélavy tarts up the fates and her dart starts the feasts.

Rrose's desire of love for ever dies of cirrhosis of the liver.

Lovers with tuberculosis, use your phthisical advantages.

The period of debauches pips the stupor of poor wretches.

In the Elysian fields, Rrose Sélavy wears deceaseful weeds.

All mankind's thoughts make some school's unkind impots.

Hurricanes have ranged over Rrose Sélavy, who reaches in no rage the age of oranges.

Jacques Baron's fun, whole bayonet-jerks on one's soul.

…merely the crystal of fops.

Morise's ideas are iridescent with obsolescent promise.

Mad broads with eyes undaubed sail through yards and yards of fire in yawls.

Thinking evil of singers opens up the Sing Sing of evildoers.

The sport of the departed is to spread and be rotted.

Assassin of harps and psalteries, have you slaughtered a saint's high hopes?

Max Ernst's cavernous eyes assess the amusement-caves of statues carved with   the maxims of his Muse: Ernestine.

On what pole does the ice-pack splinter the poets' smack?

Is a predilection for the female the dilemma of fiction and the numeral?

Rrose Sélavy knows the goblin of gloom cannot gobble the globe.

Rrose Sélavy tells us the world's rattle is the ruse of male rulers embattled in the whirl of the monthly muse.

LA RROSE DICTIONARY:

Latinity - the five Latin nations…

The magic of boule may be the jiggle of the male. [*Boule*: the lobbing game.]

Rrose Sélavy submerged the moral wheedler in a mere of mineral water.

Croesus…

ADVICE TO BELIEVERS:

Wisely await the day of faith when death shall have you enjoy the scythe.

Rrose Sélavy's going down a mine, making ready for Armageddon.

Wake up Jacob, says his pretty sister, your digit buys my birthright.

Cravan wends on the wave and his cravat waves in the wind.

In Vaché's roguish drawls, words crash like waves on rocky shores.

QUESTION:
Mystical cancer, will your long song be a canticle to mystery?

ANSWER:
Aren't you aware your misery preens like a queen of this mystery's train?
Is a watery death a wreath for the doughty?
The act of the sexes is the axis of the sects.
Sweeter than glory are the shrouds and shadows of the globe.
Our brows harbour cemeteries that a maze of boundaries on summits omits.
Will the coming of caresses reveal to us the carmine of goddesses?
Dying of perfect bone-idleness, we are dandled by perfumed blessed idols.
The militias of goddesses disregard the delights of missals.
On her trapeze Rrose Sélavy appeases the distresses of our divine mistresses.
Do poesy's Vestals take us for vesicles, Petals?
The human brood is a phantom squad with a squirt of blood.
Female phantoms perched on elephants scriven on heavens the mysterious omega that fits planetary equations.
Impatient heirs, usher your forebears into the hall of thunders.
I live where you live, urchin whose mug is the magic of journeys.
The self-regard of Rrose Sélavy forges clear as the circle closes like a shroud.
Phalanx of angels...
The gross legate from the cloister has all the éclat of a goitre.
Do you know the jolly lovely faun of folly? She is yellow.
Does your bloodstream carry cowbells at your blubbing's beck and call?
Does piety in dogma consist in pitying dogs?
For the fleshly calèche it's a long lane, will the carnal car go far?
Love's images, fishes, will your poisonless kisses make me lower my eyes?
In the land of Rrose Sélavy, males are well-matched marines, females scratch at the mange.
Swells respect tolling knells when looking-glasses reflect their longing glances.
[À tout péché, miséricorde: for every sin, let there be mercy.]...
Words, are you myths which match the myrtles of death?
Can Rrose Sélavy's arty talk alter a swan into a stork?
The laws of our desires are dice without leisure.

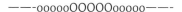

——-oooooOOOOooooo——-

5.16

No.9, February–March 1923
André Breton, Robert Desnos and Benjamin Perét
What Lovely Weather!

Translated from
the French
by Susan de Muth

To Max Ernst

In the tropical rainforest. Stage right a family tree through which a tree on a spring can be seen; the latter moves up and down throughout the whole scene. A Banyan tree takes up the whole of stage left. Enormous thoughts on all sides. The backdrop is a mirror.

Two monkeys, a leaf insect. When the curtain rises the first monkey completes the family tree with some chalk; there are already several names on it: Sade, Nouveau, Chirico, Cravan, Hegel, Vaché, Lebaudy. The second monkey dictates and the first fills in the empty escutcheons: Lautréamont, Henri Rousseau, Roussel, Néron, Apollinaire, Mongolfier, Freud, Rimbaud, Galilee, Jarry, Marat, Robespierre, Colomb, Fantomas,

Deschanel, Rosa-Josepha and lastly Silexame. Having done this, the first monkey races down the family tree and curls up on the ground.

SECOND MONKEY:

I got one hand with no hair on, I got one hand with no hair on, (*holds out his arms*) it's bigger than the other. You know them fruit, no way to get a hold of them; you can't get 'em off the trees and if you lean on them you notice that they're ringing. (*Becomes agitated*). There's water in them trees; there's water. The air is heavy it's heavy it's like something it's almost like a kind of liquid thing.

The leaf-insect, until now invisible, lowers itself to the ground.

FIRST MONKEY:

Beware of the big white face 'cos the big white face rolls along and it can squash our hands. When it passes by it attracts our dicks and it's got the power to change air into sand.

LEAF INSECT: Look how pretty I am in my mica dress made of microbes.

FIRST MONKEY: Sand is all around, all around. The trees are getting smaller. The sand is getting higher. I can feel my dick's getting longer, getting longer. Now it's just a little dot. It's disappearing like a cloud. (*Starts to cry*).

SECOND MONKEY: He's in the sand 'cos he's hanging by his tail.

LEAF INSECT: Huge swathes of time crumble on cards as silent as the grave. (*Silence.*)

An enormous worm crosses the stage and disappears.
(*Silence.*)

LEAF INSECT: In love, everything means wrinkle.

ANTEATER (*enters, shouting*): I'm asking you for maybe the thousandth time: don't explain things to me.

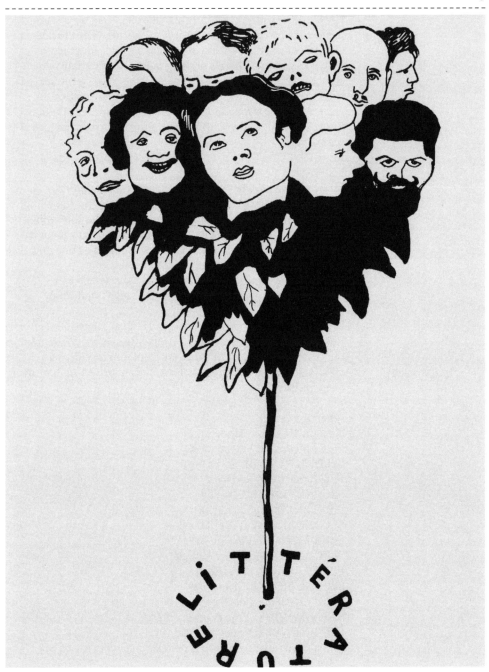

48
Front Cover
Littérature New Series
No. 8
January 1923

KANGAROO *(entering)*: That's just like me. What do you want me to say when people spin me a yarn like this: 'The President of Gourgues furnished a salon in crimson brocade for Madame Baligny-Fontaine. There's nothing more beautiful than her chimney lamps: they give off a golden light. The canopy over her bed is a mirror. Her delight in her reflection there means she never wishes to sleep. Garlands bear the inscription: "Do the right thing."' Nobody knows if this exhortation has to do with love or the gospel.

LEAF INSECT: From misery hysterical come forth words historical.

FIRST MONKEY: That's a strange sort of animal *(indicates the banyan tree)*. It looks like a clump of twisted boughs branching out to infinity. It's pale violet. I dunno its name but this animal is really sad because it's lost its sun. It shouldn't be sad about its sun though: it was a sun made of bracken. It keeps on saying: 'I've lost my sun.' It's starting to get on our nerves.

SPIDER *(enters and climbs up the tree on a spring)*: Like the Banyan tree the whole of society is just a set of intersecting interdependencies.

KANGAROO: This morning I read in *The Times* that Count Rochefort has given the great La Croix fifteen louis. In my opinion that's too much to pay for a descent from the cross. He has stipulated that she must breastfeed, like an African woman, over her shoulder.

ANTEATER: Don't mistake lemons for eggs or lemon pips for other eggs.

Don't mistake fruits for eyes.

FIRST MONKEY: Pigeon flies![1]

SECOND MONKEY: Crisis flies!

FIRST MONKEY: Red flies!

SECOND MONKEY: God flies!

FIRST MONKEY: Suicide flies!

SECOND MONKEY: Tooth flies!

FIRST MONKEY: Volcano flies!

SECOND MONKEY: United flies!

FIRST MONKEY: Sinus flies!

SECOND MONKEY: Host flies!

FIRST MONKEY: Pole flies!

SECOND MONKEY: 30 February flies!

FIRST MONKEY: Necessity flies!

An enormous white cocoon rolls on stage and comes to a halt in the middle.

SECOND MONKEY: Dirt flies!

FIRST MONKEY: Clamp flies!

SECOND MONKEY: Burying flies!

FIRST MONKEY: I don't know what flies!

ANTEATER: I'm asking you for maybe the thousandth time: don't explain things to me.

SPIDER: Bah! Stupid animal only thinks about eating, drinking and sleeping.

LEAF INSECT: Oh dear! Everything stops me sleeping. Roots give me diarrhoea, sardines set my nerves on edge. If I smoke a cigarette I start sleepwalking on the rooftops. I can't drink a cocktail without getting total amnesia. Maybe you think I could take it out on the milk? I'm afraid not – milk makes me mystical. I'm so easily influenced! I can't look at the sea where so many wonderful people are relaxing without the compulsion to get myself squashed between two pages of the Luisades turned by the wind on the reefs. I can't live in mining country without using a cane to bolster my fading strength. Statues of crystal or sulphur, the immobility that the sight of you strikes me with is possibly more absolute than your own. I've been walking with perpetual vertigo since I first met a woman. Whenever I look at myself in the mirror I cry all the tears from my body.

FIRST MONKEY: Inject yourself with gelatine for your haemophilia but take care to sterilise the needles at 120 degrees so you don't get tetanus.

SECOND MONKEY: Never let us forget that the most noble poetry is born of pain; that human suffering had brought us pity and tenderness; that sorrow has often compelled us to higher thoughts or good deeds. Nor let us forget that the brain only discerns differences and that a pleasure, which knows no end, remains unnoticed. We only register our pleasure at its onset or its end. And I understand how Tannhäuser came to experience nothing but anxiety among the perpetual delights of Venusburg, and asked to leave so that he could suffer and work like everybody else.

LEAF INSECT: Oh flea-ridden cats, when will you give the Papuans hats?

The cocoon breaks open vertically. A huge butterfly comes out which briefly flaps its wings before disappearing, leaving in its stead a large petrol lamp that is lit. The butterfly's appearance is greeted with sighs from all the animals. As soon as it disappears, the tibia insect, the snail and the rhinoceros come on.

SECOND MONKEY: That one really stinks. What a disgusting smell. What filth!

TIBIA INSECT: If I smell it's so I can speak better but what I say has no warmth and I'm off, I'm running away because a giant disc is coming down from the top of the sun. I'm sure the sun's going to fall on it.

KANGAROO: Miss Horny has changed her skin: she started out with mulatto skin and now there are lilies here and roses there. The laundry woman just found some in her linen.

TIBIA INSECT: I am the one that rings, the one that rings, the one you will never hear because the customary serpents writhe in your ears. Why do you burden yourself with serpents when it would do you so much good to hear that breathing?

Exits.

The animals gather in a circle round the lamp, the leaf insect throws itself onto the glass of the lamp: darkness, terrified shouts, silence, then in dim light the Foot appears, the sole turned towards the

49
Front Cover
Littérature New Series
No. 9
February/March 1923

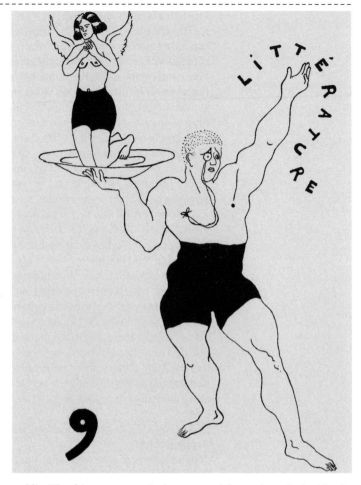

public. The rhinoceros runs its horn up and down along the inside of
the foot. The big toe flexes slowly. It goes back to normal once the
rhino has left. Then the snail comes along and stops in front of
the foot.

SNAIL:

I. In the beginning the watch chain created tobacco and coal.

II. The tobacco was shapeless and smooth. Vapours covered the
faces of the walkers and the spirit of the watch chain floated upon
the surface of alcohol.

III. Then the watch chain said: 'Let the lead weights leap'[2] and the
lead weights leapt.

IV. And the watch chain saw that the lead weights were laughing
and separated the lead weights from the vapours.

V. It gave the lead weights the name 'Love' and the vapours the
name 'Hate'. And from the evening and the morning was the last
love.

VI. The watch chain also said: 'Let the mouth be created in the
middle of the alcohol and separate alcohol from alcohol.'

VII. And the watch chain made the mouth and separated the
alcohol that was in the mouth from the alcohol that was outside

it. And thus was it done.

VIII. And the watch chain gave the mouth the name 'Kiss'. And from the evening and the morning was the last love.

IX. The watch chain spoke again: 'may the alcohol that is beneath the kiss collect in a single place and the dry element disappear'. And thus was it done.

X. The watch chain gave the dry element the name 'Coal' and all the collected alcohols it named 'Oath'. And it saw that it was good.

XI. The watch chain spoke again: 'May coal destroy the red flag which comes out of the mine-shaft and the sewer men who carry their thirst within them, each in his own way, to doze on the coal.' And thus it was done.

XII. So the coal destroyed the red flag that came out of the mine-shaft and the sewage-workers that carried their thirst within, each in his own way. And the watch chain saw that it was good.

XIII. And from the evening and the morning was the last love.

XIV. The watch chain also said: 'May tongues of lead be made in the mouth of tobacco so that they can separate love from hate and act as a funnel to mix desires and whims, loves and passions:

XV. May they shine in the mouth of tobacco and colour the alcohol.' And thus it was done.

XVI. So the watch chain made two great tongues of lead. The larger to preside over love, the smaller to preside over hate. She also created teeth.

XVII. And she put them into the mouth of tobacco to shine on the coal.

XVIII. To preside over love and hate, and to separate the lead weight from the vapours. And the watch chain saw that it was good.

XIX. And from the evening and the morning was the last love.

The snail leaves. A motor revs loudly. The foot disappears and in its place a spinning gyroscope appears. This in turn ends up falling over and disappears.

ANTEATER: I'm asking you for maybe the thousandth time: don't explain things to me.

SPIDER: Under these trees a completely unbreathable wind of poetry gusts. The skill of the artist who struggles against nature while trying hard to reproduce it will always be like that of the man who squeezed lentils through a little opening, and whom Alexander rewarded for his art with the delivery of a bushel of lentils.

RHINOCEROS: If this wind is stifling you, do the same as me. I know a lovely muddy little swamp near here.

(*He exits.*)

MADREPORE appears and sings:
The bets put on by pipette
Fool the isthmus flags
The funnel places its lips
On the sun with abbots' stains

With criminal attention
You hold up your cards to the staff
Pressed on the velvet pear
And flies off through holey hillocks

The pavement covers the snows
Promised to the equator
Rotating baptismal boxes

Soundless on the tapioca carpet
Bargains tarnish pulleys
Caresses for ancient winds

The madrepore is replaced by a horse.

LEAF INSECT: Oh horse flower of my nerves, in which channel do
you bathe in order to become green?

*The horse disappears. In its place a giant head balances on the
ground. Silence. The animals exhibit anxiety: the spider flees, the
leaf insect goes back to its original place, the kangaroo leaps from left
to right, all the leaves fall from the trees, including the ones from the
family tree, and the anteater sweeps them with his tail. Only the leaf
insect remains hanging from a branch to the end of the scene. The
first monkey falls flat on its tummy with its arms crossed and remains
completely still. The second hides behind a tree.*

SECOND MONKEY: Oooooooooooh! What is it? Ooooh it sounds
like a frog's song. And this shape that's drawing itself, it's as if it
was reflected. Oh yep, see, the clump of boughs is going back to
the soil. What a lot of sand!
KANGAROO: The girls are complaining: all the winter dresses
have been pawned for taffeta.
SECOND MONKEY: Oh! Sand, sand, the air is full of sand. Oh!
The air is full of sand. It's impossible to breathe. Now nothing can
be heard but a vast breathing *(strong wind blows)*. Have I got
thorns in my veins? I can't breathe any more. Sand. See how the
trees are liquefying.
WHITE BEAR *(runs across the stage)*: I've been watching it run
away from big polar corpses since all the unaccomplished
futures. It's coming towards us with all the speed of its
undulatory swimming strokes with the only admirable bit of
Venus's sinuses between its lips and the sperm that gets on
Minerva's nerves.
LEAF INSECT: It's something like a great anemone with the three
mixed colours sparkling on it and pierced through the middle by a
human leg. *(Silence.)* The great anemone *(panting voice)* swims
away from its underwater cage and its body brings us the
perfumes of the north.
THE KANGAROO: Colin the butcher provides for the young lady
Pelin with meat: she always asks for knickers.

SECOND MONKEY: But I can feel hairs, hairs rubbing at my face, prickly ones. Oh! And again. My limbs are being wrenched off, my limbs are being wrenched off my toes are being wrenched off. My fingers, what are they doing with my fingers, what are they doing with my fingers, what are they doing with my fingers? My skin's being cut. That vast breathing. My skin's being cut. My nerves are being ripped out. Who's ripping my nerves out? The vast breathing is making arrows from my nerves! And always, sand. All I can see is a pointed thing, spikes coming towards me, piercing my breast. Oh! I can see the fork, its breathing is appalling. No one seems to know who it is. Ah! The clump of boughs is shouting. When the air comes out of its lungs it's sand and when it breathes you can feel your skin coming away from your body, the skin passing away. Oh! My body's flown open like a door. Oooooooh! my stomach's being torn out. My intestines are all unrolling. Ooooh! my ribs are breaking. I'm going to die.
(He falls down like the first monkey.)

> *Off stage a voice recites*:
> THE GREAT ODE TO SILEXAME
> Future Minerva

The virginal greeting of flowers with no atmosphere finally finished today, 31 March 1924.

In all poets' birthplaces the antique statues in the museum are made of sugar candy. But the poets don't have fun sucking sugar candy phalluses. It's you they love, Silexame, you whom nobody has ever been able to describe, Silexame, Silexame, Silexame, Silexame. If I had to compare you to ordinary things I'd say you were like these pleasantly labelled pharmaceutical products: Silexame hystogenol, Silexame urodonal, Silexame hermaphrodite, Silexame hexamethylenetetramine, Silexame diethylmalonylurie. But in the hearts of the mistresses of those disdainful sugar candy poets there is:
An ocean of chloroform that changes the pancreas of lost seafarers into bronze. Doctors meeting in religious councils have ruined the social status of that organ, the pancreas, which would never be satisfied with the moralistic maxims they put under its name in those catechisms called natural history textbooks. The seafarers' pancreas, like the poets' pancreas, is a block of ice that doesn't melt in the heat and doesn't reflect women's faces. This unknown poet of the African peoples, this unknown poet of the white tribes, this unknown poet of astronomers – when the third terrestrial period of the sun was nigh – composed the song of the bronze pancreas of poets and seafarers which does not reflect the face of women or the degree X + 1 on the centigrade thermometer: 'Sleep greet hello. It's the song of the pancreas, salicylate appalling memory all the perfumes are sobs in the citadels of your brains. We'll dive further than blocks of bronze, Silexame, Silexame, Silexame, you who are neither the cause nor the

outcome, people who call you nothing do not do you justice because you are even less than nothing, less than less than nothing and even less than less than less than nothing. Inspire me with the song of bronze pancreas'. Matchstick eye of platinum, lovely look beautiful swimming baths, all the philanthropists are dead, murdered by other philanthropists. But those other philanthropists had been murdered by the first ones. Don't shout at the paradox, virgins have no pancreas and as a result, neither do women. But virgin men have a pancreas and the others don't have one. That's why poets and seafarers are virgins and that's why the Silexame are loved by seafarers and poets.

Between the 13th degree north and the 26th degree longitude the card game of cosmic maelstroms is found. The modern poet puts no trademark on his heart.

The Silexame in his pocket, the Silexame instead of a heart, the Silexame instead of eyes, the Silexame instead of senses, the Silexame instead of memories, the Silexame instead of sex, the Silexame instead of the navel. And off he goes on the little road, if his width is taken into consideration, on the big road if his length is taken into consideration.
Truly, Silexame, you're a very beautiful thing but is this ode worthy of you?

Silence.
Silexame comes out of the bottom of the head (its head is a fork, body made of shell, arms covered with leaves). You can only see it in the mirror.

CURTAINS

5.17

No.10, May 1923
Benjamin Péret
Bonny wants a car

Translated from
the French
by Dawn Ades

FILM
Bonny is a children's nurse. She likes cars and her great pleasure is to ride in a taxi. When she takes the children in her care for a walk, she gapes in admiration at the beautiful cars that stream past down the Champs-Elysées.

In her room she dreams of a handsome young man who owns a superb automobile. One day when she is out walking with the children of her employers she meets a young man, Gluglug, who tells her he owns a car and suggests taking her out for a drive. She agrees. Gluglug returns shortly to collect her. She leaves the children in the care of an old woman who seems respectable. Gluglug's car is an old boneshaker which constantly breaks down and when in motion moves forward in jerks. The car's occupants are terribly shaken at each advance. A gust of wind carries off Bonny's hat, which flies in front of the car. Gluglug leaps after it. A gust of wind carries it further. The car, capriciously, sets off at full speed, with Bonny at the wheel, and crushes Gluglug. The car reverses and runs over Gluglug several times. Gluglug gets up and runs after the car, which accelerates away from him. On a turning in the road the car hits another car. With the impact, Bonny is shot into the car hers has hit, while the occupant of the latter is projected into Bonny's car. The cars continue their respective routes. Gluglug, who is running to catch up with Bonny, is run over again several times as before. Bonny carries on. She turns the wheel too abruptly and runs off the road into a field of grazing cows and bulls. She is terrified of these animals. A bull rushes straight at the car and with one blow of its horn sends it to the other end of the field where another bull sends it back to the first one. This performance is repeated five or six times. In the end a third bull hits it sideways and sends it into a pond. Bonny emerges from the water covered in slime. She has drunk a great deal of water. She regurgitates a blackish liquid full of frogs. She removes the frogs' legs, which she puts in her handkerchief, and goes back into the water to fish for more frogs, whose legs she takes off. She is preparing to leave, carrying her handkerchief, when she meets Gluglug, who runs up out of breath, sweating and covered in dust. He has been looking for her and is happy to find her. Bonny is furious and hits him. Gluglug does a somersault and falls into the ditch that runs beside the road. He gets up covered in mud. They set off, on opposite sides of the road, averting their heads at each step, sadly.

As soon as Bonny left, the old woman carries the children off and telephones their parents telling them to send her a million immediately or she will kill them. The parents refuse and call the police.

Bonny comes back and looks for the children. Gone! And the old woman too. She searches everywhere and, at nightfall, in the snow, which piles up on her head and forms a cone, goes back to her employers and tells them everything. They sack her. She is determined to find the children. She meets Gluglug and tells him the whole story. Gluglug is very upset and promises to help her.

Gluglug has an idea: he will go into every house in the town and into every apartment in the houses to find the children. To guide him, Bonny gives him a photograph of the children.

In the first house where he rings the bell an old woman opens the door holding a nasty little cur in her arms. Gluglug looks in turn at the dog and at the photograph. Seeing Gluglug, the dog barks furiously and the old woman tries to calm it without paying attention to Gluglug. Another dog comes out of the house and slips past the old woman's skirt. She tries to catch it. Gluglug does too. The dog goes into the street but runs faster than Gluglug. To stop it, Gluglug snatches a sack of coal from the back of a coal merchant and throws it onto the dog. The dog is

50
Front Cover
Littérature New Series
No. 10
May 1923

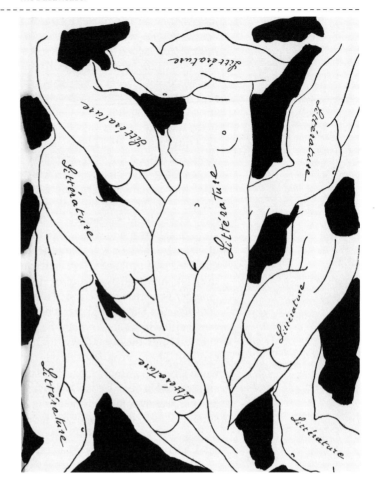

flattened like a biscuit. Its tongue still moves a little. The old
woman is furious and starts to cry. Gluglug has not forgotten the
purpose of his visit and asks her if she has seen two children. She
looks at Gluglug and the photograph, and, assuming he is mad,
beats a hasty retreat, forgetting the other dog, which runs after
her and falls into a sewer. Gluglug returns to the house and rings
another bell. This time a boxer about to enter the ring opens the
door. Holding the photo in his hands, he looks at the boxer and
the photo. The boxer, who is expecting his trainer, thinks he has
business with him. He seizes Gluglug by the hair and holds him at
arm's length. Gluglug struggles. The boxer hits him. Gluglug's
head swings like a pendulum and his face seems more and more
battered. Another blow and he is knocked out. The boxer picks
him up like a parcel and throws him downstairs. Gluglug rolls
down to the bottom and falls head first into a dustbin. When he
comes to, he has his head in the rubbish. He notices that he has a
black eye and bloody nose. Gluglug changes houses. He rings
now at a villa. A monkey opens the door. Gluglug starts back,
scared, looks at his photo and at the monkey, and sidles in,
keeping close to the wall. Nobody there ... He calls 'Boss! Boss! ... '

A parrot repeats his words and flies round him. He decides to explore the house. He opens a door. It is a bedroom in which there are two crocodiles, one on the bed, another under a table. He runs out in alarm. He opens another door. This time it's a dining room, with a camel. In the drawing room there's a sheep. In the kitchen, an ostrich, who takes his hat. He goes upstairs. He leans on the banister. The banister is a snake whose head brushes against his. Gluglug is more and more scared. Reaching the first floor, Gluglug, who is looking up, falls into an aquarium. A crab seizes his toe, and Gluglug can't dislodge it. He strokes the crab to coax it to let go. The crab grips even tighter. Gluglug takes a miniature vaporiser from his pocket and sprays the crab. The crab clings on. He is forced to empty a flask of chloroform over the crab. The crab falls asleep and loosens its grip. But Gluglug also falls asleep in the water. When he wakes up, silk worms have made a cocoon in his hair. Gluglug frees himself with great difficulty. Gluglug leaves. After entering 3,478 houses, he arrives, harassed and on his knees, at the house where the children are prisoners.

During these investigations, the children's parents have sent numerous police officers in search of the children and have promised a large reward. Every day, people who have seen the announcement of the reward lead them to different places. One day to the Morgue, next day to a circus, whence they return with mange. Another day they are taken to a barge where two strange children have taken refuge. They fall into a coal hole, from where they emerge in a pitiable state. Every day they receive an ear, a nose, a tooth, a toe, which they are told belong to their children. They are desperate.

Gluglug has learned something during his investigations. He knows that it is no use going in by the door to get the information he needs. He wants to climb via the gutter in to the roof of the house. Halfway up, the gutter comes away and Gluglug is suspended in mid-air. He carries on climbing regardless, but his weight drags him further and further back. Having reached the end of the gutter, he is a very long way from the wall. A taxi goes by. Gluglug lunges awkwardly for the roof. The gutter touches the cabman's head for a moment. The impact throws him back to the end, he clings to the roof. The gutter springs back, hits the shafts of the cab and breaks them. The horse goes on alone. The cab driver is furious, as is the occupant who thrashes the driver. Gluglug wants to go down the chimney, but there are dozens. Which is the right one? Gluglug puts his head into each chimney opening. In one he meets a chimney sweep who shoots out a jet of soot. Gluglug is as black as the sweep, whose head emerges from the chimney. In the end Gluglug draws lots as to which chimney he should descend. The one fate chooses for him is so narrow that Gluglug is unnaturally elongated when he reaches the bottom. He is in a dark, low cellar and has to walk bent double. He emerges from the cellar and enters another empty cellar whose floor is covered with a layer of mud up to his knees. The cellar has a very high ceiling but, accustomed to walking bent double he has great difficulty standing erect. He notices daylight in the distance above his head and wants to get out. He has to climb the wall using its rough surface. He falls two or three times and when, emerging through a kind of sewer, he reaches daylight, he is astonished to find himself in the street, immediately opposite the house he was trying to enter. He notices that the door is ajar. He goes in. Immediately a bell rings. Pandanleuil runs up. Gluglug hides behind a curtain. Gluglug wants to see the man and pulls back the curtain. It falls down and covers both of them. Paul struggles free and breaks a chair over Pandanleuil. Pandanleuil falls down. Gluglug dances with joy and bangs his head against the cornice. He falls down. Pandanleuil comes back at Gluglug and ties him up and then puts him into an enormous frying pan. Gluglug regains consciousness. Pandanleuil lights a fire under the pan. Gluglug is desperate and gives up hope. He weeps so profusely that he extinguishes the fire. Having lit the fire, Pandanleuil had left rubbing his hands. Gluglug uses his teeth to undo his bonds and jumps out of the frying pan. He is dirtier and dirtier. He is very hungry and gnaws the tassels of the curtain. Hunger assuaged, he moves towards the staircase. There is a thick layer of dust on the stairs. To avoid leaving the trace of his footsteps in the dust, he goes up on his hands. On the first floor he stands upright again and knocks over a vase, which breaks. A door opens and 'mother Volauvent' comes out. He notices through the half-open door a child's hand and is in no doubt that he has found the house where they are being kept prisoner. The old woman looks upwards. Gluglug takes the chance to slip under her skirts. He lifts her onto his shoulders, throws her down the stairs and enters the room. The old woman falls down the stairs, bouncing from step to step as if she were made of rubber and falls head first into the frying pan. Gluglug grabs the two children and is all ready to run away when Pandanleuil emerges from a wardrobe with an enormous club in his hand and knocks him out. He shuts the two children up in the wardrobe, leaves the room and locks it. When Gluglug comes to, the room is full of smoke and the children have cried so much that there is a long trickle of water that streams from the wardrobe, crosses the room and slides under the door. There is a fire. Gluglug smashes in the furniture before he notices that the children are in the wardrobe. He takes one under each arm and is all prepared to leave. The door is locked. The ceiling falls in. Pandanleuil rises from the ruins, with a club in his hand. After a struggle Gluglug kills him with a panel from the wardrobe. Gluglug tries to use the panel to break down the door. He holds it so awkwardly that he hits his own head and produces an enormous lump on his crown. The children cry harder and harder. Water rises in the room. It reaches Gluglug's ankles and pieces of wood start to float. Gluglug now holds the panel under his arm, but when he hits the door, the panel slides through his arm and he hits his head on the door. A new lump on his forehead. Finally he breaks down the door by kicking it, not without hurting his knees and tearing his trousers. His foot is trapped in the panel of the door. After a long struggle he manages to free himself, and falls on Pandanleuil. Because of the heat, the latter's stomach has swollen, and, when Gluglug falls on him, it explodes. The intestines come out. Gluglug takes the children and prepares to leave by the staircase, with one of the children still crying, under each arm. The staircase is on fire. He comes back quickly. He hears the fire engines approaching. Will they arrive in time? Gluglug is desperate. He searches for a way to escape death and looks all round. Suddenly he sees Pandanleuil's intestines. He unrolls them. There are metres and metres and they stretch like rubber. Gluglug attaches one end of the intestine to the balcony and one of the children to the other end and lowers it carefully; then a flame burns his hands. He drops everything. The child falls and is buried in the ground. Only its head sticks out. Two men start to pull the child out by the head. They tear off the head and fall over backwards. Piece by piece they pull it out. Then they stick it together again with glue. The child runs away as fast as it can but is caught by a policeman who, as he hurls himself forwards, loses his helmet, his coat and his white stick. The intestine rebounds. Gluglug ties the other child onto it and starts to lower it. The firemen arrive and the hoses are turned on. He lets slip the child, who is caught by the one of the hoses and dances in the jet of water like eggs in the firing range of country fairs. Another fireman has to climb up the hose, and, placing his hand over the nozzle, stops the water jet so that the child reaches the ground. It is now Gluglug's turn to hold on to the intestine, but, as he is heavy, he falls several metres very suddenly and swings vertically. The half-way down the intestine breaks between his stretched out arms. He remains suspended by one hand, with the rest of the intestine in the other. From below people pull on the intestine and Gluglug's body breaks in half. One part falls to the ground, while the other remains hanging from the intestine. With the help of pruning shears like those used by gardeners to reach the top branches of a tree, one fireman cuts the intestine, while the other seizes half Gluglug's body, like butchers unhooking a carcass of meat. The two halves are put together and fastened with the help of enormous nails which come out on the other side of his body. Gluglug, who has come to his senses, cuts them off with his penknife. Then he pulls out the nails, which he breaks and sucks like gum. He goes off with the two children, whom he returns to their parents. Joy of the parents. Gluglug smiles. They ask him to choose a reward. He wants a car. With the car, he goes off in search of Bonny, kisses her and carries her away.

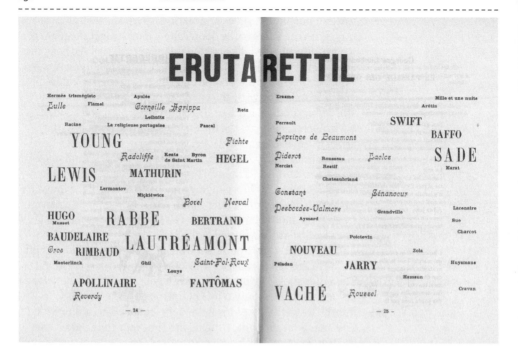

Nos. 11 and 12, October 1923
Robert Desnos
Elegant Canticle of Salome Salomon

Translated by
Timothy Adès

My miaow more maimed, my mitts may mime
Nerves knots not nicknacks. Nor, north, gnaw
My mellow marrow's amorous mammaries?
No naked knocker nun nor Ninny no.

Where's Nineveh on the Mamma Mundi?
My mates, my mer-mam murmurs me:
'One's Niles annihilate one's natally niveal nights.'
O murmur, maimed mummy, immure my Om:
Nothingness, name, nor nerve, nay, naught have I none!

N M EE   Enemies
& E M NN   Endearments
N M EE   Enemies
& E M NN   Endearments

51
'Erutarettil'
Littérature New Series
Nos. 11/12
October 1923

6.1 *Die Schammade* April 1920

Die Schammade
Emily Hage

Eager to become a part of the Dada movement, Max Ernst and Johannes Theodor Baargeld[1] produced *Die Schammade* with the help of Hans Arp in Cologne in April 1920. Only one issue was published. Baargeld's father, a wealthy local businessman, funded the publication. The title is a neologism that has been interpreted in many ways, an ambiguity no doubt intended by Ernst. *Die Schammade* includes declarations and essays by Ernst and Baargeld, Hans Arp, Walter Serner and Richard Huelsenbeck, as well as poems by Francis Picabia, Louis Aragon, André Breton and Tristan Tzara, including 'Proclamation sans Prétention' and 'Bulletin'.

The images in this Cologne publication reflect the international scope of the Dada movement after the war. On the cover is an abstract, organically shaped woodcut by Hans Arp. Inside is a mechanical drawing by Angelika Hoerle that resembles contemporary works by Ernst and Giorgio de Chirico. A photograph shows Baargeld's *Anthropophile Tapeworm*, which combines found objects such as a frying pan, springs and a bell mounted on to a piece of wood. The only image from outside Cologne is Picabia's line drawing made up of vaguely mechanical parts, entitled, *Round Eye*. What it depicts exactly is difficult to discern, and the words that label it are only somewhat helpful in determining the meaning of the drawing. Pin-up photographs of women in tight-fitting suits posing with bicycles, one of which is identified, in English, as 'the beauty American cyclist' (sic), add a popular, and at the time pornographic, flourish to the publication.

Die Schammade features two collages by Ernst from 1919 and 1920: *Dada* and *Hypertrophic Trophy*, the title of which is given in German, French and English. Ernst and Baargeld set out to make their journal an international Dada publication, evident in advertisements for Dada journals and books by Dadas in Paris and Berlin. The primary organ of the Dadas in Cologne, *Die Schammade* exhibits their desire to participate in the movement. It served as a creative venue in which they presented their distinctive interpretation of Dada after the war, a time when the movement continued to expand and diversify.

Die Schammade
Cologne
April 1920

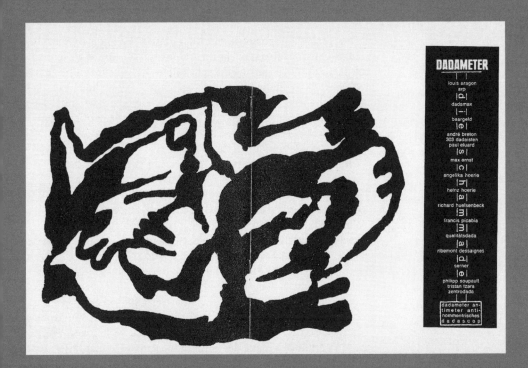

Cover (front and back)
Die Schammade
April 1920

Translated from
the German
by Jane Ennis

Johannes Baargeld
Tubular Settlement or Gothic

'asphalt is a mole'
Willi Hausenstein

Jazz, jazzband, tapeworm. The juicy boys of the Thomist Sixth
Form, or expressive speculative architects, have come up against
by-law 2333/1920 during the renovation of their continuous paid
work. At 11.30 on the morning of 15 January, the Podrekt was
personally baked by communal building apprentice moritz
remond, and the sanding of the tube system was negotiated by
the crowd outside Cologne Cathedral. After the
philopornographic bell of the bond agreement had been taken by
pumping the frozen trousers into position, the pornodidact,
currently stinging outside prison, declared in smokeless
solemnity the empathy of communal Gothic to be the dismantling
of marriage, and proceeded to the nationalisation of his wife.
Whilst albert einstein and the Socialist woman auguste rodin
crochet congratulatory telegrams, the central W/3 of the Dada
movement saws a comparison from the floor of tubular
architecture for the annual voluntary diocesan derby. The
constituencies will be allocated according to whether the vaults of
the Eiffel Tower are to be buried; this is an exposed cellar, and
contravenes the depression of the provisional business tube law.
      The cosmopolite leo sefwet has married his beloved. The
happy couple has made the acquaintance of the headquarters
W/3 for tube tincture colouring, with the help of a cop who forms
a psycho-parallel epitaph to the day by placing tubes against the
firewalls and backsides of the houses in his district. The secret
ballot of the 'location expansion' of Dada Maschke B.D.B has
erected a flat anatomical ornamental observation post in the trees
of the pet cancellation department (Nippe, Schiefersburgerweg
150-4, Tel: A4491). The Institute intends to finish chewing up the
ornamental canon of tubular aphrotecture with the addition of
outgrowths, abnormal hair-growths, filth stones and pearl
installations to the female nude. The cinema violet clever
hasenfalter has been watered by his son. Hasenwalter has been
constipated in Sylt with his son as a consequence of seducing the
Dadaist johann c. rubiner in the tubular housing scheme. As a
result of the January high tides, the vases belonging to the
Dadaist rosa meerfelt have shattered. The consumers'
association has therefore proposed the canary-isation of the head
of department by canary rollers. Nevertheless, the Propagandist
of Interjection, Prof. wilh. Fachinger-bonn has impoverished the
expressionist painting of his wife's life in the meeting of nursery
nurse diploma students. At 3.15 in the afternoon, Archbishop Dr
Shulte waved the deeply moved altar piece "my only passion"
twice through the offices of the cathedral chapter. The Satinist

hans arp, emissary of the International Committee D, has discussed the *amor intellectualis dei* with the Nitte of the philathlete Prof. Leopold von schaler. By contrast, in his next publication the amorous philathlete intends to lay a track for the mounds of the Augustinian tube synthesis. arp claims to have reached the conclusion that Gothic is an erective vomitation resulting from rotten teeth, and is travelling to a drainage outlet with the help of the tubular system. The Zurich branch of the Dadaist movement has exchanged 920 horsehair sausages with students in the Rhineland studying social compost. Tubular architecture must be on and in the tubes. Tubular limbs. annie besant stands tubes. Wieland Heartfield (misappropriated from English by the Cologne Society of Art, Edition A) stands tubes. Stand tubes! Collaborate! Standing tubes. Gothic is the grimacing exhibitionism of concrete eggs. A Gothic artist is a suicide in sexual disguise.

Collabor, drilling tube, harmful tube, röhrl, rrrrrrumpfsdada.

Translated from the German by Jean Boase-Beier

Hans Arp
From *"Superior Cockatoo"*[1]

the electric storms go put put put
and the glazing cracks off the astrolabe
the fire-gnome at the little fire desk throws his chequered die and springpromises now
the now ten spots
vast icelandscapes hang like huge silver puffs up in the dark green sky
minute medlaring minavonbarnhelm bitzbarvonbarnhelm von holzhelm helmholz huh huh
an ancient fearfully kept nuns' secret lets even the old play piano with ease
a new enormous strength
strange influence of a book on america
a stream of fire courses their veins and they say at last what I've wanted is here

tangled youths blow the horn of marvels
angels in golden shoes empty sacks of red stones into every eye every limb
and poles form and starimages
nuns show signs of aircastles goldcats foundlings steamcownips saddled
hares freshly upholstered lions
on flaming spokes birds roll across the sky
stars sneeze from their waxnosed flower sheathes
mice and men are drunk and swim on soft fingers
burning lions rush over trembling birches
those who have a tail fix a lantern to it

53
Hans Arp, wood relief,
and anon. pin-up photo
Die Schammade
April 1920

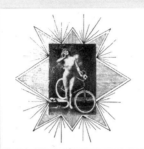

Die pensées sans langage sind der Mastarm der obersten poésie élektric und tugendübung sie enthalten die stücke die jeder Mensch kennen muß zur Erlangung der ewigen Seligkeit unaufhörlich rollen die roßapfelsinen aus dem mystischen Spund in die wassermannschen blutkloben des dörrigen lesers sie verfärben sich porfyrn du meinst es wäre ein Gletscherschis.   crest

quelles charmantes gens les artistes
attachés aus brancards de l'art
je n'ai pas un sou pour acheter une œuvre d'art

lisez mon petit livre
après avoir fait l'amour
devant la cheminée de caoutchouc
décor nouveau de dévouement
vision que la sagesse marque
de bonne cuisine
grimper dans les milieux sportifs
avec un fil de soie Tenor
bonsculer les sexes
avec un éclat de rire
l'éminent peintre moderne
sourit de son talent
ayant servi aux autres
agent de livraison
d'ameublement intrigue
dans une beauté fatale
c'est la plus belle occasion
d'alarme nouvelle
pour tourner le dos

Francis Picabia
aux pensées sans langage

arp

all night long they stand on their heads dancing mounted on
dragons climb poles and bodily wrestling fills the night with
bowwow
in the waterpulpits the acrobats shift their flags as in figure 5
adventurers with false beards and diamonded hooves went
snowing up to the platform on inflated whaleskins
the huge ghost-lion harun-al-raschid or rather harung-al-radi
yawned three times and showed his
teeth black with smoke
the mercerised rattlesnakes unravelled from their reels and
mowed their grain and buried it in stones
out of the hem of death the eyes of young stars stepped out
after flagellation on their suncheeks the hooves of a donkey
danced on bottleheads
blood and death fell like flakes from the leather towers
how many skeletons turned the wheels of the gates
when the waterfall had crowed three times the wallpaper paled
right down to the blood and the sailors' matrix burst

barriers rose from the deep and spread their anchors out
and at last the sea dared to brave the weakness of bitter
compasses
in the leafy forests the fretsaws of crashed birds chirp
the vermilion cup-animals spoon into one another like chinese
boxes
the marionette stars and flowers and figures cut their cords
the cartesian divers plunge in their morocco leather coaches into
the saltbaths that are more beautiful
than the gardens of louis the 14th
slowly I climb the milestick
and I lay my eggs in the knotholes of the milestick.

everywhere now dadas are standing up
but they are only muffled defreggers
they imitate the lisping and the tongue-twitching of the
cloudpump
a fearsome writing-on-the-wall zeppelin is prepared for them and
the dada resident band
will play for them
they will be thrown to the caterpillars to eat
and they will have beard transplants in all the wrong places
they will hang on star lassoos
THE ONLY ORIGINAL DADAISTS ARE THE SPIEGELGASSE
DADAISTS
beware of imitations
ask in bookshops only for spiegelgasse dadaists or at least for
works sprayed
with aquadadatint by the dadaist rasputin and spiritual head tzar
tristan.
though the moon hangs across from me like a mirror the angel in
my eye gives me pain
seeds collect on the tables and when you drum upon the plants
the flowers spring out
lions die in front of their sentry-boxes with diamond-filled
watering cans between their claws
the leaders wear wooden aprons
the birds wear wooden shoes
the birds are full of echoes
unceasingly the eggs roll from their little hearts
the crowns of their heads carry heaven's mast
the soles of their feet stand upon striding flames
when the snow-chain breaks then they call out to the good lord
when the wheel of heaven sinks then their hooves trample on
black grains

on the orders of the one who rests more sweetly than all the
women under the fountain the dolls were anaesthetised
then the children played at calf-park in the son-in-law's mythic halls
the song of the little ones burst open the corset that enclosed
god's genitals

with thread-thin toes they jangled the heart that hung helpless on
the tree of blood
in the cages flowers roared
the moon's white tails waved
the wooden beard sawed at the rim of a bell
stallions hung with grapes pranced across roof gardens
the pope's bann-servers turned round on their hubs gathered
sardines for sails and put a sourdine on their vocal cords
stomachs grazed over the combs of birds
night wielded its owl-spade
stars glowed through ships of wax
in the mountains baskets of gall were put out for the walkers
the electric hunts set off

seraphim and cherubim follow their leaders up and down white
ladders and do not know why
strong animals stride on balls of cotton wool sieve glowing coals
onto beds throw spears at the feathered humps and pile stones on
signposts
the children pull on their deathboots and wait for time that melts
into little black sledges and boxes and wait for the cosmetic lions
with thin wire tails full of little knots
in the injury-seats the whitewashed dead sit clap their hands and
bark huge birds bellow in chasms of wood
no-one can find the traces of their childhood shoes
the pistils fall from the stars the stars jerk in their birdhouses the
stars split and spit out fakes the muscles of the stars tear in two
the boneless princes flow like dough round the wheels of midnight
but in a metal tent sits the giantess ironhead with the false calves
a community board and an owl the giantess pulls her top hat of
fire her top hat of smoke on her head and bows and speaks so
jolly jolly jolly and so the globe will
become transparent and float as in a jar of fish with the magistri
horti deliciarum in it
the gates of the world open and close
the wax doll time flows away
unceasingly the übernothing shoots at the egg-chimer
                          arp
gross minus tare equals net

Translated from
the German
by Jane Ennis

Max Ernst
Worringer, Profetor Dadaisticus

6 a.m. The prophet listens to the seashell and hears the *furor
dadaisticus* of the new deep-drinking society. hihi
missa exhibitionalis in the invisible cathedral for intellectuals
and private prophets. titi
9.17– 9.25 *ambigente* and appreciation of the wandering
madhouse kokoschka in goose slippers. lilili
9.26–10.13 Is humanity good *a priori* in relation to the new
human contuorbine [sic] Dada? fiffi
10.14–10.14 *ubi bene ibi Dada* pippi bibbi
10.14 Photograph of the everlasting hodelie of gothic lilli in Irish
vestments. minni
Today red, tomorrow gothic mimmi. kri
10.16–11.9 with the right hand finger of empathy – Dada in, Dada
out – but!! willi
11.10 a.m.–5.23 p.m. *unio expressiva erotica et logetica* or the
mating convulsions of Brother pablo mysticus and Sister
scholastica Feiniger or Picasso's ethics. killi killi
6.pm *picastrate Eum*!

Translated from
the German by
Jean Boase-Beier

Johannes Baargeld
Bellresonance II

Soldier's letter ricocheted from a crisis sky
Blind bat starspotting crosslaid need
Berling himself keeps the mother-tongs in line
Ragrug moon and shifting shine
Moleskin trousers flag the cactus vine.

Lambs' fiddles drawn on a washing line
Washing woes draw spring and fold
Cigarrinds scrawled upon the old
Weathergnome scratching at her thigh
Till all the bellvoices die

Bergamots moth in a petrol sky
Swan candles angle masty cloud
Teleplastic the stares of the sinubic crowd
Into the wideopen heartplaces
The skybell inraces

Translated from
the French
by Timothy Adès

Tristan Tzara
Aragon house

arp and the barbered arbour
in the free night resuscitate
in the special australian kangaroo pocket edition
arp and the arc barque
are framed for semiramis
arp the arc and the arbour-barbered barque
creak – Chronometer

Translated from
French by
Timothy Adès

André Breton
All that is mysterious

the fighting Cocks of Jerome
  a breaking of bans followed by prospectus
   black sand
    mouldings from paradise
     solar inspection then real coolness
      i dream of summer in the dormitory
        they asked meWhat do you have where your heart should be

Cannibale, Z1, Projecteur and Le Cœur à barbe

Dawn Ades

A flurry of little magazines accompanied Dada's high season in Paris in the spring of 1920. Picabia produced two issues of the aptly named *Cannibale*, 25 April and 25 May 1920, one of the most ferocious Dada publications, despite its austere and elegant cover. It shared contributors with *391* but Picabia had a clear idea of the distinction between his two reviews: he seems to have regarded *391* as his personal creation and *Cannibale* rather in the nature of an official Dada production.

Two other single-issue magazines appeared, Céline Arnauld's *Projecteur* and her husband Paul Dermée's *Z1*. The format of *Projecteur* was very unusual – narrow and horizontal. It had no illustrations, while *Z1* included one drawing, an Ubu-inspired 'machine to clean out brains'.

Like *Littérature* and Tzara's *Dada intirol au grand air* the 'depository' for all these reviews was the bookshop Au Sans Pareil, run by Dada's official publisher René Hilsum. It was Hilsum who decided that a lot of little reviews would have a greater public impact than a single one, and the Dadaists responded enthusiastically.

Cannibale
Paris
No 1, April 1920

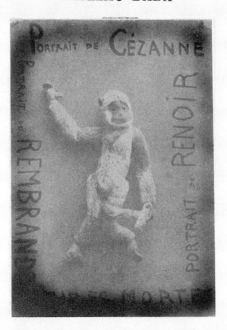

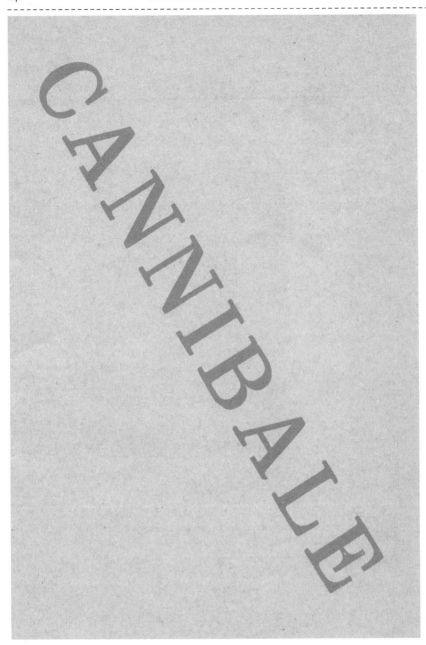

55
Front cover
Cannibale 2
May 1920

Translated from
the French
by Ian Monk

Francis Picabia
+ *AEROPHAGIA*
o *ARTERIOSCLEROSIS*
The refrain of what?

(2 male characters)

+ Your brother is a contour of eyelids.
o the eyebrow, the cheek, the revolver.
+ An unforgettable shadow.
o the image of Christ, of love, of pain against light?
+ Never! The fiancé as secret as a trickle of water, joined feet, cross yourself.
o Leave me, leave me, leave me!
+ You want some disguised body, I am now with you, victory to the dead.
o you are laughter as lukewarm as a wet dream, as a morning screw.
+ Light hurts me when I am separated from it, the crowd hurts me when I am pushed in the whirlwind by a gust, above the image of the Earth. Then, slowly, the engine reddens, thousands and thousands in the mortal play of oakum explode like a bell. Speed, speed, golden muscles, then a bloodless sting stuck with hands in a white and red machine shaped like an arch like a man for both of them.
o How pale you are beneath, your ear, your neck, your wild radiator by the new moon will never happen; it is too horrible, we will never arrive because my ankle is twisted and hurts so much.
+ It is as nervous as teeth, like the rose for another, you are the face of passion, of new expectation, when?
o I am the face with closed eyes and unknown sleep, I have the decapitated head of elation.
+ Do you want me to undress you?
I undressed myself with scissor snips for my female vulture while waiting for the car.
o Oh how beautiful!
The reminder of a fortune with its hands behind its back.
+ The smell of your cigarette hurts me, you are blowing the smoke my way, and I too smoke memories ...
+ In the darkness?
o no, in broad daylight.
+ So are you blind?
o yes, like the swallows.
+ But which are your eyes?
o the nostrils of my nose that have long hairs, you will see.
+ Everywhere, everywhere, everywhere, everywhere, *Arteriosclerosis*, elations and audacity on their knees.
o all the ground is smiling at the melancholy melody of my sobs, don't pass by!
+ I beg of you, I beg of you, I beg of you –

7.2

Z1, Paris, March 1920
Paul Dermée
What is Dada!

Translated from
the French
by Ian Monk

Everything is dada.
Everyone has a dada.
You will venerate those dadas that you have turned into gods.
The dadaists know their dadas and care not. That is the great
superiority they have over you.

Dada is not a literary school nor an aesthetic doctrine.

***

Dada is an utterly a-religious attitude, like that of the scientist
with his eye stuck on his microscope,

Dada is irritated by those who write 'Art', 'Beauty', 'Truth'
with capital letters and who turn them into entities that are
superior to man, Dada ridicules capitalisers atrociously.

Dada ruining the authority of constraints tends to liberate
the natural game of our activities. Dada thus leads to amorality
and the most spontaneous, and thus the least logical, lyricism.
This lyricism is expressed in life in a thousand ways.

Dada strips clean the thick layer of filth that has settled on
us over the centuries.

Dada destroys and limits itself to that.

May Dada help us make a clean slate, then each of us will
build a modern house with central heating and access to the
sewers, dadas in 1920.

PAUL DERMÉE
Cartesian Dadaist

Projecteur
Paris
21 May 1920

Translated from
the French
by Ian Monk

Céline Arnauld
Particulars

Tristan Tzara is never, never, never in a brown study, so ...
Louis Aragon is not liked by everyone, lucky man ...
Philippe Soupault is Paul Souday's neighbour at the theatre of Le
Vieux Colombier, that is the way with alphabetical order. The
other evening, Philippe said to Paul: 'Don't you think we'd be
better off in a b ... ?' Paul blushed and listened obstinately all the
way through the play.
   Francis Picabia kneads clay.
   Paul Dermée has made a rhymed parable with the iron
springs of armchairs. The upholsterers will once again accuse
him of theft.
   Georges Ribemont-Dessaignes is not a mute canary, and
don't forget it. Consultations: 10 francs.
   Paul Eluard is large enough to rejuvenate the Pont-Neuf.
He is Paul Draule's father.[1]
   André Breton is becoming the moralist of the dada
movement. Who will be its aesthetician?
   Céline Arnauld has already killed off two reviews:
M'Amenez-y: and Ipeca are today unobtainable.[2] Do not press
the point, Mr Doucet ... they are utterly unobtainable.[3] P.D.[4]

Translated from
the French
by Ian Monk

Céline Arnauld
Luna Park

Sinister display of that optical mirror
stuck on my shoulder
photophorous horoscope of bad days
tattoo of my enemies
submerged at the bottom of sad reservoirs
crystallised by rapid lightning

Lay hands stretch out immoderately
to grasp the flower
barge of rumours on the ocean
dreamers' bagpipes

In their fort the snails
turn the wheel of the universe

But the spontaneity of feelings
in life ...
It is the hydra sunk
on the one twaddle of racecourses
godsend of mirrors in palaces

In Luna Park one jungles
with hearts of crystal
The horoscope in beakers
listens to the mime artists speak ...

Do not distrust me
I am only the fleeting reflection
of the projector
morning song with a megaphone

Translated from
the French
by Ian Monk

Louis Aragon
White Coffee

'Hand me the red-headed diver, the spirits.'
'Dear friend, give up this delicious but deadly passion. I do not want to encourage such a singular aberration.'
'Well, believe me if you will, but I can sleep only in the labyrinth of guilloche-style mirrors where they serve refreshments and liquid flowers to idlers who have wandered for a moment into those perfidious grottoes. There, my heart turns and throws my blood like a coffee machine.'
'What fine metal.'
'The taps emit a steam that is less sad than the eyes of the woman slumped on the dancing seat. The leathers of Russia, the woods of the islands, the spheres of mistletoe, the mosaics, the best furbished stoves, the vertigos come down from heaven on rivers of liquor, the draped staircases, the counters help to create the little palace of my dreams.'
'The hanging overcoat starts looking like a reproach.'
'We have left the characters of convention in the cloakroom.'
'Play cards, that's what is healthy, exalting, highly appreciated by most men.'
'There is also the tobacco that grows on lips with beautiful scarves. The robin, my neighbour, has fine ties at 4 francs 95 and fresh smiles for one's entourage.'
'It is a dry river before its cup of hot chocolate.'
'There are no more rivers but streams of linen flower infusions which run between the happy couples of public moments devoted to lay gods or pink marble where carefully chiselled cocks are sleeping along with several naive feelings.'
'Photographs do not prevent feelings.'
'Alas, I am always afraid of the small sweet waves made by the dear breasts of two-bit Eleonores.'
'Hush, let's not talk about it. There are still branches of salvations in the florists', in the forest of Meudon. You will not get it out of my mind that the most beautiful girls in the world have not yet been given over to advertising.'
'The white gloves of proposing, what a bore.'

'A stone habit, politeness. You say hello sure enough to the dead in the street.'

'Here, no servile head movements. Welcome all the birds with cries. The dry Turin of stares. Let go blotter and die. Barman, a Kümmel! And without love, no?'

Translated from the French by Dawn Ades

Festival Dada [1]

Wednesday, 26 May 1920

1
1   *Dada's sex*
2   *painless fight* BY Paul Dermée
3   *the famous illusionist* Philippe Soupault
4   *strong manner* Paul Eluard
5   *the navel interloper* music by Ribemont-Dessaignes performed by Miss M. Buffet
6   *long-sighted festival manifesto* Francis Picabia
7   *corridor* Dr Serner
8   *the Rastaquero*   André Breton
9   *vast opera* Paul Draule
10 *the second adventure of M. Aa the antipyrine* Tristan Tzara

2
11 *you will forget me* sketch BY André Breton and Philippe Soupault
12 *American nurse* Francis Picabia
13 *baccarat manifesto* Georges Ribemont-Dessaignes
14 *chess game* Céline Arnauld
15 *frontier dance* Georges Ribemont-Dessaignes
16 *DD system* Louis Aragon
17 *I am Javanese* Francis Picabia
18 *public weight* Paul Eluard
19 *symphonic vaseline* Tristan Tzara

Le Cœur à barbe[1]
Paris
April 1922

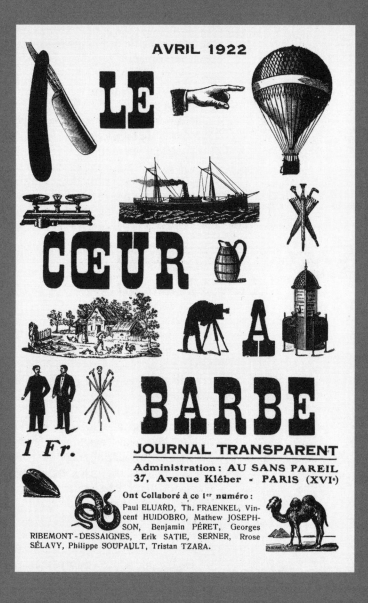

Front cover
Le Cœur à barbe
April 1922

Translated from
the French
by Ian Monk

Eluard, Ribemont-Dessaignes, Tzara
To Make the Heart Grow

These eight pages, at the dawn of the twentieth century, will open
the eyes of countless readers. The 'bearded heart' will contain no
literature or poetry. We know that divorce is a genre that
sometimes better expresses the state of mind of a minor period
such as the one we are going through in carefree ease. We do not
know why we cannot guarantee the regular publication of this
review. But the armies of occupation that we are keeping up at
great expense on the back of our activities, the spies and the
apoplectic, the wrappers and the mages, the impalers and the
enveloped, the fiancés and the false brethren will never remove
the gold from our mouths.

The faces of bankrupts attract credit like feet attract shit.

None of our contributors commits his neighbour to what he
has said here. A few people's affirmations are proof that our
omnibus is only a journal without a mudguard.

Translated from
the French
by Ian Monk

Erik Satie
A Mammal's Notebooks (Extracts)

Yes: ... The Germans take everything from France ... How
shameful! ...
As you know, Wagner was French ... He was very Franco-German
– the dear fellow – like all good Frenchmen, in fact ...
Remember ... please ... He was so wonderful! ... and so 'one of us'!
...
For he must not be confused with Strauss or Schoenberg ...
Nothing like them ... at all.
They are not wonderful, of course – or French, naturally.
At the 'Two Purists': ... Next time, it will be a painting by
Jeanneret[1] that will be lacerated ...
Wait your turn, – no? ...
Not always the same ... isn't it?

Decentralisation: ... Congratulations to Mr Rouché for having
turned the Opéra into a theatre that is absolutely provincial –
deeply provincial – and an utter success as imitations go ... You
can even picture yourself in the colonies (Djibouti) ...
Foreigners have been 'mummified' by it and 'cannot get over it' ...
How right they are! ...
What a wonder Mr Rouché is indeed!

Artful and inventive: ... Yes, it is Ozenfant who is the craftier of the
two – without overdoing it; – but do not imagine that 'the other

one' is dumb – with his low vision ...
In any case ... they are as 'Purist' as each other – more so, even.

Precision ... As regards Reims ... let us not exaggerate ...
   The cathedral was an old, outdated and uncomfortable building.
The means: ... It was Ozenfant who had the idea of using the penknife; ... As for Jeanneret, he was talking about using a sabre (this long) ...
   How young he is! – the dear fellow...

My mistake: ... Of course! ... Ravel is not a 'pawn' ... indeed not ...
He just looks like one – but only when seen from a distance ... a very great distance ...
   He is more of a 'dandy' – a tiny doddling dandy ... Indeed
     And so elegant!
     And so chic!
   We must be fair – for once.

The man of the day: ... No, my dear Ozenfant: ... you are neither ridiculous nor grotesque...
     The penknife? ... Pooh! ...
     Fear not: ... 'life' goes on.

At the Opéra: ... *L'Heure espagnole* is a real success ... Old Ravel is reaping a triumph (like at Verdun) ... The theatre is always full of Spaniards (like at Verdun)...
   A few Portuguese have had the 'cheek' to mingle in with this Hispanic crowd, ... but they were 'spotted' at once: ... their traditional merriment gave them away ... it contrasts with the beautiful Spanish sadness contained in the work of the extremely subtle composer-soldier (a true 'bore' – the extremely subtle composer-soldier! – if I might say so between brackets).

How terribly sad: ... My subscription to *L'Esprit nouveau* has just expired ... yesterday ...
     Yes ...
    I am quite 'out to sea'.

Translated from the French by Ian Monk

Tristan Tzara
Second Class Tickets

The adventurers of Adventure are just adventurers. The characteristic of adventurists is that they have had an utterly unfunny adventure. They have written as many poems as they have met in their lives.
   Eluard is my high-class whore.
   We demand a law by which articles written by Gilbert Maire and other idiotic things of the same sort will earn their author

several months' imprisonment and a considerable fine. Although it is not by laws against syntax that the genius of a race will be affirmed. Impotence has always driven people towards the worst forms of excess. But the boredom that is given off makes them harmless.

The good is to the left, evil to the right, Mr Francis in the middle.

Hélène telephones better.

How can the advertisement for a brand of cigarette papers, in Vienna, give a name to a man in Neuilly?

We know Totor. His name is Marcel Duchamp. There are people who are afraid that Totor will speak. Totor stays silent. Care is taken of him, and his name is not even printed any more without his permission. – But Totor has spoken ...

My dear Huelsenbeck, some imbeciles are dragging your name through the mud. The 'bourzouc' you mention in that book which has been so good to me has bitten their testicles. There are few things that pish me off more than the absolute, freedom of choice, the almost and

Dear Arp. We have been waiting for you a long time, but are sure that you will come along one day just as the sun comes too; there is no need for the grammar of months and trains. Like you, botanists plant pocket mirrors. To reflect the cloud of the earth in its root of darkness. We feed on it and easily spend the gallop of gazes in the wind that overtakes us.

Bleu
Emily Hage

Published in Mantua in 1920 and 1921, *Bleu* introduced the Dada movement to Italian audiences. Although its editors, Gino Cantarelli and Aldo Fiozzi, did not identify themselves with Dada directly, painter and poet Julius Evola used *Bleu* to promote the movement. He did so by contributing his own poems and essays about Dada as well as drawings and texts by recognised Dadaists. The second issue, for instance, presents two Picabia-like diagrams, Johannes Baargeld's 'The Dada Airship' and Max Ernst's 'Parafulmine giurabacca dei dada arp tzara ERNST baargeld picabia ecc', both of which are labelled with nonsensically combined German and French words. These Dada images, with their unorthodox style and subject matter, contrast with works by Italian artists that are also reproduced in *Bleu*. Examples include a drawing on the cover of the first issue, entitled simply, *Study*, by Lucio Vènna, which depicts a nude woman on a landscape, and a vaguely Cubist drawing, *Female Nude* by Ivo Pannaggi on the cover of *Bleu 3*. In addition to essays about the Dada movement by Parisian journalist Renée Dunan, *Bleu* includes many texts by Paris Dadaists. For example, an Italian translation of Louis Aragon's essay, 'Sensational Revelations', which had been printed in the May 1920 issue of *Littérature*, appears in *Bleu 2*. Although Aragon's text does not mention Dada, Evola gave it the subtitle, 'Manifesto of the Dada Movement', thus presenting it as an explanation of the movement. The second issue of *Bleu* features Georges Ribemont-Dessaignes's essay on Tristan Tzara, Paul Dermée's description of Fernand Léger, a well as various poems and texts by writers and artists associated with the Dada movement, namely Paul Eluard, Pierre Reverdy, and 'I.K. Bonset', Theo van Doesburg's Dada pseudonym. The third and final issue of *Bleu* is the most aggressively Dada. In his cover essay, Evola quotes Tzara's seminal 1918 Dada manifesto, and on a page entitled, 'Paris Rome Dada', he publishes his poem, 'Dada Paesaggio', with poems by Tzara, Francis Picabia and Walter Serner, thus linking himself with these more established members of the Dada movement. *Bleu 3* also features poems by Ribemont-Dessaignes, Eluard, Aragon and Céline Arnauld, publisher of the journal *Projecteur*. The final issue of *Bleu*, published in January 1921, launched what Evola called a 'Dada Season' of exhibitions and performances in Rome. In July 1921, however, Evola abruptly and inexplicably ceased all Dada activity in Italy. His brief, idiosyncratic engagement with Dada exemplifies how Dada journals spawned increasingly widespread and diverse interpretations of the movement.

8.1

No.2, 1920
Communications Bleu – Note 1

Translated from
the Italian
by Emily Hage

1. Ideas are the stupidest burden that hangs over humanity: when they are big they are painful – when they are small they are idiotic: all of them are the origin of and the reason for vain effort.

2. Between two types of happiness: one is eternal and the other is transient, we would not hesitate to choose the one that does not last as long: but how would you know?

3. All the desires of the suffragettes, gathered from every part of the world to the Geneva conference to claim sex rights, are contained in Mafarka's male member, natural son of F. T. Marinetti: everyone knows it, but nobody says it: why?

4. Stealing is in man as seed is in sperm, as doubt in the reasoning mind: motive power's inexorable fertilising germ. The law that punishes it is only for the coward that fears it; this cowardice created the emperor and the street sweeper, the cotton socks and the silk ones.

Only where there is no law, there is freedom of life that is freedom to steal: Nicholas II who was czar and street sweeper lived all ages and all lives, as his people who at noon ruled and at night died: what beautiful freedom!

And so: if there has never been a man who resisted the temptation of stealing, why do men create laws to punish it?

5. All human unhappiness streams from one incomprehensible truth: $2 + 2 = 4$: why? If it were not in this manner, today we would be rich enough to lie with the most beautiful woman of our country.

6. Education of all times has tried to make women an uneasy conquest object, to surround them with an allure that they do not possess naturally; remedy: possess them anywhere you run into them: and the reluctant ones condemned to chastity for life.

7. To a brother who died fighting we promised to kill who killed him: we met 10 times the assassin: 3 times we watched him, 7 times we greeted him; yesterday the assassin wore a monocle: when will we kill him?

8.2

No.3, January 1921
Either it is well or it is not well: see for yourselves Ladies, Gentlemen!

Translated from
the Italian
by Emily Hage

From the newspapers:
1. Milan, 14 January 1921 – Marinetti, the famous founder of Futurism, disappeared. His removal seems to be due to fear of being arrested for the famous Fascist anarchical conspiracy.
2. Paris, 14 January 1921 – Futurists and Dadaists clashed tonight

---

at Marinetti's conference, whose purpose was to explain to the
Parisians the mysteries of Tactilism.

We:

1. Since Marinetti is so prodigiously versatile in solving mysteries,
can he explain to us the mystery of his unexpected flight (alias
removal) from Milan, whereas days before he sent a telegram to
the Prime Minister of Italy, demanding in the name of all (?)
Italian Futurists the release of the strongest agitator and
anarchist: Errico Malatesta?

On the other hand, in Paris he exalts the beauty of the
achievements of that straw hero who is the patriot d'Annunzio ...

2. With inexpressible childishness Marinetti proposed to explain
to those present at the small theatre of Lugné-Poë the mysteries
of his new Futurist art: Tactilism: but the Dadaists accused him of
being a worshipper of the past: and why not even an exalter? As a
matter of fact, Guillaume Apollinaire in a vivacious novel entitled,
Mon cher Ludovic published in "*Almanach des lettres et des arts
1917* – Martine, Paris" wrote:

'The dry, the damp, the wet, all the degrees of cold and hot,
the sticky, the thick, the tender, the soft, the hard, the elastic, the
oily, the silky, the velvety, the rough, the granular, etc. brought
together in an unexpected way, form the rich matter where my
dear Ludovic draws the subtle and sublime combinations of
tactile art: silent music that aggravates our nerves ...'

Come on! Isn't this Tactilism? And the new art, then?
Evidently, today Marinetti is not playing fair.

— **again, from the newspapers**: 'The Dadaists enjoy
seeing that the public cannot take Marinetti's Tactilism theories
seriously: but then they protest vehemently that they would not
want to be taken seriously either, but Marinetti says in retort that
his advantage over them is that he makes the public laugh for a
much longer time ...'

We: And today? ... Always?! At any rate, everyone is DADA, is it
not, Tzara? – at 7.30 p.m: dinner is ready: the appetiser has
already been served. Goodbye for the present.

N.B. J. Evola and Christian Schaad, Dadaists, are
organising a 'Jazz-band Dada ball' event in Rome in January and
February with the involvement of the best aristocracy and with
music by Stravinsky, Casella, Auric, Defosse, etc. Among the
attractions, a 'Hésitation' with simultaneous declamations of
Dante, a 'fox-trot' for percussion instruments and revolver shots,
etc.

This is going to be the first indirect DADA demonstration in
Italy; the second will take place in March at the Bragaglio Gallery,
and painter A. Fiozzi will also participate: in the Evola opening-
conference and various declamations.

Mécano
Dawn Ades

The four issues of *Mécano* are a particularly interesting instance of the Dada-Constructivist axis in post-war Europe. Published in Leiden, Holland, the review was fully international in scope with the collaboration of Dadaists in Germany and France.

Mécano announced on its cover that its literary editor was I.K. Bonset and its 'visual arts technician' (*mécanicien plastique*) Theo van Doesburg. The latter was well known as the editor of the magazine *De Stijl*; that they were one and the same person was a surprise to many of his colleagues. It was at the International Congress in Weimar, where Van Doesburg had gone in 1922 hoping to orient the Bauhaus towards Constructivism and away from Expressionism that his double identity was revealed. The Congress was reported in Dada style in *Mécano*: 'Injection of the dada virgin microbe to Weimar and to the Bauhausians.'[1]

Van Doesburg began planning a Dada review as early as 1920, and was in correspondence with Tristan Tzara. *Mécano* described itself as an 'ultraindividualistic, irregular international review for the diffusion of neo-Dada ideas and mental hygiene'.[2] Four perfectly choreographed issues appeared: the first three were single large folded sheets, each distinguished by a primary colour – Yellow (February 1922), Blue (July 1922) and Red (October 1922). Issues 4–5 (winter 1923), was white and had a more conventional magazine format.

Mécano's title encapsulates its dual allegiances. The reference could be to Francis Picabia's machine paintings and drawings, an example of which is reproduced in the Yellow issue (*Les dents viennent aux yeux comme des larmes* – Teeth come to the eyes like tears) as well as to Constructivism – not to forget the children's construction game, Meccano. The congruence is emphasised by Bonset's choice of illustrations, with for example Man Ray's *Danger/Dancer* (1920), a glass painting dominated by cogs, and Raoul Hausmann's *Tatlin at Home* (1920) and *Mechanical Head* (1919; here reproduced simply as 'Plastique') as well as Moholy-Nagy's *Nickel-Construction* (1921). Poems, manifestos and texts speak to the common interest in experiments with language, and the final issue includes a fragment of Kurt Schwitters's *Ursonata* (Fig No. 61).[3]

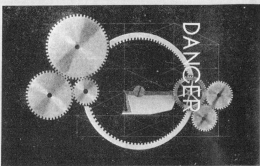

MAN RAY

NEW-YORK DADA

57
Mécano, Yellow
February 1922

Yellow, February 1922
I.K.Bonset
Antiartandpurereasonmanifesto

Translated from
the Dutch by
Michael White

Dedicated to the uneven,
floating temperature of Dada

Art and philosophy have been totally digested through the tiresome
repetition of ever one and the same theme. Europe is locked
between pure logic and the guitar. Academics and artists are bound
fast by the same rope. Each stands in his stall and above each stall
hangs a weather-beaten, creaking signboard. Imprisoned by the
spell of their fertile stupidity, artists and academics turn the worn-
out axle of the centrifugal drum of the stale, decent, bourgeois
intelligentsia. The intellectual themes clatter and turn around, spin
about, CARNIVAL of coloured slime, shit, tin and inflamed brains.
Pure logic and the guitar – the pure guitar and logic – guitarlogic –
logicguitar – logicicuitar – gicaloguitar – targuilocagi – gicaotargui –
lotarguigica – guitar, guitar, guitar, logic, logic, logic, logicanus,
ANUS. All that rattling and trotting after 'La Femme assise' and
round the 'Natures mortes', Kant-Hegel-Fichte-Schopenhauer-
Bolland-Spinoza[1] have no other significance than their own self-
inflation by means of so many difficult words and vanities, so that
for all this pretence, we should not fail to notice this appearing to be
something which is NOTHING. Nobody misses the chance to enjoy
himself at any hour without forgetting to look at the stopped clock
and thereby staining himself with decency, ethics and ALIBABA-
morality in the rock hard bedstead of his existence, he who calls
'life' a swear word. NOBODY HAS EVER SUCKED THIS SWEET
ENTIRELY without finding the temptation in it to – bite. Nicotine,
RADIO-MACARONI[2] and WHISKY-SODA are worth more to me
than the mushrooms your monks and churlish scholars grow in
their armpits. Small mouldy excrescences that they call pure reason
or spiritual aesthetic because they lack the power to turn their
heads around fast enough to see all of the world at once. It doesn't
matter if you are bremmerian,[3] bollandish or even havelaarish.[4] You
are castrated. All of you are eunuchs. Truly, you believe so strongly
and firmly in the logic of your own madness that you continually
forget the only healthy thought you may have found in your rock
hard cheesehead, to roll around for half and hour with your body
buttered (a thought that contains the idea that yes and no, full and
empty, pure illogic and impurelogic are the same thing). Dada is the
complete astringent cleansing to cure you of your art-and-logic
diarrhoea. Dada is the cork in the bottle of your stupidity. Do not
forget then, that the lead brainweight of your dialectic was not
porous enough to let even one single living and mobile thought, one
icefirethoughtpicture, through. You now know that everything is
not so. Dada knows it. And I tell you now that your intellectual
importance is of the same substance as the stony droppings you

find on your pillow each morning. And now that we have spoken the truth to each other, from anus to anus, I would like you to accept these small daggers from me as presents (I bought them in CALICANOURO). Do not strike the rivets of your soul with them. Rather slide them under the nail of your right index finger, like a bayonet in its sheath. You lick your lips in anticipation of a pornographic double entendre (what do you take me for?) that you thought you spotted and you carry off the well-packed rotten mackerel under your coat, already pleased with your imaginary catch. The rosy STUBBLEHEATHERBLOSSOMJAWBONE, which you have given a crystal clear humble thrashing for 20 centuries, sticks so far out over your flat chest that in future I will allow myself to use you as Dada's walking-stick.

Holland 31.1.1921

9.2

Blue, July 1922
I.K. Bonset
Dada Holland: Manifesto 0,96013

Translated from the Dutch by Michael White

I am without name without trunk without importance
I am everything and nothing without sex and without any
ambition
I am Rasta-failure[1] Bandit and isolated
With my feet my pipe and my cigar and
my shoes
I **spit** on all the youths who are imbecilic enough to
Believe in love art or science I hate these dimensions
of stupidity of vacant worlds and precocious
children with their **celluloid** skulls
I spit on all the phylosophers these **syphilosophers**
I spit on God-Jesus-Marx with their prayers
the **bamboo** eunuchs more irritating than
the small corpses of cats in the Dutch canals
I spit on all moralists
Christianity's urinals
I spit on artists papier-maché trinkets who
want to make a world of soft chocolate and of
perfumed shit
I spit   I spit   I spit
on all the revolutionary cockatoos with their nickel
brains

The World is a small Sperm Machine
Life – a venereal disease
All my prayers are dedicated
To Saint Venerica

Translated from
the Dutch by
Michael White

Blue, July 1922
I.K. Bonset
Archachitektonica[1]

(Inscription for the museum of Dr Berlage in The Hague)[2]
(very fast) hear hear how the architectonic swans sing their song in the ponds[3] on which floats the debris of Moorish Romanesque gothic baroqueroccocostyles nesting the rainbowrudiments (with and without tail) not already the monstered of the spoutknittingmachine of the **spoutknittingmachine** in the Capital of the capital[4] of the hotchpotchberlagestyle? The unwashed lousysnouts of unsurprisingly sensitive snotnoses (hey hey where is the toilet!) stick out of the Peekaboohatches bookapeephatches of this Moorish charnelhouseinstitute (echo: charnelhouseinstitute) the stockingbremmermaidens[5] (hirsute, bearded echo: tail) walk without winking blinking amidst this entrenched stupidity pretentious of impotence sleekly combed and weighty of paving slabs which they find behind their small barren skulls (hey hey where is the toilet then!).

      Oh architectonic skunks who grub your noses between the pylons of petrified waterlilies and the camouflaged font spouts architectonic firewater into the hall from which exudes the smell of the male Vagina.

Oh who here does not long for a buffet in this temple space (Café-Expresse!)[6] a mammoth hollow where every conceivable insanity of human artliverpaté lies heaped, around which are grouped the architectonic horsedroppings the architectonic horsedroppings because this is holland's great stone tombharmonica

	JAZZ
toot	B
toot	A
toot	N
	D

tick-tock – tick-tock

this is Holland's petrified cheesegable (one is requested before leaving to take this opportunity to put one's clothes in order) inflated and closed up tight edammer interrupted by the Windowpanecurrantloaf of

Widow of De Jong and Co.

Oh! The hall hall hall hole hole holecheese cheesehole cheese hat St Peter in which tactile hermaphrodites go pining for van Goghles.

Oh tropical corpse composed of skeletons and mummies of every bagpipe pasted bags. **BAG**

Nothing, apart from Dada, is strong enough to stamp this sleepy cucumberarchitecture into the ground.

Yes Yes

DADA

58
Mécano, Blue
July 1922

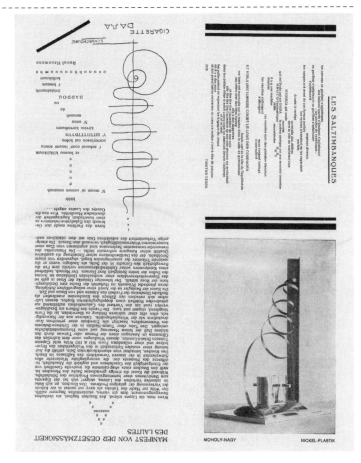

Red, October 1922
ChRoNIEk-MECANo

Translated from
the Dutch by
Michael White

Cablogramme
Weimar – Paris – Zurich – Budapest – Moscow
**International Congress of Constructivists and Dadaists
in Weimar 1922**
19. Sept. Tristan Tzara in Weimar – Soft temperature – Saint-
Siegenzack-arp's[1] flute is missing – 20. Sept. eighteen telegrams.
– 21. Sept. Tzara visits the house of sick artists 'Bauhaus' (Many
sick with the pip of Mazdaznan[2] and wireless expressionism) –
observation: Of the direction of 'De Stijl' in all creative domains.
Observations of the absolute impotence of the 'Masters'
(exclusively the director,[3] poor baby of his catastrophic impulses!)
– The students more endowed than their 'masters' – – 22. Drink –
drink – drink – drunk – 23. Schwitters's arrival – buys a postcard
at the Bauhaus and disappears up the chimney – In the Residenz
Café Kuwitter[4] is christened 'Sonniermerz' – In the evening a

general storming of Van Doesburg's studio. – Arp is still floating – somewhere 24. Arp arrives in Jena – Great move cross-country – Extra train with food and drink wagons. – Great expectation at the station The Jenarites have taken up position under the command of Dr Dexel[5] – Greeting from Jazz-band-Arp. Procession through the city. – 25. Return to Weimar. Injection of the virgin microbe dada in Weimar and in the Bauhausians.[6] – Bortniyk[7] has struggled for Dadaism in Hungary. Lissitzky-Moscow says to Dadaism: 'You have cut the bellybrain of the bourgeoisie from the inside.' – Rain of champagne. Madame – madame – madame – madame – madame – madame – madame – madame – madame – madame – madame – madame – madame – madame[8] – Arp has lost his flute in the Chat-noir – 26. After much pressure, the first Constructivist egg is laid by the international chicken. Moholy's dynamic egg is simultaneously a chicken. – 27. Pétro[9] is unanimously declared Europe's unmistakeable Dadaistic musical instrument. – Military march for a crocodile[10] in front of the museum. – Jena-hygiene-hyena-dada. Destruction of Jena by Kuwitter's scarf[11] – 28. dada tour of Germany from Munich to Hanover – The great Pra[12] travels back to Zurich on his flute.

Translated from the French by Ian Monk

Red, October 1922
Benjamin Péret
The child with the blond belly

It is when he discovers America and slips
road signs and nuns
It is because all these woes support one another
around his sunny greatness

The president of purchases buys 13 for 15
wears out his whiskers like glass
eats like a cat
pisses like a hotel

at the time when the youngest carburettor
uses the last bulrushes
for the last cake
The female hides in a flag
around a belly
beneath spectacles.

SAVANTS

Celui qui mange une purée d'yeux bleus
　　pour voir plus loin dans le ciel
Celui qui nourrit ses poissons rouges
　　avec du guano de perroquet et com-
　　prend leur langage
La sueur de cheval a la vertu du beurre
　　pour frire des gardenias
Celui qui se nourrit de verge de soute-
　　neur pour s'occuper de balistique
Les araignées et les abeilles utilisant les
　　artistes
Les artistes modernes et les artistes
　　modernes

GEORGES RIBEMONT-DESSAIGNES

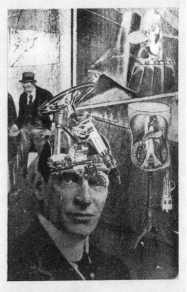

Raoul Hausmann
Tatlin lebt zu Hause

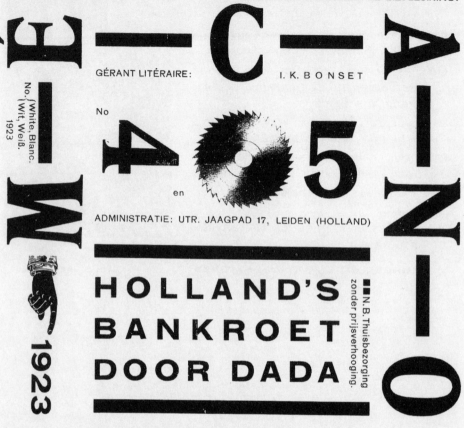

Et je trouve qu'on a en tort de dire que le Dadaïsme, le Cubisme, le Futurisme, reposaient sur un fond commun. Le deux dernières tendances étaient surtout basées sur un principe de perfectionnement technique ou intellectuel tandis que le Dadaïsme n'a jamais reposé sur aucune théorie et n'a été qu'une

Protestation

(Tristan Tzara)

Dada est la force désintéressée, ce n'est pas une maladie, pas une énergie pas une vérité.

Evola

Waar het hart leeg van is loopt de neus van over.

Bonset

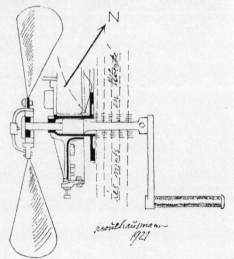

9.4

White, January 1924
The White Lacquered Little Black Paper Bag:[i] *'Souvenir from Holland' by Kurt Schwitters*[ii]

Translated from
the Dutch[1]
by Michael White

i I emphasise that the bag
in question is made of paper,
such as that used for spices.
ii Pseudonym of Josef Merz,
Hanover.

It was cream, as Amalia, a 'smoking forbidden'… in every respect: a teetotaller. Why should there be any hesitation.

Amalia suffered sauerkraut. Like burping strawberry lemonade. Despite that, the tablecloth was scoured white. It could and should not go any further. Amalia was certain of that.

Finally, the saving thought rose up in her…she bought some black lacquer. A small, empty bottle full. Suddenly she took a hatchet in her hand and hacked the bottle open with it. She now had no time to lose. So she left the tablecloth white and took the bust of Venus in her hand. It was a beauty of a bust. Covered in marble. Naked. A real beauty.

Amalia lacquered it – for the hell of it – black. Then the canary was lacquered black and, once Amalia had put the canary back in its cage, the dear little bird sang nothing but Negro songs.[2] It was downright amazing how much comfort the lacquer appear to provide!

The whole family was hypnotised by the black lacquer. Then the man of the house was lacquered. First his fingers were lacquered black. However his feet were convulsively turned inwards. His fingernails were pulled out. That made such a funny impression that mother had to laugh out loud.

Then Amalia took the brush in her hand again and lacquered his earlobes.

The ears themselves were painted cherry red.

I make particular note of this although it was only a temporary measure.

60
Front cover
Mécano, White, Nos. 4-5
1923

SONATE

					Tata	tata	tui	E	tui	E
					tata	tata	tui	E	tui	E
Grim	glim	gnim	bimbim		tata	tata	tui	E	tui	E
grim	glim	gnim	bimbim		tata	tata	tui	E	tui	E
grim	glim	gnim	bimbim		Tillalala	tillalala				
grim	glim	gnim	bimbim		tillalala	tillalala.				
grim	glim	gnim	bimbim		Tata	tata	tui	E	tui	E
grim	glim	gnim	bimbim		tata	tata	tui	E	tui	E.
grim	glim	gnim	bimbim		Tillalala	tillalala				
grim	glim	gnim	bimbim		tillalala	tillalala.				

Tui tui tui tui tui tui tui tui
te te te te te te te te
tui tui tui tui tui tui tui tui
te te te te te te te te.

bum	bimbim	bam	bimbim
bum	bimbim	bam	bimbim
bum	bimbim	bam	bimbim
bum	bimbim	bam	bimbim

Tata tata tui E tui E
tata tata tui E tui E.
Tillalala Tilla lala
tillalala tilla lala

| grim | glim | gnim | bimbim |
| grim | glim | gnim | bimbim |

Tui tui tui tui tui tui tui tui
te te te te te te te te
tui tui tui tui tui tui tui tui
te te te te te te te te

grim	glim	gnim	bimbim
bum	bimbim	bam	bimbim
bum	bimbim	bam	bimbim
bum	bimbim	bam	bimbim
bum	bimbim	bam	bimbim

O be o be o be o be
o be o be o be o be.

KURT SCHWITTERS

Tila	lola	lula	lola
tila	lula	lola	lula
tila	lola	lula	lola
tila	lula	lola	lula
Grim	glim	gnim	bimbim
grim	glim	gnim	bimbim
grim	glim	gnim	bimbim
grim	glim	gnim	bimbim
bem		bem	
bem		bem	
bem		bem	
bem		bem	

61
Kurt Schwitters 'Sonate'
Mécano, White, Nos. 4-5
1923

10.1 *Dada-Tank*, June 1922
10.2 *Dada Jazz*, September 1922
10.3 *Dada-Jok*, 1922

Dada-Tank, Dada Jazz and Dada-Jok

Emily Hage

1922 marks the year of Dada's short but active period in Zagreb, led by poet Dragan Aleksić. Aleksić became a supporter of Dada, which means "yes yes" in Serbo-Croatian, as a student in Prague, and after his return to Zagreb in the spring of 1921, he contributed articles about Dada to the new journal, *Zenit* (1921-1926). Edited by Ljubomir Micić and Branko Poljanski, *Zenit* (zenith) was the main organ of the Zenitist movement in Croatia. Differences between Aleksić and Micić about Dada became increasingly divisive, and in May 1922 Aleksić stopped contributing to *Zenit.* The following month he published his own, single-issue journal, *Dada-Tank*, with the support of a group of artists and writers in Zagreb. Aleksić included only two illustrations in *Dada-Tank*, both abstracted linocuts by the young Russian painter and graphic artist Mihailo S. Petrov. A poet, he was primarily interested in Dada writing, and he solicited contributions to *Dada-Tank* from recognized Western European Dadaists. In an enthusiastic letter to founding Dadaist Tristan Tzara from May 14, 1922, he identifies himself as part of the Dada movement in Zagreb and announces *Dada-Tank*, which he describes as an international Dada review. After reporting to Tzara about his Dada activity in Prague and his contributions to *Zenit*, he asks him for Dada reviews and books. *Dada-Tank* features Tzara's poem, "Zanzibar," Kurt Schwitters's as yet unpublished "Poem no. 48" (c. 1920), and an excerpt from Huelsenbeck's introduction of *Dada Almanach* (Berlin, 1920), all of which Aleksić translated into Serbo-Croatian. *Dada-Tank* also features poems by Aleksić, which he published in German, presumably so that foreign readers could read his poetry. His verse mimics the nonsensical tone and disregard for grammar and syntax that Aleksić had found in other Dada poems. Like Dadaists before him, he inserts neologisms and English words referring to capitalism and the entertainment industry such as "trademark" and "ragtime" into his poems.

In September 1922, Aleksić produced a second Dada journal, *Dada Jazz*, whose lively cover promotes the journal as a "Dadaistic review" in English, French, Italian and Croatian. *Dada Jazz* features only a few texts by Aleksić and Tzara; these include Aleksić's Dada manifesto (printed in *Zenit* the year before) and his essay on Archipenko, as well as a few previously-published texts by Tzara, printed in the original French. *Dada Jazz* is best understood as a footnote to Aleksić's Dada performances the previous summer.

Poljanski and Micić responded to Aleksić's promotion of Dada in Zagreb with the anti-Dada review, *Dada-Jok*, published at around the same time as *Dada Jazz*. This single issue betrays a close familiars set out parody. One could easily mistake it for a Dada journal. The articles in *Dada-Jok* are by Poljanski, Micić and his wife, Anuska, under the pseudonym "Nina-Naj." The images in particular resemble Dada works. "Anti-Dada Zagreb," for example, is a reproduction of a painting of people gathered in Zagreb's city square by tailor and self-taught artist Petar Bauk, to which the editors added the words, "Anti-dada" and "Zenit." *Dada-Jok* also features two Dada-like collages by Poljanski: an "anti-dada construction" featuring the words, "Dada," "Dada jok," and "Poljanski," and another that combines randomly chosen images with the word, "dada," "I am a Dadaist," "Are you a Dadaist?" and, "Every shoemaker (Schuster) is a Dadaist," written in German.

In October 1922, Aleksić abruptly declared an end to Dada until 1999. He continued to advance his unflagging campaign to bring Dada to Zagreb, however. He went by the name "Dada" and maintained an archive of Dada activity (now lost) until his death in 1958. Although short-lived, Dada in Zagreb had a lasting influence on art and literature there, and *Dada-Tank*, *Dada Jazz*, and *Dada-Jok* reflect the understood centrality of the journal medium to the Dada dialogue that continued to develop in the early 1920s.

Dada-Tank
Zagreb
June 1922

Translated from
the Croatian by
Celia Hawkesworth

Architecture

Who says that it won't be stable. it will be. we need skyscrapers to frighten a prehistoric jehovah, we know that we have to give the world a factory-made spur, but churches and other dwelling premises (a lot of the holy momentary, here we have to put machines, besides you'll see that our church, under the signature Schwitters, is full of wheels and we shall bring it into being, go and pray to batteries and linotypes.

apartments can be taken with our paintings, for what do you want with an apartment that has been decorated by some house-painter with a feather-duster, contact the DADA head office and for less money you will wonder at the colossal range of DADA paintings, to change your life every day we will acquire for your boudoirs tents à la Bedouin for your simple entertainment. We are for growing younger not the scoundrel Steinach.

dada absorbs contemporaneity

dada cabarets above you

dada saves youth

dada brings unhappiness to problems.

dada beats axioms: old and new.

dada makes pleaseyourselfness of the world-circus.

dada beats poets energetically.

Dada has an international (worldman) character: dada is the product of international hotel foyers, dada is as much at home in the Boulevard Sebastopol, and the Calle Arenal, Unter der Linden and Zrinjevac.

dada against meliorism, against utilitarianism, against the aesthetic ethical principle: a true dadaist does not go for the improvement of anything.

the problem of love and death is considered by dada quiet conciliation, but it can come to an agreement in that as well, for suicide unfortunately he lacks motivation.

Dada Jazz
Zagreb
September 1922

Translated from
the Croatian by
Celia Hawkesworth

Dragan Aleksić
Dadaism (club dada bluf)

Art was dreary, boring. The time filled up and came into being, it
was a part, a detail of a blow and it revolted. Art is all that is the
expression of nerves. Nerves are primitivism. Feeling comes into
being when the body accepts, and is on the way to thinking.
Feeling is not a nerve. Nerves are the original, uncorrupted
notknowingoneself well. Primitivism has a base.

The realism of truth keeps circulating. Truth is my concept
($2 \times 2 = 5$), and the contrast delusion is my concept. Therefore the
objectivity of truth is inaccurate. Morality is a sunken version of
truth and all today's kinds of truth will sink. Morality (Over here,
over here is salvation!) is chain commerce, and truth has begun.
Let us take the world and look at it as at a cow at a fair.
(Cometophobia threatens!) That is why DADA tends towards
pleaseyourselfness. Joy is delusion and truth, joy, the basis of
everything. It needs to last a long time.

Everything is a symptom. Speech is a symptom, as are its
results. (Absolute algebra!) It is used most sincerely. There is no
madness therefore, because otherwise the Cosmos is a factory of
real madnesses; at the final point of madness = fury, but not yet
reason. The sincere fury of the most sincere person. To act not to
know what you are doing means to give yourself. Not the staging
of truths, reality, demonics – the soul does not limit; it is not a
dam but rather expansion. A drawn-out concept. Do not narrow-
gauge yourselves. You need to elasticate yourself. We do not live
for years, but rather for minutes, seconds. Let every second be
something new. Boredom threatens with age; we need to die
interesting. That is why there is no style of constancy, that is a
gesture of the opportunity, a moment of the deepest structure of
joy.

==========

The reality of expression boring, over-full, stupid (400 years
they have been beating: donkeys). Art is not only the expression of
an event, reproducer and banterer (sons!), that is how art as
language comes into being as the transference of optical or (tick
tick) cardiac endeavours, fictionalized or (sup sup sup)
experienced. The transference of experience (cheeps Marzynski)
always also undervalues the artistic. To see art does not mean to
return to the event (surrogate without competition), the alteration
of the events of réalité is abstraction. Abstraction is the sense of
great essentials, not trivial ones. That is the sense of
interpolation. Not romanticism (gentlemen, I've had recourse to
yellow paper!), Dadaism is a primitivistic secondary-abstract with
denial of everything in tradition. (Learn to talk baby-talk!)

The abstract effect of art is the postulate of occultnerved
person. Clanking clamour banging din advertising
(ppppapapapapa trtrtrtrlitititi huhuhuhuhuhu) are indications of

the abstract for the whole complex of conglomerates. A person does not start to remember, rather the process of that Before is set vibrating in him. A second does not have a long beginning, that is why it gives the abstract effect of unconsciousness about some image as tableaux Now-images. It is as though it gives a chiselled-out dash through the whole artist: the Artist has a nerve for art, feeling is the longfeeling of thoughts, the nerve resonates, pounds. (Box-ton, jujitsu-quickscale.) To understand. The eternal sphinx. Homo has bitten into that concept (Sumatra = I am black!) Who is going for understanding? The motor components of seconds are so over-knotted that they are cut through by surprise. To have a nerve, less a brain. (Spiraloid caravan). To understand the detail of some art (oh the superficiality of arrogance!) is the plan of madmen or professors.

To be general. That is you DADA.

Join in childishness, prove phenomenality. A phenomenon is a special thing for a psychologist, to strengthen his position in a group. (Quo-quotes Marzynski). The expressionist is the half-general observer. The DADAist a panoramic abstractivist.

==========

The expressionists already affirmed that beauty was generally decorative – superficial – spirituality. Absolute beauty is the will. Boredom is lack of will chance non-art. Abstraction is hypertension and will power. The artist creates secondaryexpressive allusions. (Cover yourselves, symbolists!) A naked man in the first year is a Dadaist. Life in itself is an image of the present, abstraction is also contemporaneity. In the main the future has to open tones.

The poetry of abstraction. Speech is a device. I am reducing it to secondness. What is comparison other than dissection (the W. and Cl. Pitt Clinic). An overflow of abstraction takes the place of a handful of comparisons (Schwitters Kurt, Kurt, Kurt!!) The concordalist Mind weeps for clarity, while drowning in snivelling barberous powdery glacations. (Pisspisspisspissication of S. T. R. K. electroluminations.) Throughfact line and form do not exist (Ducic, cut off your nose!) Form has greatly dispersed, the concept of form has to disperse as well. Abstractions live in the last outshrieking of form. (Serner Lugano Last Diffusion of Peanuts 1° - 78°)[1]. The expressionist shouts after the departure of completingness with abstraction. Poetry moment. Poetry circulus of wonders changes. Poetry is noendinsightness.

Dada-Jok
Zagreb
September 1922

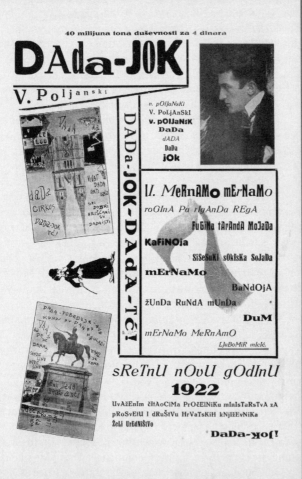

Translated from
the Croatian by
Celia Hawkesworth

Virgil Poljanski
Dada Antidada

Dada is the last consequence of the europeisation of cabaret cerebrality.

Dada is the activity of all disarmed minuses, who have settled down on the border of a new epoch.

I am a Dadaist, because I am not!

If you buy an afternoon newspaper in Berlin you have bought a dada outlook on the world. If you travel along a street in Moscow you see nothing but Dadaists. Every coolie on the streets of Peking is a Dadaist. And precisely for that reason all these people are at the same time also antidadaists, because they are Dadaists. (Don't confuse yourself, citizen!)

Why are Dadaists not dadaists. They are always travelling further. I became a Dadaist and at the same second I ceased to be dada. Always onward.

Dada! Pandada! Ultradada! Hyperdada! Whoever has not yet met you does not know of your leggy nonchalantness, Dada Europe hereditary lues! Who is the first dada! Tristan Tzara! A Romanian! Degenerate intellectual little suckling pig. And that is why I love dada, because I love fresh suckling pigs roasted on the spit! I am a Dadaist!

Antidada is winning. I am antidada, because I violated Ana Blume in a Prague park.

To think. To unthink. To rethink. To freethink. To afterthink.

DADA

ANTIDADA

ZENITH

Mankind has had a good cry and become a Dadaist. The whole world is

Dadaworld

And so one fine fresh morning there drove up in a car the great master of all the Dadaists within the borders of the Kingdom of Serbs, Croats and Slovenes, full of explosive haughtiness and thunderousness

Antidada

in the form of

Ljubomir Micić.

All fingers were pointed at him.

All eyes were staring at him.

All curses fell on him.

All the girls made faces at him.

All the Begovices were horrified

All the Krlezas flushed red

with shame.

All the Vinavers fell on their knees.

All the hermetic journalists

stilled

their drumming.
All the citizens vociferated
All the café tables became stoned
The whole of Zagreb plunged into an ocean of laughter
And the great master of all the Dadaists
the first great Antidada
Contradada
Zenithist
Contrapseudozenithist
THE GOD OF DADA
LJUBOMIR MICIC
collected all the laughter in a copper jug and guards it calculatedly,
laughter for the time
when the antidada terminator
reveals
a hurricane
Crocodiles have made good friends with the kings of all literatures
and have devoured by agreement all copies of *Zenit* (Zenith) so that
no single idea
should ever again see the light of day
out of crocodile bellies.
And the European agency for advertising
DADA
has come and offered itself to Zenithism for carrying out all its
advertising
business. There were printed prospectuses in all languages, living
and dead:
What is Zenithism?
Zenithism is nevertheless the best method for perfecting
intellectual
nosecleaningmachines!
Zenithism is the best tried and tested method for curing
rheumatism
of the skull.
Zenithism-powder is nevertheless the best means of cleaning the
stomach
if you have gorged yourself on glass.
Swallow a whole sausage factory and take Zenithism drops then
you will
recover.
Zenithism is the best method for curing stiff necks,
if you can't think zenithistically.
What is Dada?
What is Antidada?
How can you become 'ein echter' Dadaist?
You must become an
Antidadaist.
Get into a wheelbarrow, hug an aeroplane, sail through the town
sewers, enter the stomach of Eugen Demetrovic, and disembark in
New Zealand. That's the best route to Dadaism.
DADAIST.

DAdA-aNtI
EN AVANT
DADA ANTIDADA
ZENIT

DADA ZENIT SLEPAC broj 52

Halo!
Lubanja.
Boli me broj
52
Stepac o ponoći stoji
čeka
prelom ulica
ugao
kabaret
orgijska muzika
Kad će sinuti dan
kroz crna stakla
slepčevih očala.
Čarobnjaci ruski carski generali
po večeri za dinara
10.
Sena moja vampir moj.
Pokvariti časovnik
vreme stati
ceo svet preobraziti
u glupi vašarski
idiotomanski
pan
pan
pan
pantoptikum
kum
um
m.

ANTIDADA KOnstRukcIJA
V. PoljanskI

DAda KaUzA/ dAdA

1, 2, 3 i t. d.
Svako podne zvoni prelom imaginacija
na poluzi moga kažiprsta.
Ljubim te u u u u u
utopiju
39° topline.
Raskuštrane su tračnice željeznice za Rusiju.
Reći ću svome učeniku S e n e k i da je
Kurt Šviters pobegao iz Hanovera
da ne mora platiti cipelaru
        Fridrihu Niče
račun za prave Dadacipele.
1, 2, 3, 4, 5, 6, 7, 8, 8, 10, 11, 12 . . .
Marš kurvo kauzalnosti!
Kakokakokakokakokako . . .
kokokokokokokoko
ooooooooooooooooo . . .

ZENIT Br 16 ! RUSKA NoVA UMETNOST
Erenburg - Hlebnikov - Jesenin - Kusikov - Lisicki - Majakovski - Malevič - Pasternak - Tairov - Tatlin

2

Translated from
the Croatian by
Celia Hawkesworth

Virgil Poljanski
A Panopticon Travels In a Mirror

'Do not despair shoe I shall put you on. Is it not fine to watch the battle of bulls and the arrogance of the picadors. That is reality.'

Such words fell from who knows whose lips and whose ears.

The day before yesterday they hanged a man for completely justified reasons; on the one hand. But every man has two hands, unless he happens to have been in a fight for his home and righteousness, and instead of a hand he wears an original prosthesis. A man with two healthy hands seeks also on the other one to know the reason why that man was hanged. But the one who reasons from the point of view of those who are being hanged, never had another hand in his life. The surgeon prophesied a bad future for it and cut it off. There is no other hand to seek its rights, it is not a hand, it is a — prosthesis. Hypothesis.

*

In the afternoon a lot of people, dogs, horses, etc. were taking a walk.

Everything entered into the bright level of a mirror. Everything was reflected in the imagination and everything perished.

In the bright level of the mirror there entered:
churches and nuns
cars and phaetons
newspapers and builders
suns and moons
stars and notorious prostitutes
editors of reviews and kangaroos.

When they crossed the frame of the mirror everything suddenly changed! Boom! Something broke. It was the blockhead of the American king of potatoes.

*

The song of the whirlpool is great. The whirlpool is the first and last sense of sense. Can anyone drum the word:

Senselessness.

Consequently sense exists too!

What is the sense of senselessness? Senselessness! And what is its sense?

That is a very fine concept of something, which it is impossible even for the hellish mind of man to recall.

But senselessness makes sense!

Its sense is to occupy such a wonderful place in the world of our concepts. What is beyond conception?

Merz
Emily Hage

Kurt Schwitters produced twenty-five issues of *Merz* in Hanover between 1923 and 1932. This journal reflects Schwitters's negotiation of Dada and Constructivism and his determination to develop and disseminate his single-member movement, 'Merz.' Although the only images in *Merz* by Dadaists are two drawings by Hannah Höch and Francis Picabia, the texts in the first two years of the publication feature many contributions from Dadaists and Dada enthusiasts. The primary descriptions of the Dada movement are an interview with Tristan Tzara and a two-part essay, 'Dadaism', by 'I.K. Bonset', the Dada pseudonym of Theo van Doesburg. Other Dada texts include those by Picabia, Raoul Hausmann, Philippe Soupault, Paul Eluard, Walter Serner and Georges Ribemont-Dessaignes. *Merz* also highlights Russian Constructivists' innovations in architecture and painting with contributions such as a photograph of El Lissitzky's 'Proun (City)' and a drawing of Vladimir Tatlin's *Monument to the Third International*. In addition, *Merz* showcases many of Schwitters's 'Merz Pictures'. Examples include his *The Circle (Merz Picture)*, reproduced in *Merz* 2, in which six circles float around a canvas divided by the prongs of the compass, and *Merz Picture* in *Merz 6*, which is made up of scraps of mesh and paper and pieces of wood and metal stacked on top of one another, with a small ladder-like piece dividing the composition diagonally. These collages reflect the importance of Dadaist and Constructivist art to Schwitters's work. His essays in *Merz* also reveal his simultaneous affinity towards these two movements. In 'Banalities', for example, he compares Dada and Merz, and in 'Watch Your Step' he describes the differences between 'style' and 'imitation'. *Merz 8/9*, 'Nasci' (April–July 1924), co-edited by Schwitters and Lissitzky, reflects a shift towards a distinctly Constructivist style of typography and graphic design. In 1925, the journal began to have much closer links with Constructivism and was no longer in direct contact with the Dada movement. *Merz* reflects Schwitters's eagerness to enter into dialogue with contemporaries in other cities, and it succeeded in expanding the international network that earlier Dada journals had established.

Inhalt: DADA IN HOLLAND. KOK: GEDICHT. BONSET: GEDICHT; AAN ANNA BLOEME.
PICABIA: ZEICHNUNG. HANNAH HÖCH: ZEICHNUNG; WEISSLACKIERTE TÜTE

MERZ

1

DA
DA   DA
DA

HOLLAND ■

DADA

JANUAR 1923
HERAUSGEBER: KURT SCHWITTERS
HANNOVER · WALDHAUSENSTRASSE 5"

65
Front cover "Holland Dada"
Merz, No. 1
January 1923
Collection of the International
Dada Archive, the University
of Iowa Libraries

No.1, January 1923
Theo van Doesburg
Dadaism

Translated from
the Dutch by
Michael White

Dada forms itself.

Dada was born from resistance to what humanity has for
centuries developed as important and valuable for life.
Speechless and without any systematically formed conviction,
this resistance expressed itself in some or other senseless
behaviour. This senselessness was of course deliberate. The
young and apparently intelligent people (such as Hugo Bal [sic],
Tristan Tzara, Hans Arp, Richard Huelsenbeck et.al.) 'individuals
of unique edition', knew of no better way to express their cool
contempt for existence as a whole. Each struggled for
independence in the most independent manner. Enough was had
of the laboratories where ideas are examined under the
microscope and put in acid. What is art made for? To caress the
dear bourgeoisie? Do not the sonnets of our 'famous' poets sound
as hollow as the coins with which they are bought? Is not art not
like a bank where every generation is deposited to be speculated
on, just as the bourgeoisie does?

This is the spirit in which the public was initiated into
dadaism at the 'Cabaret Voltaire'. A sense of how riotous these
soirées were can be gleaned from the Zurich Chronicle 1915–19.

'One shouts in the hall, one fights, the first row approves
the second declares incompetence the rest shouts, who is quickly
one brought a large cash register, Huelsenbeck against 200, Ho-
osenlatz accentuated by the very large cash register and the bells
where left leg – one protests, one shouts, one breaks windows,
kills oneself, one destroys, one fights the police intervention.'

Was this determined opposition from the public justified?
Was it merely a matter of a brutal elitism? And where did
dadaism come from and what did it want?

Dadaism represents the chaos in which we live. Dada
existed in the atmosphere. It did not come into being, it was not
created – it simply was; there was no expression at the time to
distinguish this general spiritual condition from all the other
spiritual attitudes. And indeed this word: DADA, which was
found accidentally in a dictionary, means nothing. It was
constructed from the sensitivity to a particular moment. One
needs a slogan that suddenly calls up an entire world in the
imagination.

No, dadaism did not emerge from a brutal elitism. Quite the
opposite, from the complete and deep devotion of people who
busied themselves in quiet isolation with the most important
problems.

Dadaism was first brought from its vague situation to clarity
following the return of the painter Francis Picabia (formerly a

cubist) from America. In Picabia's favourite journal *391* (subtitled *le raté*) deep meaningfulness, weak aesthetics, religious nonsense and philosophical seriousness were ridiculed in the wittiest fashion. The dadaists, in their certainty of the relativity of existence, do not recoil from also ridiculing themselves.

Thus Picabia sometimes calls himself a *rastaquouère* (that is, someone who lives the high life without any obvious means) and at other times *le raté* (the failure).

In his dadaistic-philosophical work 'Jesus-Christ Rastaquouère' Picabia

gives the following definition of 'rastaquouère'.

'The Rastaquouère is possessed by the desire to eat diamonds. He owns some disparate glad rags and naive sentiments: he is simple and tender: he juggles with all the objects that fall into his hands: he does not know how to use them, he only wants to juggle – he has not learned anything, but he invents.

'The rastaquouère is just a kind of equilibrist.'

This definition completely characterises the dadaist.

Translated from the German by Michael Kane

No. 1, January 1923
Kurt Schwitters
Dadaism in Holland

DADA

in Holland is a novelty. Only one Dutchman, I.K. BONSET, is a Dadaist. (He lives in Vienna) And one Dutch woman, PETRO VAN DOESBURG, is a Dadaist. (She lives in Weimar.) I also know a Dutch pseudo-Dadaist, but he is not a Dadaist. But Holland,

HOLLAND is DADA.

Our arrival in Holland was like a tremendous triumphal march. The whole of Holland is now dada, because it was always already dada.

Our audience feels that it is DADA and believes that it must shriek dada, shout dada, whisper dada, sing dada, howl dada, curse dada. Hardly has one of us representatives of the Dadaist movement in Holland stepped onto the platform than the dormant Dadaist instincts in the audience awake and it welcomes us with a Dadaist howling and chattering of teeth. But we are the dadaist resident band and we're going to blow one for you. A dreadful portent will be prepared for them, we are pouring out the Spiegelgasse-Dadaist spirit of the great URDADAS: hans arp and TRISTAN TZARA, and on all heads a bluish flame is burning, in the mirror one can clearly read the name PRA. We blow one, we present DADA, *the public did* DADA.[1] We wake, wake, wake. Dada awakes.

We awake the dormant Dadaism of the masses. We are

3

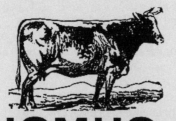 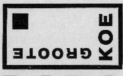

DADA

ISMUS IN HOLLAND

DADA

in Holland ist ein Novum. Nur e in Holländer, I. K. BON-
SET, ist Dadaist. (Er wohnt in Wien.) Und e in e Holländerin,
PETRO VAN DOESBURG, ist Dadaistin. (Sie wohnt in
Weimar.) Ich kenne dann noch einen holländischen Pseudo=
dadaisten, er ist aber kein Dadaist. Holland aber,

HOLLAND IST DADA

Unser Erscheinen in Holland glich einem gewaltigen Sieges=
zug. Ganz Holland ist jetzt dada, weil es immer schon dada
war.

Unser Publikum fühlt, daß es DADA ist und glaubt, dada
kreischen, dada schreien, dada lispeln, dada singen, dada
heulen, dada schelten zu müssen. Kaum hat jemand von uns,
die wir in Holland Träger der dadaistischen Bewegung sind,
das Podium betreten, so erwachen im Publikum die ver=
schlafenen dadaistischen Instinkte, und es empfängt uns ein
dadaistisches Heulen und Zähneklappen. Aber wir sind die
dadaistische Hauskapelle, wir werden Ihnen eins blasen.

66
Kurt Schwitters
'Dada in Holand'
Merz, No. 1
January 1923
Collection of the International
Dada Archive, the University
of Iowa Libraries

prophets. As from a flute, from the masses of our listeners we coax sounds of Dadaist beauty. Like a sea. Like a goat without horns. Even the police inspector, here today not as a mere spectator, but as a representative of the order of the state to the order of Dada, is shaken by the power of dada. A smile shivers over his officially appointed face when I say: 'DADA is the moral seriousness of our time!' Like horns without a prophet. Only momentarily he smiles, but we have seen it, we, the representatives of the Dadaist movement in the Netherlands.

May I introduce us? *Watch out, we are* Kurt Schwitters, not dada, but MERZ; Theo van Doesburg, not dada, but Stijl; Petro van Doesburg, you won't believe it, but she calls herself dada; and Huszar, not dada, but Stijl. You will ask in astonishment: 'Why are Dadaists not coming to show us dada?' *Watch out*, that is precisely the *Refined in our culture*, that a Dadaist, just because he is a Dadaist, cannot wake the dormant Dadaism in the audience and purify it artistically. *Do you understand?* And all udders ring. *Watch out*, the present time is, in our opinion, dada, nothing but dada. There has been a classical antiquity, a Gothic middle ages, a Renaissance, a Biedermeier period and a Dadamodernity. Our time is called dada. We live in the dada period. We experience in the period dada. Nothing is so characteristic of our time as dada.

For our culture is dada. At no time have there been such tremendous tensions as in ours. There has been no time that has been as lacking in style as ours. DADA is a DECLARATION OF BELIEF in the LACK OF STYLE. Dada is the style of our time, which has no style. *Do you understand?*

So now you think, Holland could not be dada, because Holland is not as lacking in style as Germany. Isn't that so? But you are mistaken. Holland is dada too, and our audience is even attempting to prove that Holland is far more Dadaist than Germany. Only Holland is still asleep, and Germany already knows how lacking in style it is. When, for example, I am moving past the lyrical windmills in the fast train, first-class compartment, and below a lad is moving manure, but over us the plague is moving through the air, then this is a tremendous tension. I send from the moving train a telegram to my new impresario in North America, while a small dog barks at the moon. Just then a dogcart knocks a car down. Do you see? That is Dada. I have, for example, a child's pistol with a cork on a string. I load by pulling out the butt and can fire 300 shots a second, and in Helder there are big cannons. And the intellectual tensions? Here, as everywhere, living side by side as members of the same community and on friendly terms with one another we find Anarchists, Socialists, Monarchists, Impressionists, Expressionists, Dadaists. And Beauty, Art, as it were? Where do you find traces of it? *Kijk eens*, houses, for example, are there for inhabiting. Houses are not advertising pillars. But the empty gable is the underpants of the house. And here in Berlin the underpants of the houses are painted with advertising. Is that supposed to be beautiful? Is it really? It is dada when one is wearing Dadaist advertising in one's underpants. Or is the house supposed to be a Janssen's meat vol-au-vent? For so I must believe, when it is expressly written on its gable end. Is it not crazy, houses, that we all know to be not flesh as we are, to call such houses made out of stone and iron a Janssen's meat vol-au-vent? I find that idiotic. A house is not a Janssen's meat vol-au-vent, and he who writes on a house that it is a Janssen's meat vol-au-vent, is either very deluded himself, or he takes us for fools. But I say to you, your houses are mostly dada, but very rarely Janssen's meat vol-au-vents. Advertising is a sign of our times. Our times are functional, practical, or un-functional and impractical, as you like it. Isn't that so? Our times allow advertising to proliferate even at the expense of beauty. And then you have kitsch, conscious and unconscious. In Amsterdam I saw a lunchroom that was decorated with the remains of old stalactites to look like an artificial dripstone cave. And I ask myself in amazement: why? Do you find a stalactite grotto in Amsterdam stylish? Yes? Well, then I am quite right, the style of Amsterdam is a lack of style. But that is dada. Just like in Berlin. And if there must be a dripstone cave, why does it have to be magnified to infinity by these gigantic mirrors? The little room in Amsterdam that says: 'The whole world is an infinite lunchroom in the form of a dripstone cave,' this little room is dada *complet*. And when this stalactite room lets flowers and leaves entwine and drip and reflect each other to the extent that one begins to think that one is sitting in an eastern infinite drip-lunch-stone-grotto, well then you have garnished dada. A dada *hors d'oeuvre varié*, as it were. Or do you perhaps find the bottle of Ems water on the roof of a house in The Hague stylish? I even doubt whether that is a bottle, as it is rather big for one. And what a waste it would be to put so much precious soda water on the roof, instead of on the table. Forgive me, but I for one consider this kind of thing to be advertising. But if you want to see what good and functional architecture looks like, take Line Three to the terminus and take a look at the *Papaverhof* [2] and the *Kliemopstraat*.[3] An oasis in the desert of misunderstood architecture. These are houses that grow out of their materials and their time with a consciousness of their purpose, like a flower grows and blossoms. Flowers are always beautiful. Have you ever seen a violet advertising for the zoological gardens?

We representatives of the Dadaist movement will now try to hold a mirror up to the time, so that the time may clearly see the tensions. I remind you of the song: 'And when you think the moon is going down, it isn't going down, it just seems like it.' And now I will explain why we, who are not Dadaists, are precisely the most capable of being representatives of the Dadaist movement.

We have come together here by chance. As often happens. But nothing is pure coincidence. A door can close, but even that is not a coincidence, but rather a conscious act of the door. Nothing is pure coincidence. We found ourselves, after we had found ourselves, working together. Our audience gave the movement direction. We reflected and were the echo of the audience before us, boisterous with Dadaist enthusiasm. And now you see why we do not want Dadaism. The mirror that deflects and indignantly throws your worthy visage back at you, this mirror does not want you, it wants the opposite. And we want style. We mirror Dada because we want style. For this reason we are the representatives of the Dadaist movement. Out of love for style we are putting all our weight behind the Dadaist movement.

Our arrival in Holland was like a tremendous triumphal march, the like of which was never heard of before. While the French were occupying the Ruhr with cannon and tanks, we were occupying artistic Holland with dada. The newspapers write endless Dada-articles and short treatises about the Ruhr and reparations. While the French found great resistance in the Ruhr, Dada triumphed in Holland without resistance. For the enormous resistance of our audience is dada and is therefore disarmed. This resistance is 'our' weapon. The press, which understands things better than the masses, has recognised that and has joined our side with flags flying. It offers resistance to us by expressing its open enthusiasm for the Dadaist movement. The whole of Holland learned the word 'dada' in 24 hours. Everybody knows it now, everybody is familiar with a nuance of the word, how he can shout it out stupidly, as stupidly as possible. That is an enormous success. The otherwise so worthy-seeming modern man of culture suddenly realises how stupid he can be, and how stupid he is at the bottom of his soul. That is an enormous success. For now the man of culture suddenly sees that his great culture is perhaps not so great as it appears. It was a powerful moment in Utrecht when the audience suddenly ceased to be an audience. A worm-like movement surged through the corpse of the variously constituted audience. Worms came creeping up onto the stage. A man with a top hat and a frock coat read out a manifesto. A colossal, old laurel wreath from the cemetery, rusty and weathered, was donated to Dada. A whole Groenten-action was established *on the stage*. We could light a cigarette and watch how our audience was working in our stead. It was a sublime moment. Our proof was complete.

In the foreseeable future we hope that our enlightening activity concerning the enormous lack of style in our culture will awaken a strong will and a great desire for style. Then the most important activity begins for us. We will turn against Dada and will then fight only for style. Our activity in this regard began long ago, even before we recognised Dada and its significance. We are attempting to reach this aim in various ways. Style is the result of collective work. Have we done this? The magazine *De stijl* has been in existence for 7 years under the direction of Th. V. Doesburg. There one can be persuaded of the work and the success of the Stijl artists.

I print here a poem by J.K. Bonset: from *De Stijl*:

LETTERSOUNDIMAGES (1921)

IV (in dissonanten)			
U^l	$J—$	m^l	n^l
U	$J—$	m^l	n^l
$V—$	$F—$	K^l	Q^l
F^l	$V—$	Q^l	K^l
X^l	Q^l	V^l	W^l
X^l	Q^l	W	V
U^l	$J—$	$m—$	$n—$

$$g^l$$

$A—O—$		P^l	B^l
$A—O—$		P^l	B^l
$D—T—$		O^l	$E—$
d t		o	e

$$O^l\ E^l$$
$$B^l\ D^l$$

$$Z^l\ C\ S \qquad B\ P\ D$$
$$j$$

Now I come to my topic, to the significance of the Merz idea in the world. If you see things differently, that is a matter of indifference for Merz, but MERZ, and only Merz, is capable of sometime, in a yet unforeseeable future, transforming the whole world into a massive work of art. You may ask: 'Why?' *Watch out*, MERZ reckons with all the facts as they are, and that is its significance, both practically and ideally. Merz is as tolerant as possible in relation to its material:

And if the work still looks a fright,
MERZ will make it all right.

Merz even reckons with materials and complexes in the work of art that it is itself not capable of fully assessing and judging. However, if we ever want to turn the whole world into a work of art, we must be prepared for the fact that there are powerful complexes in the world that are unknown to us, or that we do not control, because they do not lie within our power. But from the perspective of

MERZ

that is of no importance. What is important in the work of art is only that all the parts relate to each other, and are given a value in relation to each other. And even unknown quantities can be given a value. The great secret of Merz consists in the giving of a value to unknown quantities. Thus Merz controls that over which one can have no control. And thus Merz is larger than Merz. The secret consists in knowing that when you have a known and an unknown quantity together that you also change the unknown quantity when you change the known one. As the sum of known and

67
Kurt Schwitters
'Dada in Holland'
Merz, No. 1
January 1923
Collection of the International
Dada Archive, the University
of Iowa Libraries

unknown always remains the same, always must remain the same, and indeed in absolute balance. *Watch out*, if one has mills, then one can also pump the land under the surface of the sea dry. (Proof of this: Holland.)

For the moment Merz is making preliminary studies on the collective world formation, on the general style. These preliminary studies are the Merz pictures.

The only important thing in painting is the tone, the colour. The only material for it is the paint. Everything in the picture comes about as a result of the paint. Bright and dark are values of the colour. Lines are borders of various colours. Therefore in the picture nothing is important but the values of the paint/colour. Everything that is unimportant disturbs the consistency of the important. Therefore a logically consistent picture must be abstract. Only giving a value to the colour. How the colour material came about is of no importance in the picture. What is important is only that the characteristic balance of the work of art comes about through giving values to all the colours in relation to each other. Every means is appropriate, if it is to the purpose. Whether the artist recognises the colour tones used in the picture or not is irrelevant, as long as the balance is produced. What the material used meant before its use in the work of art is irrelevant, as long as it has received its artistic meaning in the work of art through being given a value.

So I first started to construct pictures out of the material I happened to have conveniently to hand, such as tram tickets, cloakroom tickets, bits of wood, wire, string, buckled wheels, tissue paper, tin cans, bits of broken glass, etc. These objects are fitted into the picture either as they are or after they have been altered, depending on what the picture demands. Through being given a value in relation to one another they lose their individual character, their own poison, are dematerialised and are material for the picture. The picture is a self-sufficient work of art. It does not refer outside of itself. A logically consistent work of art can never refer outside of itself, without losing its reference to art. It is only by the reverse process that someone from the outside can relate to the work of art: the viewer. The materials of poetry are letters, syllables, words, sentences, paragraphs. Words and sentences in poetry are nothing more than parts. Their relation to each other is not the usual one of colloquial speech, which has a different purpose: to express something. In poetry words are torn out of their old context, emptied of formulas and brought into a new, artistic context, they become form-parts of the poetry, nothing further.

I do not want to go into the blurring of the boundaries between the art forms here, such as that between poetry and painting. I must write a long treatise on this, maybe in MERZ 2 or 3. There are no art forms, they have been artificially separated from each other. There is only art. But Merz is the general work of art, not a speciality.

The most inclusive work of art is architecture. It includes all

8

art forms. MERZ does not want to build, MERZ wants to rebuild. The task of Merz in the world is:

To even out differences
And distribute centres of gravity.

Architecture pays too little consideration today to habitability, it takes too little account of the fact that people alter a room by their presence. If a room is well balanced, a person walking into it will disturb the artistic balance. Only MERZ can and must reckon with new occurrences of a chance nature. I will write more about this in one of the coming Merz issues. In the meantime I am only suggesting that one could, for example, create weights, that could be mechanically turned on and off by walking into a room, in order to bring the person into absolute balance. But one can manage without mechanics, if not so perfectly. One must create an intensive relationship between man and space. And that can be achieved by including tracks of movement in architecture. This is a completely new idea that will be able to eradicate the uninhabitability of houses. I will write about this in detail. But even now I can tell you that experiments are being conducted in secret with white mice that are living in Merz pictures specially constructed for the purpose. For the moment the tracks of the mice are being studied. There are however Merz pictures in the hangar that will mechanically balance out the movement of the white mice. Some contacts trigger various lights mechanically in relation to the movement of the mice. However, the mechanical room is the only logical space that is artistically formed and is still habitable.

11.2

No.2, April 1923
Theo van Doesburg, Kurt Schwitters, Hans Arp, Tristan Tzara, Chr. Spengemannd
Manifesto Prole Art

Translated from
the German
by Michael Kane

There is no such thing as an art that refers to a particular class of people, and if it did exist, it would not be important for life.

We ask those who want to create proletarian art: 'What is proletarian art?' Is it art made by proletarians themselves? Or art that only serves the proletariat? Or art intended to awaken proletarian (revolutionary) instincts? There is no such thing as art made by proletarians, because a proletarian who makes art is no longer a proletarian, but becomes an artist. The artist is neither a proletarian nor a bourgeois, and what he creates belongs neither to the proletariat nor to the bourgeoisie, but to all. Art is a spiritual function of man, with the purpose of delivering him from the chaos of life (tragedy). Art is free in the use of its means, but bound to its own laws, and only to its own laws, and as soon as the work is a work of art, it is sublimely raised above the class differences of proletariat and bourgeoisie. If art were intended exclusively to serve the proletariat (apart from the fact that the proletariat is infected by bourgeois taste) then this art would be limited, and indeed would be just as limited as specifically bourgeois art. Such art would not be universal, would not grow out of the world nationality feeling, but out of an individual and social perspective restricted to a particular time and place. If art is now supposed to awaken proletarian instincts in a tendentious manner, it then essentially uses the same means as church art or national socialist art. As banal as it may sound, whether somebody paints a red army led by Trotsky or an imperial army led by Napoleon is essentially all the same. Whether it is intended to arouse proletarian instincts or patriotic feelings is of no significance for the value of the picture as a work of art. From an artistic point of view both are fraudulent.

Art should only arouse with its own means the creative power of man, its aim is the mature person, not the proletarian nor the bourgeois. With a limited perspective, lacking in culture, only those of little talent can make something such as proletarian art (i.e. politics in painted form), as they have no appreciation of greatness. But the artist refrains from [treating] the special area of social organisation.

Art as we want it to be is neither proletarian nor bourgeois, for it develops powers that are strong enough to influence the whole culture rather than letting itself be influenced by social affairs.

The proletariat is a condition that must be overcome, the bourgeoisie is a condition that must be overcome. However, by imitating the bourgeois cult, the proletarians with their proletarian cult are themselves supporting this depraved culture of the bourgeois without realising it; to the detriment of art and to the detriment of culture.

With their conservative love for old, outmoded forms of expression and their utterly incomprehensible distaste for the new art, they are keeping alive the very thing they claim they want to fight: bourgeois culture. Thus it is that bourgeois sentimentalism and bourgeois romanticism, despite all the intensive efforts of the radical artists to annihilate them, continue to exist and are even cultivated anew. Communism is already just as much a bourgeois affair as majority socialism, namely capitalism in a new form. The bourgeoisie is using the apparatus of communism, which was invented not by the proletariat, but by bourgeois men, only as a means of renewing their own degenerate culture (Russia). As a result, the proletarian artist is fighting for neither art nor for the future new life, but for the bourgeoisie. Every proletarian work of art is nothing more than a poster for the bourgeoisie.

That which we, on the other hand, are preparing is *Gesamtkunstwerk*[1] that is sublimely superior to all posters, whether they are made for sparkling wine, Dada or a communist dictatorship.

Translated from
the German
by Michael Kane

No.2, April 1923
Kurt Schwitters
P...Pornographic – i- poem

The g-
This bleat is
Sweet and placid
And she will
With her horns

The line shows where I have cut down through the harmless little
poem out of a children's picture book. The goat thus became
'the g-'.

And she will	not get furious
With her horns	become injurious

The only act of the artist in **i** is the removal of set phrases by the
restriction of a rhythm.

A doctor friend of mine took, for scientific purposes
unknown to me, photos of revolving bodies and X-rays. I am
publishing 2 of them here as **i** pictures, see above. Now the doctor
who took the photographs is no longer the creator of the work of
art, but I am, as it was I wh**o** recognised their artistic content. I
am also the arti**s**tic creator of the Hague t**r**am ticket, at least of the
right corner. For if you cut a square off the right corner you have
an **i**-drawing.

If any**o**ne thinks that it is easy to create an **i**, he is **m**istaken.
It is **m**uch more difficult than forming a **w**ork by giving **v**alues to
the parts, as the world of appearances resists being art and one
seldom finds somewhere where one has only to reach out one's
hand to get a work of art.

X
Y
Z

MERZ is comprehensive, **i** is a special form of MERZ. **i** is the
decadence of Me**r**z.

Het dynamische ei van MoholyIs tegelijk een kuiken.
(BAUHAUS WEIMAR,
New professors' department)

A R T I S T S!
declare your solidarity with art!

11.3

No.6, October 1923
Kurt Schwitters
Watch Your Step!

Translated from
the German
by Michael Kane

Believe it or believe it not, the word MERZ is nothing more than the second syllable of *Commerz*. One can see the Merz picture that gave rise to the name on pages 56 to 64. The city gallery in Dresden has now acquired the work. The word came about organically as the picture was 'merzed', not by chance, for in the artistic assigning of values nothing is merely chance, which is consistent. At the time I named the picture after the legible part the 'Merz picture'. And when I was looking for a generic term for my art, when it became clear to me that I was working outside of the usual genres, I named it after the most typical picture, the Merz picture MERZ. The term Merz was untranslatable, and thus could be developed in the direction the Merz picture had given.

By pursuing the idea consistently I worked into the term Merz its current meaning and gave it to the general public with the magazine Merz.

Merz aspires to rise from the individual to the universal by thoroughly getting rid of all old prejudices, e.g. in relation to the material, that in itself is unimportant for the artistic creative process, and in relation to the composition through the creation of a new order and through selection. In every artistic genre, materials, means and laws correspond to a very particular will to form and a very particular, constantly changing time. Art lives by the life of time. As it says in *G* magazine: 'Just no eternal verities, please!'[1] There is only the truth of our time, as there has been the truth of past times. Merz is concerned to help find the truth of the time. And thus Merz arrives at endeavours in communal artistic activity, such as have already been partly realised in e.g. Holland (Stijl) and Russia. The word style is outmoded, and yet it best describes the aspirations of artists who are typical of our time. Normalising the means and alignment of the intentions to a common will to form, that is what I call style. Today the desire for style is greater than the desire for art. One must clearly distinguish between STYLE *> and artistic composition. Style is an expression of the common will of many, in the best case of all, democracy of the will to form. As, however, most people, and even some artists here and there, are mostly idiots, and as the idiots are the most convinced of their arguments, and as an agreement of all can only happen on a middle line, style is mostly a compromise of art and non-art, of play and purpose. Artistic construction knows of no purpose. The work of art is composed only out of its means. The means of art are clear. Art is exclusively balance through the assignment of value to the parts. Only if the artists agreed on this principle could a style come about that would also be art. But there are too many idiots. I do not call the highly developed collective art of the Stijl artists in Holland style,

*> See Sturm 14, 5 p74, "From the world of Merz", article on the meaning of the Merz stage.

as it is not general enough in its scope. Indeed a strong push to a general style can come from here, one has only to think of the extraordinary influence of the Stijl artists on Germany, especially on the BAUHAUS.

MERZ wants the centre, wants to mediate, wants to rescue artistic composition as much as possible for the general style. Merz does not want the club of the Idiots or the club of the geniuses. Merz wants the club of everybody, the club of the normal people for the normalisation of the catarrhs.

> NICOTINES
> Lovely nicotines grow
> On the land
> For they are flowers of the land
> The villages let them grow
> But the farmer eats them up
> How nice when we have them first
> Ernst Lehmann. 18.12.22.

MERZ is open to all, to the idiots as to the geniuses. I recall my collections of banalities. If everyone fulfils his own laws very conscientiously, and knows the laws of art well at the same time and also critically examines from his own perspective the forms of expression of other creative artists, he can then slowly and by constant work prepare the capacities in himself to be able to contribute to create style. Let him always only criticise the others in order to learn, not in order to teach and to copy. As the plant grows out of the ground in which it is rooted, so should the artist be rooted in the ground on which he grows. The artist grows to collective composition out of the circumstances in which he lives.

Diagram for style: Diagram for imitation:

Style is creation out of normalised forms according to individual laws. Imitation is an uncritical copy of any forms, e.g. also of normalised forms, without any laws. One should not let oneself be deceived by the claim of the imitators that they are striving for style, nor by the imitator's attempt to conceal his imitation, by slyly mixing several different models. Such a mixture is not style, but fraud. The imitator is not rooted at all. As he is artistically dead, he does not need any nourishment. He lives only as a more or less decent mirror lives, that reflects something living. As he is not rooted, anyone can knock him over. As the imitator doesn't grow, he cannot help to create style, as he is himself withering away. And finally the undigested, borrowed forms of others rot in his stomach and he decays from within. That is why there is always a stink around imitators. Some wear perfume, but to a sensitive nose no smell can outstink or kill the putrefaction of their bowels.

Imitators, watch [your] step!

Now the imitator will cheekily claim that he surveys everything from a lofty viewpoint because his soul is not involved in his work, and for that reason precisely HE is more important than the creative artist himself. But it is a mistake to accept that the imitator is more objective than the artist. The imitator is caught in external formulas because he does not understand the core. And as his observation of the art of the other can only skim the surface, his imitation remains only superficial.

THE IMITATOR is a scourge, a PLAGUE. Imitators are scoundrels with no consciences, dishonourable cheats, caterpillars and stupid as sheep, pushers, pigs, idiots and insurgents, athletes of the economy, base wallahs and there is no decent swearword that doesn't suit them. The subscribers will please extend the list of swearwords according to their own capacity and taste, my pencil is foaming. Only the honorary title 'critical person', not to be confused with 'critic', is not suitable. The critical person judges in order to learn, the critic condemns in order to teach. The artist of our time is the creative, critical person. For only the critical person can mature internally enough to be able to prepare somehow for the coming **STYLE**, without imitating.

The critical artist will always create new composition forms, in the spirit of the time, the imitator, on the other hand, will repeat used up forms of expression, without meaning, without any intellectual content, purely decoratively. The critical artist is always consistent, the imitator extreme. The artist has his laws in himself; that is why he can be logically consistent. The imitator rescues himself by resorting to a fanatical extreme, because he can follow no laws of his own and is therefore uncertain. Consistency is more important than inconsistency or extremes. Certainty is more important than hidden uncertainty. And thus we come to look at the term CONSISTENCY.

This would be the place to write the article 'dada complet 2', figure 'Untertaille' page 37 in Merz 4. However, for reasons of lack of space I refer you to the following Year II, 1924.
Happy New Year!

8 MERZ 9

DIESES DOPPELHEFT IST ERSCHIENEN UNTER DER REDAKTION VON
EL LISSITZKY UND KURT SCHWITTERS

REDAKTION DES MERZVERLAGES
KURT SCHWITTERS, HANNOVER, WALDHAUSENSTR. 5"

TYPOGRAPHIE ANGEGEBEN VON EL LISSITZKY
K. SCHWITTERS
HERAUSGEBER

NATUR VON LAT. **NASCI**

D. I. WERDEN ODER ENT-

STEHEN HEISST ALLES,

WAS SICH AUS SICH

SELBST DURCH EIGENE

KRAFT ENTWICKELT

GESTALTET UND BEWEGT

KLEINER BROKHAUS

BAND 2, Nr. 8/9
APRIL
JULI
1924

Nature, du latin **NASCI** signifie devenir, provenier, c'est à dire tout ce qui par sa propre force, se développe, se forme, se meut.

68
Front cover "Nasci"
Merz, Nos. 8/9
April-July 1924
Collection of the
International Dada
Archive, the University
of Iowa Libraries

69
Kasimir Malevich,
Black Square, *Merz*,
Nos. 8/9
April-July 1924
Collection of the
International Dada
Archive, the University
of Iowa Libraries

74

K. MALEWITSCH

Alles, was schafft, sei es die Natur, der Künstler, oder überhaupt jeder schaffende Mensch, hat die Aufgabe ein Fahrzeug zur Ueberwindung unseres unendlichen Weges zu bauen. Nur durch die optische Wahrnehmbarmachung unseres Schaffens bringen wir uns vorwärts und befreien uns vom vergangenen Tag. Unser Bemühen, die Schönheit der Natur festzulegen, ist und wird immer erfolglos bleiben, denn wir sind selbst Natur und immer bestrebt die optische Erscheinung der Natur umzubauen. Die Natur selbst kennt keine ewige Schönheit, ändert in ständigem Ablauf ihre Formen und baut in dem Geschaffenen Neues und Neues. — Die moderne Welt ist die andere Hälfte der Natur, die aus dem Menschen wächst.

Tout ce qui crée, que ce soit la nature, l'artiste ou n'importe quel individu, est tenu de construire, disons, un véhicule pour triompher de l'infini de notre route. Nous n'avançons et nous ne nous éloignons du passé que par la réalisation visible de notre oeuvre. C'est pourquoi, créant toujours du nouveau, la beauté éternelle n'est qu'un mythe. Toute la peine que nous nous donnons et donnerons pour fixer la beauté de la nature reste et restera sans résultat, car étant nous mêmes nature, nous nous efforçons de changer la face du monde. La nature même ne veut pas de beauté éternelle, par changement continuel de ses formes elle fait naître incessamment du nouveau dans sa création. — Le monde moderne est l'autre moitié de la nature, celle qui vient de l' homme.

Everything creative, whether it be nature, the artist, or any individual whatsoever, has to construct a medium in order to triumph over our unending road. We only move forward and distance ourselves form the past by the visible realisation of our work. That is why, always creating anew, eternal beauty is just a myth. All the trouble we give ourselves to fix the beauty of nature is and will remain fruitless, for, as we are nature ourselves, we struggle to change the face of the world. Nature itself does not want eternal beauty, for by the continual alteration of its forms it gives birth incessantly to the new. – The modern world is the other half of nature, that which derives from man.

70
Hans Arp
Geometric Collage
arranged according
to the laws of chance
Merz, Nos. 8/9
April-July 1924
Collection of the International
Dada Archive, the University
of Iowa Libraries

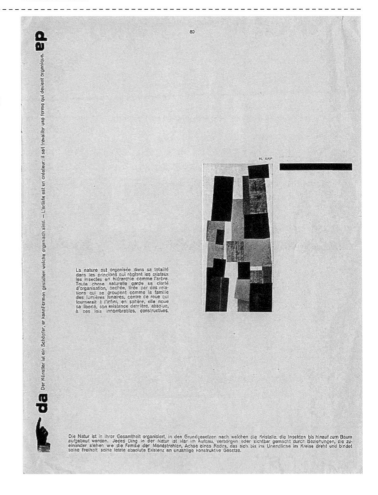

Translated from
the French by
Michelle Owoo

Nature is organised in her totality by principles that rank crystals
and insects in hierarchy like the branches of a tree. In nature all
things have this imperceptible clarity of organisation, united in
kinship, bound together like children of lunar light, the axis of a
wheel infinitely turning, its freedom, its absolute existence,
bound to these innumerable laws of progression. The artist is a
creator who knows how to bring into being forms that are
organic.

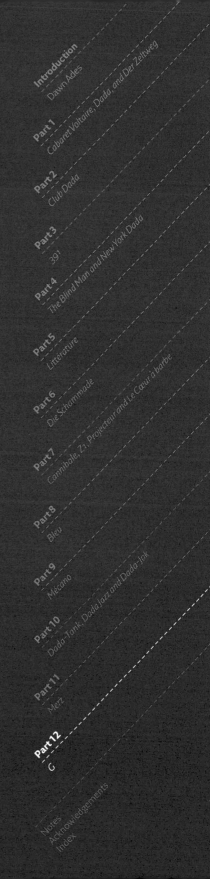

12.1   No. 3, June 1924

G

Dawn Ades

Although not a Dada magazine, G is an interesting example of the cross-fertilisation of Dada and Constructivism in the early 1920s, often overlooked in favour of the Surrealist legacy of Paris Dada. G's editor, Hans Richter, had been a member of Zurich Dada and many of his former associates appear in its pages. The Russian Constructivist El Lissitzky, who had earlier produced his own review, Veshch-Objet-Gegenstand (1922–3), and was on the editorial board for the first issue, had also collaborated with Kurt Schwitters on Merz Nos. 8–9 (1924). Subsequently the architects Mies van der Rohe and Kiesler joined Richter as editors.[1]

G's first two issues consisted of a large folded sheet with just four pages, but from June 1924 it became a more conventional magazine. The first rubric changed, with the third issue, from 'Material zur elementaren Gestaltung' (Material for Elementary Construction) to 'Zeitschrift für elementare Gestaltung.' (Journal for Elementary Construction). International in outlook, the magazine was primarily interested in modern constructive form, including buildings, aeroplanes, cars and town planning, and it drew into its orbit film and photomontage. The illustrations in the third issue, from which the text below is taken, included woodcuts by Hans Arp, a Rayogram by Man Ray, photomontage by John Heartfield,

paintings by Mondrian, drawings by George Grosz and a photograph of Schwitters's Merzbau (1933). This conjunction cuts across the normal divisions imposed by art history and unites work usually labelled 'Dada', 'Surrealist', 'Constructivist', 'De Stijl' and 'Expressionist'. This highlights the great variety of abstract forms in the visual arts at the time, and acknowledges Zurich Dada as an important precursor. The special issue devoted to film (4–5) discussed both Léger's Ballet mécanique and René Clair's Entr'acte (both 1924) with a photo of Francis Picabia as ballet dancer. Marcel Duchamp's Rotary Demisphere (Precision Optics) of 1925 is reproduced and both its spiral form and its link to the moving image are noted.

On the back page of the first issue, G advertised the four contemporary magazines with which it had most in common: Mécano, Merz, Ma and De Stijl. By the third issue it had added most of the avant-garde magazines of the time, such as Disk and Devetsil from Prague, Contimporanul from Bucarest and Zwrotnika from Warsaw.

George Grosz's text translated here forms part of the important book he and Wieland Herzfelde published in 1925, Die Kunst ist in Gefahr (Art is in Danger), which argued that short-lived Dada had been the only serious art movement for centuries.[2]

G
Edited by Hans Richter
Berlin 1923–26

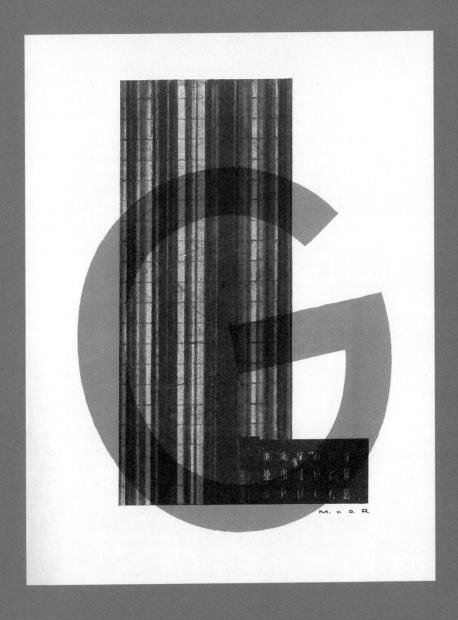

Translated from
the German
by Christina Mills

No. 3, June 1924
George Grosz
George Groß

No era has ever been more hostile to art than our own. And this is true for the average type of man when it is claimed that he could live without art. I have no desire to explain what art is. The most celebrated bigwigs of our time have offered us definitions of varying degrees of cleverness and we are all familiar with them. It is clear that the average type of person is hungry for art and that this hunger is being satisfied as never before, though not with anything that we, with our narrow-minded views and our empirical showcase concepts, term Art. Illustrative photography and cinematography are directed at this need. The dawn of art began with the discovery of photography.

Art has forfeited its role as commentator. All the romantic yearnings of the masses are satisfied by cinema. There you will find love, ambition, the yearning for the unknown and nature sufficiently nourished. And those with an interest in current affairs and historical splendour are also well catered for. The sovereign, with and without his top hat ... Grossmann the robber and murderer ... gymnastics festivals, celebrations of monuments, our dear old countryside – it's all there. It is not Rembrandt or Dürer who bring the face of Hindenburg, etched through with sorrow, to the people. It is not Michaelangelo who bears witness to Dempsey's muscles. It is film that captures the splendour of the Alps.

When I began to experience the world in a conscious fashion, I soon discovered that for all its colour and glamour – and especially taking into account my fellow human beings – it just didn't add up to much.

I hated human beings.

I began with drawings, which at that time were the basic expression of my mood of hatred. For example, I might draw a scene of one of the tables reserved for regulars at Siechen's where men and women sat huddled together in ugly grey rooms like fat red masses of flesh. To achieve a style that would give full expression to the desperately hard, ugly, unloving and unlovable nature of my subjects, I studied examples of the drive for artistic expression. I copied folkloric drawings in urinals because these seemed to me to be the most concise expression of strong feelings. Children's drawings also excited me because of their clarity.

To sum up my feelings in those pre-war days, let it simply be said that my knowledge came down to this: Human beings are pigs. Any talk of ethics is deception, directed at fools. Life has no other meaning than to satisfy the hunger for food and women. There is no soul. The main thing is that one has what one needs. Elbowing one's way through life was necessary, albeit disgusting. What expressed itself most clearly in my work was a deep disgust for life that could only be overcome by an interest in events. And, should that disgust prove too overwhelming, one could always drink oneself to death.

When war broke out, it became clear to me that the vast majority of the people had no will of their own. There they would be, walking enthusiastically along the streets, each and every one mesmerised by the will of the army. I too felt this will being exercised over me but took no joy from it because I could see that the individual freedom that I had enjoyed until then was being threatened. At that time I had felt a kind of anarchistic remoteness from other people ... now I was in danger of being forced to join the society of people I most hated. My hatred directed itself for the most part towards those who wanted to coerce me in any way. I viewed this war as a monstrous and denatured manifestation of the ugly struggle for ownership. In close-up it was repulsive to me ... from a distance, even more so. That did not stop me becoming a Prussian soldier. I discovered, to my astonishment, that there were others who shared my lack of enthusiasm. I hated these people a little less. My feeling of isolation was slightly diminished. The beautiful soldier's way of life inspired me to turn to drawing. It was clear that my drawings gave pleasure to some of my comrades for they shared my feelings. And this occupation was dearer to me than any recognition from this or that art collector who, in any case, would only view my work from a speculative position. At this time I began to draw, not only because it gave me pleasure but also in the knowledge that other people shared my way of thinking. I began to perceive that there was a better aim than working only for myself and for the art dealer. I wanted to be an illustrator. High art did not interest me because it sought to represent the beauty of the world ... what interested me were those largely scorned moralists and 'Tendenzmaler' ... artists who reflected currents of thought ... Hogarth, Goya, Daumier and the like. I drew and painted out of protest and I tried through these works to convince the world that this world was ugly, sick and untruthful. I had no noteworthy successes nor did I have any particular hopes yet I felt like a revolutionary and had traded in my resentment for knowledge.

The war had brought about no radical changes in my way of thinking. I remained distrustful of my friends. The very concept of comradeship was alien to me because I wanted to be free of illusions. I began to hear about revolutionary trends but remained sceptical – one needed only to look at the Socialist Party of Germany ... a huge brotherhood that had financed the war. That was the reality. There were no more demonic powers for me, no Schwedenborg hell ... I had started to see my own devils and princes of darkness – men with long trousers and beards, with and without medals. I considered any hopes for peace or revolution expressed by some of my friends as unfounded. I was a civilian again when I first experienced the beginnings of the Dada movement in Berlin.

This German Dada movement had its roots in the knowledge (that came simultaneously to me and several comrades) that it was madness to believe that The Spirit or indeed any spirits ruled the

72
Front cover
G, Nos. 5-6
April 1926

world. Goethe in the drumfire ... Nietzsche with his knapsack ... Jesus in the trench ... there were still people who believed that spirit and art had power.

Since we are speaking about art, let us add a few words about Dadaism, the only artistic movement in Germany for centuries. No, don't laugh – this movement has relegated all 'isms' in art to the status of outdated workshop projects. Dadaism was no ideological movement but an organic product that came into existence as a reaction against the cloud-cuckoo-land tendencies of so-called sacred art. This art mused upon cubes and the Gothic period while military leaders painted in blood. Dadaism forced art lovers to show their true colours. What did the Dadaists do? They said what does it matter what art is produced ... a sonnet from Petrarch ... or Rilke? What does it matter if you spend your time gold-plating the heels of boots or carving Madonnas? People are being shot. There is mass profiteering. And hunger. People are being lied to. What is the point of art? Was it not the height of deception that they were pulling the wool over our eyes with these 'sacred' works? Was it not utterly ridiculous that they were taking themselves seriously? But no, they wouldn't have it. 'Hands off holy art', screamed the opponents of Dadaism. Why did these gentlemen forget to scream when their artistic monuments were being shot at, their colleagues raped and murdered? Why were they blathering on about Spirit when there was really only one spirit ... that of the press ... which wrote 'Sign up now!' Today I know, along with all the other founders of German Dadaism that our only mistake was to have taken so-called art seriously in the first place. Dadaism was our wake-up call from this self-deception. We saw the end products of the prevailing structure of society and burst out laughing. We still did not see that this insanity was built upon a system.

The coming revolution brought to light the recognition of this system. There was no longer any cause for laughter because there were more important problems than art to consider. If art was to make any sense at all it had to rank lower than these problems.

Today I no longer hate people arbitrarily but I hate their corrupt institutions and those in power who defend these institutions. And if I have any hope at all, it is that these institutions and the kind of people they protect, disappear. My art serves this hope. Millions of people share this hope with me. They are not experts in art, not mercenaries, not those with purchasing power. And whether my work is henceforth called art is entirely separate from the question of whether there is a future for the Working Class.

G. Grosz déteste les exploiteurs mais aime les producteurs.
G. Grosz hates exploiters but likes producers.

Жорж Гросс ненавидит выживателей а любит творцов.

One can only hope that the new art has experienced all forms of neurosis and that some time remains where we can be spared any more 'isms'.
Robert Bereny

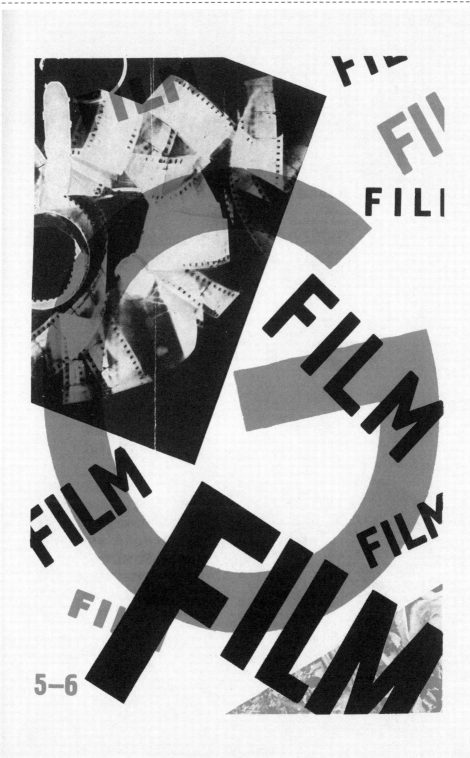

Notes

GENERAL INTRODUCTION

1 Hugo Ball, *Flight out of Time: A Dada Diary*, ed. John Elderfield, New York 1974, p.63. There were rival claims between Tzara and Ball for the discovery of the word; Ball's claim to have found it in a French-German dictionary is most plausible. Meanings proliferate: as well as those mentioned it is the French name of a board game known in English as Ludo.

2 Ramon Jakobson, 'Dada' (1921), cited in T.J. Demos, 'Circulations: In and Around Zurich Dada', *October*, no.105, summer 2003 (Dada special issue), p.149.

3 Hugo Ball, *Flight out of Time*, ed. John Elderfield, New York 1974, p.62.

4 Robert Motherwell, *Dada Painters and Poets: An Anthology*, New York 1951, p.xi.

5 Ibid., p.xii.

6 Ibid., p.xi.

7 *Times Literary Supplement*, London 1951.

CABARET VOLTAIRE
Cabaret Voltaire by Dawn Ades

1 *Cabaret Voltaire* was published in June 1916 in an edition of 500. Fifty special copies, hand-coloured, contained 10 woodcuts each by Hans Arp, Marcel Janco and Artur Segall, and etchings by Max Oppenheimer and Marcel Slodki.

2 Entry for 16 June 1916, in Hugo Ball, *Flight out of Time: A Dada Diary*, edited by John Elderfield, New York 1974, p.67.

3 Hans Arp, 'Dadaland', *On My Way: Poetry and Essays 1912–1947*, Documents of Modern Art, New York 1948, p.39.

4 Press notice, quoted February 1916, in Hugo Ball, *Flight out of Time: A Dada Diary*, edited by John Elderfield, New York 1974, p.50.

5 Entry for 11 April 1916, in Hugo Ball, ibid., p.60.

6 Entry for 6 August 1916 in Hugo Ball, ibid., p.73.

7 Hans Arp: 'I became more and more removed from

aesthetics' in *On My Way: Poetry and Essays 1912–1947*, Documents of Modern Art, New York 1948, p.48.
Cabaret Voltaire
1 This is the opening text for *Cabaret Voltaire*, a type of editorial.
'Song to the Dawn'
1 Die Rote Hanne or Red Hannah was a legendary femme fatale, variously a hangman's daughter or wife of a poacher. In the horror film of 1918 *Alraune*, based on the novel (1911) by Hans Heinz Ewers, an insane scientist artificially inseminates a prostitute with the semen of a hanged man. The child becomes a beautiful but evil woman who turns against her creator.
'A Musical Puking'
1 The Muse of Music
DADA 3
'Dada Manifesto 1918'
1 In Robert Motherwell, *The Dada Painters and Poets: An Anthology*, New York, 1951, pp. 76-82
'Marcel Janco'
1 Neologism, by analogy with and in contrast to 'mobile'.
DER ZELTWEG
'In-between Painting'
1 Originally translated into German by Walter Serner
2 The first Dada exhibition took place in January and February 1917 at the Galerie Corray, Bahnhofstrasse19, Zurich, later the home of the Galerie Dada. Tzara noted the success of the exhibition in his *Zurich Chronicle*: 'Van Rees, Arp, Janco, Tscharner, Mme van Rees, Lüthy, Richter, Helbig, Negro art, brilliant success: the new art.' (*Dada Painters and Poets* 1951 p. 237)

CLUB DADA
Club Dada by Emily Hage
1 Published as a prospectus for the Verlag Freiestrasse, *Club Dada* was sixteen pages long. Fifty normal copies cost 5 marks, and the ten copies with a handwritten poem by Huelsenbeck could be purchased for 10 marks.
'Foreword to the History of the Age'
1 Ludwig Rubiner (1861-1920), politically committed expressionist poet, opposed to the war; from 1917 edited *Zeit-Echo* from Zurich.
2 Franz Pfemfert, founder of the expressionist –political weekly *Die Aktion* in 1911.
3 John Philip Sousa, (1854–1932), American bandleader and composer of popular marches.
4 Round we go.
5 Brocken is a region in the Harz

Mountains notorious for supernatural happenings. It has the highest mountain in North Germany.
6 The holiest mountain in Nepal, Gaurisankar is sacred to both Hindus and Buddhists.
'American Parade'
1 Franz Jung (1888–1963), Berlin writer, activist and co-founder of 'Club Dada'. An editor of pre-war *Die Revolution*, arrested after anti-war demonstration and sent to the front, deserted and given spurious medical certificate by Dr Walter Serner. Signed Berlin 'Dada Manifesto' drawn up by Huelsenbeck; close friend of Grosz, involved in 1918 German Revolution. Contributed *The Red Week* to the 'Red Novel Series' published by Herzfelde's Malik-Verlag, 1921.
DER DADA 1
'Year 1 of World Peace'
1 Johannes Baader was known as the *Oberdada*, Chief Dada.
'Alitterel'
1 The Alitterel, Delitterel, Sublitterel: Litterel, bogus adjective from *Littérature*. A-, De-, Sub-: prefixes of negation or abstraction, detraction and subtraction.
DER DADA 2
'Join Dada!'
1 Walter Mehring (1896–1981), poet, cabaret and song writer, social critic; contributed to Club Dada activities in Berlin, including manning a typewriter in a race against a sewing machine operated by Grosz. In 1920s wrote for Piscator's theatre company in Berlin
DER DADA 3
1 Hausmann was known as the 'Dadasoph', the Philosopher Dada or Dada Sage.

391
391 by Dawn Ades
1 See Chapter 7, '391 and Cannibale', in Dawn Ades, *Dada and Surrealism Reviewed*, London 1978, pp.137-59.
2 The story was told that a chess game between Picabia and Henri-Pierre Roché, co-editor of *The Blind Man* with Duchamp, determined the fate of the magazines. Picabia won, and *The Blind Man* ceased publication. See *391*, no.7, August 1917, p.3.
3 Alice Bailly, the Swiss painter (1872–1938).
4 See Michel Sanouillet, *Dada à Paris*, Paris 1965.
No.1 'Whispers from Abroad'
1 Pharamousse is one of Francis Picabia's several pseudonyms.
No.8 'Automatic Text'
1 Picabia and Tzara apparently

wrote these automatic texts while seated opposite one another, hence their orientation.
No.9 'The Autumn Salon'
1 Frantz Jourdain (1847–1935), President of the Autumn Salon, the architect of, among other Parisian buildings, La Samaritaine department store, as well as a critic and writer.
2 Othon Friesz (c.1879–1949), a French Fauvist painter.
3 In French the phrase *le violon d'Ingres* is also an idiom for a hobby.
4 Picabia's paintings had been hung in shadow under the stairs.
No.10 'Letter from Mr Ribemont-Dessaignes to Mr Frantz Jourdain'
1 The review of the Autumn Salon by Ribemont-Dessaignes, which insulted and mocked most of the artists, had appeared in *391*, No.9 (see p.38). Picabia had exhibited at the Salon his 'machine anti-paintings', which, although hidden at the bottom of the staircase, caused a scandal exacerbated by the Ribemont-Dessaignes review. The President of the Salon, Frantz Jourdain, then summoned Ribemont-Dessaignes to account for himself and requested his resignation. Picabia was delighted to report the affair in *391* and print Ribemont-Dessaignes's response.
2 'National' and 'Institute' are references to the great institutions of French political and academic life. The implication is that Maurice Denis, who had become a conservative, Catholic painter, would lose little if he resigned from the Salon.
No.12 'Dada Manifesto'
1 'Viens Poupoule' ('Come on Darling') is a popular French song dating from the early part of the nineteenth century.
No.12 'First and Final Report of the Secretary of the Golden Section: The Excommunicated'
1 *La Section d'Or* was a group of Cubist painters who first exhibited together at the Galerie la Boetie in Paris in 1912. It also published a short-lived magazine entitled *Section d'Or*. The start of the First World War in 1914 saw the temporary end of the group's activities until this revival in 1920.
2 Henriette Caillaux (1874–1943) was a Parisian socialite who murdered the editor of *Le Figaro* in 1915 so that he would not fight a duel

with her husband. She was acquitted on the basis that it was a crime of passion.

3 Roch-Grey, Baroness d'Oettingen, companion of Serge Férat and close friend of Apollinaire, who contributed to his pre-war review *Les Soirées de Paris*.

4 Marie Wassilief or Vassilief (1884–1957), the Russian painter.

5 Larionov and Vassilief were among the painters whom Gleizes attempted to rally to the revived *Section d'Or*.

No.14 'Interview with Jean Metzinger about Cubism'

1 This is a completely untranslatable pun. Albert Gleizes (see below) is the subject of this 'conversation'. The original French text refers to *une capote en gleizes*, which sounds exactly like *une capote anglaise*, slang for a condom.

2 Albert Gleizes (1881–1953) was the co-author with Jean Metzinger (1883–1956) of *Du Cubisme*, which was published in 1912 shortly before the celebrated *Section d'Or* exhibition that had established Cubism as the leading avant-garde movement. Gleizes's attempts to revive the *Section d'Or* in 1919 were regularly pilloried in *391*.

No.15 '391'

1 Instead of the fifteenth issue of *391*, Picabia produced *Le Pilhaou-Thibaou*, as an 'illustrated supplement to *391*'. *Le Pilhaou-Thibaou* in fact consisted entirely of texts.

2 This is a form of myrrh, used in medicine and perfume.

3 Roger de la Fresnaye, French Fauvist/Cubist painter (1885–1925).

No.15 'Letter from Georges Auric to Francis Picabia'

1 Georges Auric (1899–1983), composer and member of 'Les Six'.

2 Dr Faivre's tablets were first produced in 1897 to combat 'all types of pain'.

No.17 'The Star on his Forehead'

1 Raymond Roussel (1877–1933) was a wealthy writer of 'magnificent originality' (to quote André Breton in *Anthologie de l'humour noir* of 1940) whose books and plays were generally greeted with hilarity and mockery by the critics. Roussel's method, in *Impressions d'Afrique* (first performed in 1911), of constructing a dramatic narrative through linguistic puns, which produced bizarre characters and irrational episodes, had fascinated Marcel Duchamp (1887–1968).

'Etoile au front' ('The Star on his Forehead'), first performed in Paris in 1924, was received with the usual incomprehension; it was defended here by Desnos and again by Paul Eluard in *La Révolution surréaliste* (no.4, 1925). Desnos contrasts Roussel with several then popular playwrights, authors and journalists.

No.17 'A Mammal's Notebooks (I)'

1 The neologism 're-laloise' might refer to the music critic Pierre Lalo (1866–1943), the son of the French composer Edouard Lalo (1823–92). Lalo senior stopped composing for ten years, disgusted at the French public's lack of interest in music other than opera. 'Laloy' may be a misprint for Lalo.

2 In French this is a musical pun: *grave (& assez bas) – grave* can mean deep in tone.

3 Another pun: *conseil de famille* also means board of guardians.

4 Another pun: *pompes* can mean vanities and also pumps. The descriptive words in brackets also have a double meaning, as they refer to pumps.

5 A ballet written by Auric based on a work by Molière.

No.17 'Letter from my Grandfather'

1 This letter from André Breton to Picabia is in response to the reappearance of *391* in May 1924, after a three-year gap. The sixteenth issue of *391* was subtitled *superréalisme* and full of scabrous drawings and texts referring to Breton and his group, who were shortly to announce the formation of the Surrealist movement. They were already using the term *surréalisme*, invented by Apollinaire. Breton sharply rejected Picabia's cynical invitation and condemned his journalism and involvement with the ballet, two particular *bêtes noires* of the Surrealists.

2 Jacques Rigaut (1899–1929) was an enigmatic, dandyish Dadaist, obsessed with suicide and death. He committed suicide in 1929.

No.18 'A Mammal's Notebooks (II)'

1 In French a pun: *lettre ordurière* means hate mail, but here he says *lettre, gentiment ordurière*.

2 Francis Poulenc (1899–1963) was a self-taught composer who joined the circle around Satie and was part of the group 'Les Six', together with Milhaud, Auric and Honegger. His music was witty and anti-

conventional and his ballet *Les biches* (1923) incorporated monotonous, repetitive and popular elements.

No.18 'Letters from Paris'

1 The 1924 ballet *Mercure*, commissioned by Comte Etienne de Beaumont for Massine's company, had an eight-minute score by Satie and sets and costumes designed by Picasso. The abstract choreography and radical designs by Picasso were controversial; Picabia is obliquely referring here to the paradoxical position of Breton & Co. towards the ballet.

2 The group around André Breton and *Littérature*: see the signatories to 'Homage to Pablo Picasso'.

3 The poet and novelist Louis Aragon (1897–1982) was one of the founders of Surrealism.

No.19 'Opinions and Portraits'

1 André Gide (1869–1951) was an already established if controversial writer; his participation in the very first issue of *Littérature* in 1919 was a spectacular coup for the young group. 'Clean sheet. I've swept away everything,' he announced. For Breton, Gide's anti-hero Lafcadio was akin to Vaché.

2 Jacques Vaché (1896–1919) was a charismatic figure idolised by Breton, who published his *Lettres de Guerre* in 1920, soon after Vaché's death from an overdose of opium.

3 This is a distortion of Philippe Soupault's name. In French, *couper* means to cut, 'Coupeaux' then could be translated roughly as 'Cutters'.

4 Lucien Guitry (1860–1925) was an actor renowned for his versatility but obviously not at his peak at this time – just one year before his death.

5 Herman Bernstein (1876–1935) was a prolific playwright who lived in Berlin.

6 Yvan Goll (1891–1950) published the single issue of a review entitled *Le Surréalisme* in 1924, complaining that the 'Surrealism' of Breton had nothing to do with the ideas of its inventor, Apollinaire, and arguing for the importance of film. However, it was Breton's Surrealism that took root and lasted.

7 Jean Eugene Robert-Houdin (1805–71) was a famous magician and illusionist.

No.19 'Why Pay?'

1 Life is a fine lavatory.

2 In March 1925 E.L.T. Mesens (1903–71) and René Magritte (1898–1967) published the

review *Oesophage* in Brussels, the nearest to a Dada review in Belgium. Contributors included Arp, Tzara, I.K. Bonset (1883–1931) and Picabia, among others. They became leading members of the Belgian Surrealist group.

NEW YORK DADA
The Blind Man and *New York Dada* by Dawn Ades

1 Marcel Duchamp, *Entretiens avec Pierre Cabanne*, Paris 1967, p.101.

LITTERATURE
Littérature by Dawn Ades

1 'Two Dada Manifestos', *Lost Steps* [1924], trans. Mark Polizotti, Nebraska 1996, p.44. The versions published by Breton in his summary of Dada, *Les Pas perdus* [Lost Steps] differ from the originals in *Littérature*, May 1920. The phrase 'Dada is a state of mind' is from the first 'Manifesto' in the former, which does not appear in *Littérature*. The second 'Manifesto' in *Littérature*, 'Dada Geography', is not included in *Lost Steps*.

2 Breton, 'After Dada', *Comoedia*, 2 March 1922 [*Les Pas Perdus*, 1924].

3 See Michel Sanouillet, *Dada à Paris*, Paris 1965, pp. 102–4.

4 Jacques Vaché, *War Letters*, London 1993.

5 André Breton, *Entretiens*, Paris 1952, p.56.

6 Philippe Soupault is named sole editor for this issue alone.

No.1 'Review of Dada'

1 'R.L.' was Raymonde Linossier, friend of Adrienne Monnier and inventor of 'Bibisme', which shared some of Dada's 'primitivism'. She warmly welcomed Tzara's 'Dada Manifesto 1918' **(see p.43)**.

2 The 'Review of Reviews' was a staple item in artistic and literary reviews.

No.2 'A New Work'

1 Auric here celebrates Satie's cantata *Socrates* (1919), which, according to the *New Oxford Companion to Music* (Oxford 1983), 'takes creative humility almost to its limits'.

2 Cocteau, Satie and Picasso collaborated on the ballet *Parade*. Audiences had been outraged by Satie's score, which included noises from a typewriter, a revolver and a football rattle, and also by Picasso's 'Cubist' set and dancers, hampered by huge geometric structures. They were a nasty shock after the gentle Neo-classical scene he had painted on the stage curtain.

No.5 'A Philosopher'

1 Rousseau often wrote short texts or poems to be displayed together with his paintings; a painting entitled *Un Philosophe* was exhibited at the 1896 Salon des Indépendants.

No.7 'Factory'

1 This fragment was the first example of automatic writing in *Littérature*. Excerpts from *Les Champs magnétiques* (*The Magnetic Fields*), the major collaborative experiment in automatism, by André Breton and Philippe Soupault, started to appear in the issue October 1919.

No. 7 'Opium!'

1 Press coverage of the death of Breton's friend Jacques Vaché from an overdose of opium.

No.13 'Twenty-three Manifestos of the Dada Movement'

1 German aeroplanes in the First World War.

2 René Bazin (1853–1932), French novelist of provincial life, known for his love of nature and simple values.

3 *Colique* meaning diarrhoea. This was a small tin toy figure, popular at the beginning of the twentieth century in France, of a man squatting with his trousers down.   When ignited, the rear end excreted a brown substance.

4 Presumably baseball. In French this is pun on *se mettre en boule*, to fly into a fury.

5 Musée Grevin is a famous waxworks museum in Paris.

6 Jean Eugène Robert Houdin (1805–71) was a French magician, born in Blois, France, where he also died. The stage name of Harry Houdini was taken in tribute to him.

7 The French, *feux d'artifice de la beauté*, is an untranslatable play on words.

8 Possibly a reference to the scandalous 'orgasmic' statue of Apollonie Sabatier in the Musée d'Orsay, Paris.

9 Dr Walter Serner, a German doctor of law, who was active in Zurich Dada.

10 Pierre Rosenberg was a contemporary dealer in Cubist painting in Paris.

11 Père Lachaise is a famous cemetery in Paris; Père la Colique was a tin toy that excreted diarrhoea (see above).

12 The tour Nesle, which stood in Paris, was reputed to have been the scene of some scandalous orgies involving Queen Marguerite, two princesses and various lovers who were usually executed in the morning.

13 Céline Arnauld, the only female writer represented in this edition of *Littérature*, was a member of the Paris Dada movement. She was married to Paul Dermée.

No.17 'Minutes'

1 René Hilsum, director of the bookshop *Au sans pareil*.

No.17 'Projected Habitation Reform'

1 Pseudonym evoking "small-town cousin".

LITTERATURE NEW SERIES

No.7 'Rrose Sélavy'

1 Marcel Duchamp invented Rrose Sélavy as a female alter ego and credited her with his first intricate, spooneristic, poetic tongue-twisters. From October 1922, Desnos wrote or uttered two hundred more, evidently in some kind of trance akin to sleep or self-hypnosis. The periodical *Littérature* published 174 sentences in December 1922. A few omissions are indicated by dots ... The translations have been done very freely in the hope of catching the poetry, originality and mystery of the original.

No.9 'What Lovely Weather!'

1 This is a classic problem pun. In French, *voler* can mean to win all the tricks in a card game, as well as to fly.

2 In French, *sauter les plumbs* can also mean to blow the fuses.

DIE SCHAMMADE

Die Schammade by **Emily Hage**

1 'Baargeld' (meaning 'cash' in German) was the pseudonym of Alfred Gruenwald, son of a banker and a leading member of the International Socialist Party in Germany.

'Superior Cockatoo'

1 In the original German the title 'Superior Cockatoo' was in French. Arp was bilingual and often translated his own work between French and German.

PROJECTEUR

'Particulars'

1 'Draule' is 'Eluard' backwards.

2 Arnauld had previously considered *M'Amenez*-y, the title of a Picabia painting, and 'Ipeca' (a plant that induces vomiting) as titles for her review.

3 Jacques Doucet was a couturier and collector, not only of pictures but also of reviews. The Bibliothèque Doucet in Paris is now the most important collection of avant-garde and Dada

manuscripts and documents.

4 Paul Dermée.

'Festival Dada'

1 Programme of the performances at the Dada evening held at the Salle Gaveau, Paris

LE COEUR A BARBE

Le Cœur à barbe

1 *Le Coeur à barbe: journal transparent* was an eight-page pamphlet on pink paper, decorated with ready-made vignettes, produced by Tzara and his group. Dada was in the process of splitting apart acrimoniously, a process accelerated by a planned 'Paris Congress', against which *Le Coeur à barbe*'s invectives are aimed. While Breton was anxious to separate himself from Dada, Tzara was dedicated to continuing it. The Congress was to have brought together the main avant-garde groups, including the Cubists and Purists (Ozenfant and Le Corbusier), and had been named by Breton 'Congress to determine the directives and defence of the Modern Spirit'. For a brief period Tzara found himself pitted against both Breton and Picabia, who had rallied to Breton's support with the publication of another ephemeral journal, *La Pomme des pins*, in March 1922. Tzara was joined by Ribemont-Dessaignes, Eluard, Soupault, Satie and Rrose Sélavy, among others. Most of the pamphlet is concerned with the immediate incidents surrounding plans for the Congress (which never took place.) Tzara had originally planned to call his little review *L'Oeil à poils* (The Hairy Eye). *A barbe* can mean 'untrimmed', as with the pages of de luxe books of poetry: so the title could be translated as either the Bearded or the Untrimmed Heart.

'A Mammal's Notebooks'

1 Jeanneret (Le Corbusier) and Ozenfant were editors of *L'Esprit nouveau* (1920–5), a rationalist, post-Cubist review opposed to Dada.

MECANO

Mécano by **Dawn Ades**

1 'Chroniek-Mécano', Red, 1922.

2 Nos. 4–5.

3 Here entitled *Sonata*.

'Antiartandpurereasonman ifesto'

1 G.J.P.J. Bolland (1854–1922), the Dutch Hegelian philosopher, was professor at the University of Leiden. His most widely read book was

Zuivere rede en hare werkelijkheid (Pure Reason and its Reality) of 1904. Mondrian became familiar with Bolland's writings around 1916 and they form one of the many influences on Neo-Plasticism.

2 The radio pioneer Guglielmo Marconi (1874–1937). The first domestic radios, made by the Marconi company, were brought out around 1920.

3 Hendrik Bremmer (1871–1956), an artist, critic and collector who gave lessons in art appreciation to the well-to-do, including Hélène Kröller-Müller, the most important collector of modern art in the Netherlands.

4 The famous nineteenth-century Dutch novel, *Max Havelaar*, written by Multatuli in 1860, which contains an indictment of Dutch colonial policy.

'Dada Holland'

1 A reference to Francis Picabia's *Jésus-Christ rastoquouère* (Paris 1920).

'Archachitektonica'

1 The untranslatable title inserts 'ach' meaning 'oh!' or 'alas!' into architectonic.

2 Between 1919 and 1924 the celebrated Dutch architect H.P. Berlage (1856–1934) drew up plans for a new municipal museum in The Hague. His first design was never realised but a second plan devised in 1927 was eventually built and opened in the 1935 as the Gemeentemuseum.

3 There are two ponds in front of the Gemeentemuseum.

4 The first 'capital' (kapiteel) refers to the decorative top of a column, the second (kapitaal) to The Hague, which was – and still is – the capital city of the Netherlands.

5 Reference to Hendrik Bremmer (1871–1956), an artist, critic and collector who gave lessons in art appreciation to the well-to-do, including Hélène Kröller-Müller, the most important collector of modern art in the Netherlands.

6 Ironically the Gemeentemuseum, when it opened in 1935, was ahead of its time by including a purpose-designed café space.

'Chroniek-Mécano'

1 Hans Arp (1887–1966). Siegenzack does not mean anything but may be a Germanised version of Segonzac (capital of the Grande Champagne district in France), making a pun on Arp's Alsatian origins and Franco-German identity. He

later called himself Jean Arp. If spelt Ziegensack, this would mean 'goat's balls'. The invitation card for the Dada Soirée on 25 September 1922 at the Hotel Fürstenhof in Weimar contains the line 'Sankt Zigenzack wird aus dem Ei springen' (Saint Zigenzack will jump out of an egg).

2 Eastern religion followed by Johannes Itten, who taught at the Bauhaus between 1919 and 1913 with particular responsibility for establishing the preliminary course. Theo van Doesburg, who probably wrote this chronicle, savagely criticised the mystical tendency Itten promoted among students. The blue issue of Mécano included a satirical drawing of Van Doesburg and Itten confronting each other as a 'mechanical' and 'natural' man respectively.

3 Walter Gropius (1883–1969). Van Doesburg was supported in his stay in Weimar by the partner in Gropius's architectural firm, Adolf Meyer. There had always been the suggestion that Van Doesburg expected to be offered a post at the Bauhaus but it never happened and he felt a great deal of resentment towards Gropius thereafter.

4 One of Kurt Schwitters many versions of his name.

5 Walter Dexel (1890–1973). An artist and art historian who was at the time exhibition organiser at the Kunstverein in Jena, where he staged several significant constructivist exhibitions and also hosted lectures such as Van Doesburg's 'Der Wille zum Stil' (The Will to Style) in March 1922.

6 Tristan Tzara's lecture, given in Weimar at the congress, ended with the sentence: 'Perhaps you will understand me better when I tell you that Dada is a virgin microbe that penetrates with the insistence of air into all the spaces that reason has not been able to fill with words or conventions.'

7 Sandor Bortnyik (1893–1976) was a Hungarian artist associated with the journal MA, like Moholy-Nagy. He spent the years from 1922 to 1925 in Weimar, where he met Van Doesburg.

8 Tristan Tzara's poem 'An Petro' (To Petro [Nelly van Doesburg]) is simply the repetition of the word 'madame'. See Merz No.7, January 1924, p.71.

9 Nelly van Doesburg (1899–1975), an accomplished pianist.

10 Piano composition by Vittorio Rieti probably played by Nelly van Doesburg at the Dada Soirée in Weimar. Rieti's piano pieces were a standard feature of the Dada Tour of Holland in 1923.

11 Some photographs of the Congress of Dadaists and Constructivists show Schwitters wearing a very large, striped scarf.

12 Schwitters frequently refers to Arp in this way.

'The White Lacquered Little Black Paper Bag'

1 Theo van Doesburg's translation of Schwitters' text Die Weisslackierte Schwarze Tüte.

2 The German version published in Merz 1: Holland Dada, January 1923, pp.14–15 has an additional sentence at this point, missing in the Dutch version, that says: 'Emilie's mother glowed with enthusiasm like fat'.

DADA-TANK, DADA JAZZ AND DADA-JOK
Dada-Tank, Dada Jazz and Dada-Jok by Emily Hage

1 The cost of this single issue, eight-page journal is given only in Croatian currency (five dinar) and texts are primarily in Serbo-Croatian, indicating that it was intended for a local audience.

2 The texts by Tzara were 'Comment je suis devenu charmant, sympathique et délicieux', the beginning of 'Manifeste de Monsieur Aa l'antiphilosophe' and 'Sillogisme colonial'.

3 'Jok' means 'no' in Turkish, so the title of the journal can help translated to mean 'Dada no' or, using the Serbo-Croatian translation of 'Dada', 'yes, yes, no'.

'Dadaism (club dada bluf)' in Dada Jazz

1 Serner Lugano refers to Zurich Dada, to Walter Serner and Lugano, where Ball lived.

MERZ
Merz by Emily Hage

2 Published in Hanover, Merz was distributed in over sixteen countries, including Germany, France, Norway, the United States and Japan, indicating Schwitters's international ambitions.

No.1 'Dadaism in Holland'

1 The italicised phrases are in Dutch in the original. The reference is probably to the Dada tour of Holland in January 1923 by Schwitters and Van Doesburg. In Utrecht the audience invaded the stage.

2 A new estate in The Hague built by De Stijl architect.

3 Address in The Hague where Van Doesburg's second wife, Nelly van Doesburg, lived. She was the agent for De Stijl and assisted at the 1923 Dada tour of Holland.

No.2 'Manifesto Prole Art'

1 Synthesis of the arts.

No.6 'Watch Your Step!'

1 The first two issues of Hans Richter magazine G appeared in July and September 1923.

G
G by Dawn Ades

1 Frederick Kiesler (1890–1965) was an architect and radical exhibition designer. He moved to New York in 1926 and was closely associated with the Surrealist refugees during the war, and with Peggy Guggenheim, whose Art of this Century Gallery, New York, he designed in 1942.

2 Wieland Herzfelde (1896–1988), the writer and publisher, brother of John Heartfield (Helmut Herzfelde).

Acknowledgements

We would like to thank the following for their help with and contributions to the *Dada Reader*:

Atlas Press,
www.atlaspress.co.uk
Emma Berry
Alastair Brotchie
Branko Dimitrijevic
Jasna Jovanov
Richard Sheppard
International Dada Archive,
University of Iowa Libraries

Translators
Timothy Adès
Rebecca Beard
Jean Boase-Beier
Caitríona Ní Dhubhghaill
Jane Ennis
Emily Hage
Celia Hawkesworth
Michael Kane
Christina Mills
Ian Monk
Susan de Muth
Michelle Owoo
Michael White
Kathryn Woodham